S0-BRF-168

WILLIAM F. RUSKA LIBRARY
BECKER COLLEGE

Michael Shernoff, MSW
Editor

AIDS and Mental Health Practice
Clinical and Policy Issues

Pre-publication
REVIEWS,
COMMENTARIES,
EVALUATIONS . . .

"**M**ichael Shernoff has made an important contribution to the professional literature on AIDS by editing this rich collection of current practitioners' insights on the AIDS pandemic. The writers fill an important void by addressing the changing character of the pandemic characterized by long-term survival and new medications that do not always work or live up to expectations. The chapters are well written and are full of up-to-date examples direct from practice. I do not know how any clinician working with persons with AIDS and their loved ones can fail to benefit from reading it."

George S. Getzel, DSW
Professor,
Hunter College School of Social Work,
City University of New York

"**M**ichael Shernoff has truly mastered the fine art of opening the door to all the real clinical problems you work with everyday, are burning to talk about with your colleagues, but may feel you must keep to yourself because of conventional and political considerations. This is the most courageous, outspoken teaching manual that I know of in the field of AIDS and mental health. It not only names the issues, e.g., HIV discordancy in couples and in groups, homelessness, racism, neglect of women, homophobia, etc., but it provides the evidence you need to deal with them and frankly describes others' experiences in trying to cope with them. A stunning eye-opener!"

Bertram Schaffner, MD
Medical Director,
HIV Service,
William Alanson White Institute,
New York, NY

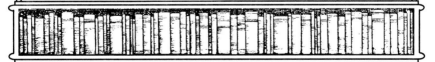

More pre-publication
REVIEWS, COMMENTARIES, EVALUATIONS . . .

"**T**his book is the answer to an HIV/AIDS educator's prayer— a timely, thoughtful, challenging collection that conveys to newcomers what mental health practice in the field is really like. Clinical and policy issues are not treated as theoretically discrete, but linked as they are in real life; individual and group interventions are not cloaked in generalities, but described in sufficient detail to replicate; and the persistent undercurrents of racism and homophobia that bedevil service delivery are not merely lamented, but addressed with practical suggestions as to how they can be overcome. What's more, previously underexplored HIV-related topics such as decision making on antiviral medication, rational suicide, and neuropsychiatric difficulties are accorded overdue attention. In a word, this book is authentic. Rich in the case examples that mark the work of authors who preach what they practice, the text is a welcome addition to the library of anyone who wants to know where we are now, and where we are headed, in the rapidly changing field of AIDS care."

Ann Burack-Weiss, DSW
Adjunct Associate Professor,
Columbia University School
of Social Work,
New York, NY

"**T**his book fills a substantial void in the current body of AIDS/HIV knowledge. Michael Shernoff, a contributor, has exquisitely edited this real-time collection of insightful and practical perspectives for *all* health professionals dealing with HIV. A wide range of challenges are addressed by practitioners who are working on the cutting edge of 'meeting clients exactly where they are.' This text makes a significant contribution in reducing the suffering of those of us challenged with HIV/AIDS in sharing how the issues being presented today are effectively addressed.

AIDS and Mental Health Practice: Clinical and Policy Issues synthesizes what we know through the wisdom of actual current clinical experience and is buttressed with theoretical frameworks. This book is a companion guide that we can rely on. I need such a resource. Great work!"

Michael Picucci, PhD, MAC
Co-Founder, the Institute
for Staged Recovery;
Author, *The Journey Toward Complete Recovery: Reclaiming Your Emotional, Spiritual & Sexual Wholeness*

More pre-publication
REVIEWS, COMMENTARIES, EVALUATIONS . . .

"**A**s the AIDS epidemic approaches the millennium, Michael Shernoff's edited volume surveys its changing landscape for mental health practitioners. No longer an automatic death sentence, HIV/AIDS is now a medical diagnosis that requires new ways of living and relating for patients, and new ways of intervening for professionals.

Shernoff's book reflects the diversity of the epidemic. It includes chapters on the new populations affected by HIV (women, children, the homeless, minority groups, immigrants, transsexuals), new dilemmas (helping AIDS patients prepare to return to work), and new efforts at prevention, particularly with HIV-positive gay men. This book will help professionals keep abreast of the new challenges."

Gil Tunnell, PhD
Family Therapy Supervisor,
Beth Israel Medical Center,
New York, NY

"*A IDS and Mental Health Practice* is an incredibly valuable addition to the literature of the second decade of AIDS. Michael Shernoff has collected a wide variety of perspectives and topics that will greatly assist newcomers as well as veteran professionals in the war on AIDS. Many of the chapters exhibit both academic expertise and compelling storytelling. I will recommend this book to my mental health professional staff."

Gerard Ilaria, CSW
Director,
Center for Special Studies,
The New York Hospital,
Cornell Medical Center,
New York, NY

The Haworth Press
New York • London

NOTES FOR PROFESSIONAL LIBRARIANS AND LIBRARY USERS

This is an original book title published by The Haworth Press, Inc. Unless otherwise noted in specific chapters with attribution, materials in this book have not been previously published elsewhere in any format or language.

CONSERVATION AND PRESERVATION NOTES

All books published by The Haworth Press, Inc. and its imprints are printed on certified pH neutral, acid free book grade paper. This paper meets the minimum requirements of American National Standard for Information Sciences-Permanence of Paper for Printed Material, ANSI Z39.48-1984.

AIDS and Mental Health Practice
Clinical and Policy Issues

AIDS and Mental Health Practice
Practice
Clinical and Policy Issues

Michael Shernoff, MSW
Editor

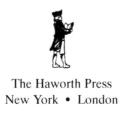

The Haworth Press
New York • London

© 1999 by The Haworth Press, Inc. All rights reserved. No part of this work may be reproduced or utilized in any form or by any means, electronic or mechanical, including photocopying, microfilm and recording, or by any information storage and retrieval system, without permission in writing from the publisher. Printed in the United States of America.

The Haworth Press, Inc., 10 Alice Street, Binghamton, NY 13904-1580

Cover design by Jennifer M. Gaska.

Library of Congress Cataloging-in-Publication Data

AIDS and mental health practice : clinical and policy issues / Michael Shernoff, editor.
  p. cm.
  Includes bibliographical references and index.
  ISBN 0-7890-0464-X (alk. paper)
  1. AIDS (Disease)—Patients—Mental health. 2. AIDS (Disease)—Psychological aspects.
3. HIV-positive persons—Mental health. I. Shernoff, Michael, 1951- .
RC607.A26A3455533 1998
616.97′92′0019—dc21   98-39347
                                                                                       CIP

This book is dedicated to the memory of
Willis Green Jr.
(May 21, 1947–December 19, 1997)

Another casualty of the disease he spent the last years of his professional life dedicated to fighting. He was a pioneer, who worked valiantly and tirelessly to provide quality comprehensive services to all people with AIDS, but especially to African Americans living in Harlem, who are among the most underserved population affected by the HIV/AIDS epidemic. His commitment to fighting racism, homophobia, and discrimination against people with HIV, combined with his dedication, love, and integrity, will long be remembered and remain an inspiration.

CONTENTS

POLICY ISSUES

ABOUT THE EDITOR

Michael Shernoff, MSW, is a psychotherapist in private practice in Manhattan and an adjunct faculty member at Hunter College Graduate School of Social Work. His recent publications include editing *Gay Widowers: Life After the Death of a Partner*; *Human Services for Gay People: Clinical and Community Practice*; and *Counseling Chemically Dependent People with HIV Illness*; an entry in the nineteenth edition of *The Encyclopedia of Social Work*; and four entries in the forthcoming *Encyclopedia of AIDS*. He is co-editor of *The Sourcebook on Lesbian/Gay Health Care*, Volumes 1 and 2 and co-editor with Walt Odets of *The Second Decade of AIDS: A Mental Health Practice Handbook*. In addition, he co-authored three brochures on AIDS that are widely used throughout the world, as well as the earliest AIDS prevention intervention for gay and bisexual men on eroticizing safer sex, which is also used worldwide.

He has served on the boards of the National Social Work AIDS Network (NSWAN) and the National Lesbian/Gay Health Foundation. He is a past member of the NASW National Committee on Lesbian/Gay Issues, NYC Department of Mental Health, Mental Retardation and Alcoholism Services Lesbian and Gay Advisory Committee, and cochaired the AIDS Task Forces for the American Orthopsychiatric Association and the Society for the Scientific Study of Sex. Currently, he is a senior consulting editor for the *Journal of Gay & Lesbian Social Services,* contributing editor for *In The Family* magazine, and the founding editor of the NSWAN Journal, *Readings & Writings.*

He can be reached either at his Web site, http://members.aol.com/therapysvc, or via e-mail at mshernoff@aol.com.

CONTRIBUTORS

Eduardo J. Baez, MSW, was Assistant Director of the Volunteer Department, Gay Men's Health Crisis, NYC, at the time "Spiritual Issues and HIV/AIDS in the Latino Community" was written. Correspondence can be sent to 436 Ft. Washington Avenue, Apt. 5A, New York, NY 10033.

Steven Ball, MSW, is a psychotherapist in private practice in New York City. He is also a consultant to Gay Men's Health Crisis in the Prevention Department. Correspondence can be sent to 626 Washington Street, Apt. 3B, New York, NY 10014.

Mary Beaudet, MS, CSW, is a social worker in the AIDS Center Program at St. Luke's Roosevelt Hospital, 1111 Amsterdam Avenue, New York, NY 10025.

Miriam Bernson, MS, CSW, was a social worker in the AIDS Center Program at St. Luke's Roosevelt Hospital, 1111 Amsterdam Avenue, New York, NY 10025.

Michael Bettinger, PhD, MFCC, is a psychotherapist and family therapist in private practice in San Francisco and works primarily with gay men. He also teaches a course titled "Work and Leadership Issues for Bisexuals, Lesbians, and Gays" at San Francisco State University. He can be reached by e-mail at mcpsycle@well.com or at 1726 Fillmore Street, San Francisco, CA 94115.

Evelyn Blackburn, MSW, is a social worker at the Community Health Network, 758 South Avenue, Rochester, NY 14620; phone: (716) 244-9000.

Stephan L. Buckingham, MSSW, ACSW, is in private practice and consultation in Manhattan and is the former Director of Mental Health, AIDS Project, Los Angeles.

Chris Carlson, MSW, CSW, is a social worker in the AIDS Center Program at St. Luke's Roosevelt Hospital, 1111 Amsterdam Avenue, New York, NY 10025.

James Cassese, MSW, CSW, is a psychotherapist in private practice in New York City, specializing in the treatment of gay male survivors of childhood sexual trauma; and former clinical supervisor in the Group Services Unit of Gay Men's Health Crisis. He is adjunct faculty at New York University's Graduate School of Social Work.

Martine Cesaire, CSW, is a social worker and case manager working with HIV-infected adults and family members at Brookdale Hospital and Medical Center, Brooklyn, New York.

Maria R. Derevenco, PsyD, has been Supervising Psychologist for the HIV/AIDS Center Programs at St. Luke's Roosevelt Hospital in Manhattan since 1988. She is also Assistant Clinical Professor of Medical Psychology (in Psychiatry) at the College of Physicians and Surgeons at Columbia University and Assistant Clinical Professor of Psychology at New York University. She maintains a private practice of psychoanalytic psychotherapy and neuropsychological diagnosis in Manhattan.

Roy Ferdinand, BA, CSAC, is a case manager working with HEAT (Health Education Alternative for Teens) at Kings County Hospital Center in Brooklyn, New York. The HEAT Program is part of the Brooklyn Pediatric AIDS Network.

Hank Flacks, MSW, ACSW, is senior social worker in the Immigrant Program at St. Vincent's Hospital and Medical Center, New York, NY 10014; he also has a private psychotherapy practice in Manhattan.

Ronald J. Frederick, PhD, was Director of Clinical Services at Housing Works 9th Street Adult Day Health Care Program for people living with HIV/AIDS at the time "Internalized Homophobia in the Psychotherapy of Gay Men with HIV/AIDS" was written.

Larry M. Gant, CSW, PhD, is Associate Professor at the School of Social Work, University of Michigan, Ann Arbor, MI 48109-1285; phone: (313) 763-5990; e-mail: lmgant@umich.edu.

James Grimaldi, MSW, is a multilingual social worker at the Center for Special Studies of New York Hospital Cornell Medical Center, who has created and implemented specialized case management models and support groups for HIV-positive MTF pre-op transsexuals and for HIV-positive non-English-speaking undocumented alien mothers. He can be contacted at the Center for Special Studies, New York Hospital, Baker 24, 525 East 68th Street, New York, NY 10021.

Arnold H. Grossman, PhD, CSW, is Professor, Department of Health Studies, and Project Director, NYU AIDS/SIDA Mental Hygiene Project, School of Education, New York University. Correspondence can be sent to the Department of Health Studies, New York University, 35 West 4th Street, Suite 1200, New York, NY 10012-1172; phone: (212) 998-5615.

Barbara Halin-Willinger, MS, CSW, is Social Work Supervisor in the AIDS Center Program at St. Luke's Roosevelt Hospital, 1111 Amsterdam Avenue, New York, NY 10025.

Michael E. Holtby, LCSW, BCD, is a licensed clinical social worker who has been serving Denver's gay community as a full-time private practitioner since 1977. He also writes a regular column, titled "Shrink Rap," in Colorado's HIV/AIDS newsletter, *Resolute!* He has testified before the Colorado state legislature on physician-assisted suicide. Reactions are welcomed by the author via e-mail: MHoltby@aol.com.

Ken Howard, LCSW, is a psychiatric social worker for Los Angeles County Department of Mental Health and is in private practice in Beverly Hills. Correspondence can be sent to 9033 Wilshire Boulevard, Suite 406, Beverly Hills, CA 90211; or via e-mail at KBHMSW@aol.com.

Annette "Chi" Hughes, MSW, is Director, Community Health and HIV Services Division at Prototypes Centers for Innovation in Health, Mental Health, and Social Services, in Culver City, California.

Hillary Kallor, CSW, was a case manager with the Brooklyn Pediatric AIDS Network working at Long Island College Hospital at the time "'Storytelling' in a Bereavement Support Group" was written.

John Kleinschmidt, MSW, CSW, is a social worker in the AIDS Center Program at St. Luke's Roosevelt Hospital, 1111 Amsterdam Avenue, New York, NY 10025.

Lorna Lee, MS, CSW, is a social worker in the AIDS Center Program at St. Luke's Roosevelt Hospital, 1111 Amsterdam Avenue, New York, NY 10025.

Carl Locke, MSW, was Coordinator of Counseling Services at the David Geffin Center for HIV Prevention and Health Education at the Gay Men's Health Crisis, New York City at the time "Finding Their Voices in Group: HIV-Negative Gay Men Speak" was written. He is currently Director of

Client Services, NYC Gay and Lesbian Anti-Violence Project, 240 West 35th Street, Suite 200, New York, NY 10001-2506. He can be contacted via e-mail at carllocke@aol.com.

Gerald P. Mallon, DSW, is an Assistant Professor at the Columbia University School of Social Work and is the Associate Executive Director at Green Chimneys Children's Services. Correspondence can be sent to him at Columbia School of Social Work, 622 West 113th Street, New York, NY 10025.

Dale V. Miller, BA, is a graduate of New York University, where he studied race, gender, and sexuality. He was the Prevention and Education Materials Coordinator at Harlem United Community AIDS Center.

Dorothy Moore, CSW, is a Brooklyn Pediatric AIDS Network case manager at Woodhull Medical Center in Brooklyn, New York.

Peter A. Newman, MSW, is a doctoral student at the School of Social Work, University of Michigan, Ann Arbor, Michigan, and is a board member of the National Social Work AIDS Network.

Craig Podell, LCSW, is a clinical social worker in private practice in Brooklyn, New York, and consultant to the Brooklyn Pediatric AIDS Network at SUNY Health Sciences Center, 450 Clarkson Avenue, Box 49, Brooklyn, NY 11203.

Martha Powers, MS, CSW, was a social worker in the AIDS Center Program at St. Luke's Roosevelt Hospital at the time "Social Work with Hospitalized AIDS Patients" was written.

Robert H. Remien, PhD, is Principal Investigator of The Couples Project, a psychological intervention and research study of male couples of mixed HIV status, at the HIV Center for Clinical and Behavioral Studies at the New York State Psychiatric Institute. He is also an assistant professor in the Department of Psychiatry at the Columbia University College of Physicians and Surgeons and was Principal Investigator of an earlier study of serodiscordant male couples at the HIV Center. He co-authored *Good Doctors, Good Patients: Partners in HIV Treatment* (1994). Correspondence can be sent to The Couples Project, NYS Psychiatric Institute, Unit 74, 722 West 168th Street, New York, NY 10032.

Raymond A. Smith, MA, MPhil, is Project Director of The Couples Project, a psychological intervention and research study of male couples of mixed HIV status, at the HIV Center for Clinical and Behavioral Studies at the New York State Psychiatric Institute. He is also a doctoral candidate in the Columbia University Graduate School and editor of the *Encyclopedia of AIDS: A Social, Political, Cultural, and Scientific Record of the HIV Epidemic* (1998). Correspondence can be sent to The Couples Project, NYS Psychiatric Institute, Unit 29, 722 West 168th Street, New York, NY 10032.

Edith Springer, ACSW, is Clinical Director of the New York Peer AIDS Education Coalition. Her work focuses on HIV prevention and harm reduction with marginalized populations.

Patricia A. Stewart, MSS, ACSW, LSW, is a social worker with an independent psychotherapy and consulting practice in Philadelphia, Pennsylvania. She is an adjunct faculty member at La Salle University, where she teaches a course on HIV/AIDS. She serves on the boards of the AIDS Law Project of Pennsylvania and National Social Work AIDS Network. She is also an associate at the National Research and Training Center on Social Work and HIV/AIDS. Correspondence can be sent to P.O. Box 1154, Lansdowne, PA 19050; or via e-mail: StewartLSW@aol.com.

David Strug, PhD, CSW, is a social worker and medical anthropologist. He is Assistant Professor in the Department of Pediatrics at SUNY Health Sciences Center, Brooklyn, and is Case Management Coordinator with the Brooklyn Pediatric AIDS Network, SUNY HSCB, 450 Clarkson Avenue, Box 49, Brooklyn, NY 11203.

Susan Taylor-Brown, MSW, PhD, MPH, is on the faculty of the School of Social Work, Syracuse University, Syracuse, NY 13244; phone: (315) 443-5550; e-mail: stbrown@social.syr.edu.

Mark Thomas, PhD, is a psychotherapist in private practice in Manhattan and, until April 1, 1998, was the coordinator of Group Services at Gay Men's Health Crisis.

Wilfred G. Van Gorp, PhD, is Associate Professor of Psychology in Psychiatry and Director, Neuropsychology Assessment Services, Cornell University Medical College, New York Hospital, Cornell Medical Center, New York, NY.

Josephine Walker, BA, is a Brooklyn Pediatric AIDS Network case manager working in the Division of Pediatric Immunology at State University Hospital in Brooklyn, New York.

Lori Weiner, PhD, is coordinator of the Pediatric HIV Psychosocial Support Program at the National Institutes of Health. Her mailing address is NIH, Building 10, Room 13 N240, Bethesda, MD 20892.

Darrell P. Wheeler, PhD, MPH, is Assistant Professor at the School of Social Work, Columbia University. Correspondence may be sent to him at Columbia School of Social Work, 622 West 113th Street, New York, NY 10025.

Ednita Wright, PhD, CSW, MSW, CAC, is on the faculty of the School of Social Work, Syracuse University, Syracuse, NY 13244; phone: (315) 443-5550; e-mail: nwright@social.syr.edu.

Introduction

Michael Shernoff

In early 1982, a small group of gay men met in response to some of their friends becoming ill from a mysterious new disease. At this meeting, they formed what was to become Gay Men's Health Crisis (GMHC), the world's first community-based AIDS service organization. That summer I was asked by Diego Lopez, the social worker coordinating mental health services for the fledgling GMHC, to become a volunteer and donate my time and clinical skills to help the men in my community who were sick with what was then known as GRID (gay-related immune deficiency).

Diego was one of the first mental health professionals in the United States to respond to AIDS. Others in that first generation of AIDS mental health professionals were Dr. Stuart Nichols, Dr. Bertram Schaffner, and Dr. Robert Remien in Manhattan; Dr. Lori Weiner, then at Memorial Sloan-Kettering Cancer Center in Manhattan; Gillian Walker and Dr. John Patten at New York's Ackerman Institute; Mel Rosen, Dr. Michael Quadland, Dr. Ken Wein and Peter Seiford at GMHC in New York City; Caitlin Ryan, then in Atlanta; Dr. James Dilley, Barbara Faltz, John Acevedo, Dr. Peter Goldblum, Dr. Leon McKusick and Judy Macks in San Francisco; Bill Scott in Houston; Paul Clover in Austin; David Aronstein and Dr. Marshall Forstein in Boston; Dr. Gary Lloyd in New Orleans; Dr. Wilfred Van Gorp and Steve Buckingham in Los Angeles; Bill Bailey at the American Psychological Association in Washington, DC; and Anthony Hillin in London. Among the first individuals to begin educating and counseling injection drug users about AIDS were social workers Luis Palacios-Jiminez and Edith Springer, while working at the Van Eten Methadone Maintenance Treatment Center in the Bronx. Some of these individuals are still working with people with HIV/AIDS, but too many others are now dead, themselves casualties of AIDS.

Although these men and women were among the original pioneers of identifying and serving the mental health needs of people living with HIV/AIDS and their loved ones, by now, well into the second decade of this epidemic, there are thousands of other dedicated mental health professionals ensuring that the emotional and psychological needs of all people living with and affected by HIV/AIDS are met in sophisticated and sensitive ways. From the early 1980s, when AIDS was known as GRID, it became clear that serving affected individuals and populations would require an integrated biopsychosocial approach. Today, even with the encouraging news about HAART (highly active antiretroviral therapy) on which triple combination therapy is based, the impact of HIV on an individual's, a family's, and a community's psyche needs to be continuously evaluated and addressed. It is precisely this professional work with the emotional and psychological issues related to living with HIV that the following chapters describe so eloquently.

Once it became clear that individuals who had shared intravenous drug-using paraphernalia were also contracting AIDS, those of us who had experience in the drug treatment field began to train the staff and volunteers of AIDS service agencies in the issues and dynamics of drug addiction, recovery, and working with active and recovering drug users. These issues became incorporated into the professional trainings that were offered to agencies, hospitals, and other facilities. By 1984, drug treatment centers were regularly requesting training on AIDS for their staff and clients.

As the HIV pandemic has spread in developed countries and in Africa and Asia, it has highlighted all of the social ills and inequities in contemporary society. In Western countries such as the United States, people infected with HIV who are privileged enough to be educated, sophisticated consumers of medical care with private insurance are living longer than poor uninsured people, who all too often are women and people of color. In undeveloped countries where medical care has never approached the standards of twentieth-century medicine, people with AIDS die much faster than those living in developed countries with health insurance and access to the most sophisticated diagnostic and treatment procedures. In the United States, the disparity in AIDS care—who is dying from the disease and how quickly they are dying—is a mirror of the ever-increasing class, race, and economic inequities in this country. For most poor and all uninsured people in the United States, AIDS is a third world illness, with women and children of color dying sooner than middle-class people with access to sophisticated treatments. From the outset, social workers, psychologists, and psychiatrists have been on the vanguard of developing and providing services for all people with HIV and AIDS, including advocating for the underserved client populations ravaged by AIDS worldwide. In his ground-breaking chapter, James Grimaldi discusses issues for one of the populations of people with HIV/AIDS that remains grossly underserved: male to female pre-operative transsexuals.

In the United States, the largest AIDS service organizations (ASOs) were founded by and for middle-class gay (predominantly white) clients who were not being adequately served by existing health and social service organizations. They are now the AIDS establishment and unfortunately often are in competition for shrinking funds with smaller community-based organizations that specifically serve communities of color. By the late 1980s, several years into the epidemic, the large ASOs, such as AIDS Project Los Angeles and Gay Men's Health Crisis in New York, began to develop services for the newer faces of AIDS: women, people of color and injection drug users, while continuing to serve their original constituency.

Initially, the community-based AIDS service organizations were not prepared for all of the cultural differences that arose from serving nongay and nonwhite clients. Almost all of the AIDS service organizations in the major cities reported conflicts and clashes between different groups of clients. Although recognizing that the poor, nonwhites, and injection drug users with HIV/AIDS needed services also, many gay men resented sharing with nongay people the organizations they had started and funded. Often these middle-class white gay men were quite racist. In addition, there were middle-class, nonwhite gay men who, similar to their white counterparts, resented having to share "their organizations" with heterosexuals and intravenous drug users.

One reason so many gay men with AIDS resented the expansion of services by ASOs to nongay people was rooted in the reality that prior to the development of ASOs there were few gay-identified health care services available. Before AIDS, the delivery of health care in the United States was almost exclusively dominated by homophobic professionals and institutions. Thus, gay men with AIDS were scared—often with good reason—that they would soon be excluded from the ASOs which they had helped begin for themselves, their friends, and their community.

Contributing to the tension among clients at the ASOs was that nongay clients were often verbally and aggressively homophobic. What the evolving realities of AIDS created was an immediate need for the staff, volunteers, and clients of the existing community-based organizations to learn about cultural diversity. Trainers from communities of color were brought in to provide education on racial and ethnic differences and how to be sensitive to the unique issues faced by these populations. Ultimately, the community-based organizations realized that they needed to hire people who reflected the diversity of clients they were now serving. In his chapter, Larry Gant provides numerous suggestions for attempting to address racism within ASOs.

Now well into the second decade of the HIV/AIDS epidemic, exciting breakthroughs have occurred in antiretroviral combination therapies that include protease inhibitors and continuously improved treatments and prophylaxis for opportunistic infections. The chapter by Darrell Wheeler and Michael Shernoff explores how mental health professionals can be useful to clients concerning issues pertaining to protease inhibitors. Michael Bettinger poignantly discusses how issues of work and returning to work can be dealt with therapeutically, and Mark Thomas describes how the new treatments are affecting support groups for people with AIDS.

Yet there is no indication that either a cure or vaccine is in sight or that prevention efforts will stop new infections. A second wave of infections is occurring among educated, middle-class urban gay men, for whom infection rates had dropped dramatically as a result of the initial AIDS prevention efforts in the early days of the epidemic. Infection rates for young gay men, especially among black and Latino gay adolescents, are still high and show no indication of slowing down. (See Peter Newman's and Edith Springer's chapters for discussions of prevention efforts aimed at this group.) New infections among injection drug users are also not abating. AIDS is continuing to decimate inner-city neighborhoods: three generations of some families have been infected or have died from AIDS. (The chapters by Ednita Wright, Evelyn Blackburn, and Susan Taylor-Brown; Patricia Stewart, Annette Hughes, and Lori Weiner speak eloquently to these issues.) Recent years have shown how living in the midst of this ongoing plague has a psychosocial impact on even those who are not infected, and new prevention efforts are targeting these populations. Steven Ball's and Carl Locke's chapters discuss a group model specifically targeting uninfected gay men.

In developed countries, current medical breakthroughs have resulted in a dramatic increase in the number of people who are long-term survivors. "As of 1990, the Centers for Disease Control (CDC) defined a long-term survivor as any person living for more than three years following a diagnosis of an AIDS-defining opportunistic infection" (Remien and Wagner, 1995, p. 180). Remien and Wagner (1995) also discuss a subgroup of long-term survivors known as "long-term nonprogressors." These are HIV-positive individuals who have a confirmed exposure for at least ten years and show minimal or no signs of being immune compromised. There is now a category of people labeled "slow progressors" who, similar to the nonprogressors, have a confirmed exposure to HIV for at least ten years. These people have never had an AIDS-defining condition, but blood work shows evidence of a compromised immune system. Many of these people now show no detectable levels of viral activity due to the new combination "cocktail" therapies. In his chapter, James Cassese discusses clinical issues that arise in practice with long-term survivors and nonprogressors from a self-psychology perspective. Despite these breakthroughs, many people with HIV will die from the disease. Michael Shernoff's chapter, "Dying Well: Counseling End-Stage Clients with AIDS," provides a framework for working with clients at the very end of their lives. Michael Holtby's two chapters will seem controversial to many—he advocates for all counselors and therapists to be professionally supportive to clients who choose to end their own lives because they have neither the stamina nor the will to continue to fight.

With incubation rates of up to ten or fifteen years from infection to onset of disease, even if a vaccine were discovered today, people living with HIV and AIDS will be served by the mental health professions for at least another generation. The cost to society in terms of medical and social services and entitlements is staggering, but these costs pale in comparison to the cost in human lives lost and shattered by AIDS.

Both the gay community and communities of color are overwhelmed by the number of people who are sick and who have died. Entire families and friendship networks have been wiped out. Some AIDS workers and other service providers working at agencies, hospitals, or in private practice have worked with literally hundreds of individuals who have died. The term "bereavement overload" was coined as a result of the AIDS epidemic. The effect of working with large numbers of people who later die has only recently begun to be addressed. How do we prevent these skilled clinicians from burning out? One of the best ways is through appropriate training and preparation for working in the field of AIDS. Another way is by creating time for staff support groups and additional mechanisms whereby professionals can process all the feelings that are a natural by-product of AIDS work, including grieving their losses. The chapters by Barbara Halin-Willinger and her colleagues and David Strug and his colleagues speak eloquently to these issues. In addition, unique issues arise when providers themselves are seropositive or become symptomatic and have to struggle with whether or not to continue working in the field.

This book is not meant to be an introduction to the basics of HIV and AIDS, either medically or psychosocially. It is rather one effort in continuing to provide professionals in the field and students in training with the most current practice information about mental health practice and HIV/AIDS. The authors are all experts seasoned by their many years of working with people with HIV and AIDS. They share their expertise about cutting-edge clinical and policy issues in the pages that follow. The chapters reflect the diversity of people affected by HIV disease. Yet there are still many faces of HIV/AIDS that could not be included in this book due to space limitations.

Most of the chapters in this book were originally published in a journal, of which I was founding editor, titled *Reading and Writings,* published by the National Social Work AIDS Network, a national organization of HIV/AIDS social workers. All people living with or affected by HIV/AIDS have enormous and complex mental health and social service needs due to the harsh realities of HIV disease, racism, homophobia, poverty, and the ever-growing mean-spiritedness that is so prevalent in the repressive political climate of diminishing social services for the neediest people in our society. Historically, some mental health professionals have made critical differences in the lives of people. As the chapters in this book demonstrate, many are still on the front lines of working to ameliorate social injustice, only now in the era of AIDS. The work reflected in this book is a large part of why I am proud to have been one of the legions of professional social workers, psychiatrists, psychologists, and counselors surrounded by inspiring colleagues in the fight against AIDS.

REFERENCE

Remien, R. and Wagner, G. (1995). Counseling long-term survivors of HIV/ AIDS. In W. Odets and M. Shernoff (Eds.), *The second decade of AIDS: A mental health practice handbook* (pp. 179-200). New York: Hatherleigh Press.

CLINICAL ISSUES

Chapter 1

The Role of Mental Health Professionals in Medical Decision Making Regarding Protease Inhibitors

Darrell P. Wheeler
Michael Shernoff

INTRODUCTION

The advent of the new class of antiretroviral drugs known as protease inhibitors has revolutionized care for people living with HIV/AIDS (PWAs). The four protease inhibitors that have been approved by the FDA are indinavir (brand name Crixivan), saquinavir mesylate (brand name Invirase), ritonavir (brand name Norvir), and nelfinavir (brand name Viracept). Reports at the International AIDS Conference held in Vancouver, Canada, in June 1996, documented that a regimen of therapy with one or more of these new drugs in combination with two of the older class of antiretroviral drugs, known as nucleoside analogues—zidovudine (AZT), didanosine (ddI), zalcitabine (ddC), stavudine (d4T), and lamivudine (3TC)—can significantly reduce the amount of HIV to undetectable levels in the bloodstream and result in patients feeling better, having improved quality of life, and ultimately living longer (James, 1996; Waldholz, 1996; Markowitz, 1996).

"For the first time in the epidemic, there has been a marked decrease in deaths among people with AIDS. During the first two quarters of 1996, the estimated number of AIDS deaths (22,000) was 12% less than the estimated number of AIDS deaths during the first two quarters of 1995; AIDS deaths declined in all four regions of the United States" (Centers for Disease Control and Prevention, 1997, p. 2). This decline has been associated with many biomedical advances, including the FDA approval and practitioners' use of antiretroviral drugs. Protease inhibitors used in combination therapies have brought numerous individuals back from the brink of death, sharply reducing, and in some cases eliminating, any detectable levels of virus from the blood of thousands of others. "It's emotionally satisfying to test undetectable, but we have no idea what that really means," said Sally Cooper, executive director of the PWA Health Group, an organization in Manhattan that provides treatment information to people with HIV (Jacobs, 1997, p. 12). "I'm excited by these drugs, but at the same time, I'm terrified by them," she explained. Protease inhibitors have changed the landscape of AIDS but not always in predictable and expected ways. To work effectively in this field, social workers need to be educated about the issues that have accompanied the arrival of protease inhibitors and the combination "cocktail" therapies of which they form one crucial component. All therapists and counselors have a prominent role to play in ensuring that their clients are knowledgeable about the medications they are considering, the limitations of their effect, and the implications for choosing or not choosing to use them. Social workers in particular can, and must, work with client groups to translate many of the complicated issues surrounding the arrival of these biomedical break-throughs into useful components that may be readily incorporated by and into the lives of the clients with whom we work.

MENTAL HEALTH PRACTICE
AND PROTEASE INHIBITORS

Therapists working with people with HIV and AIDS should be well informed about these new developments to assume the traditional variety of social work roles to best assist clients who are faced with the issues surrounding this new therapy. This is no simple task. Biomedical advances, as underscored by the rapid introduction of new medications and our emerging understanding of the effects of these drugs, are constantly being refined and updated. Beyond the traditional roles of discharge planning and the provision of acute care services, hospital social workers and psychologists must incorporate goals of health promotion, health maintenance, and a participatory relationship in the treatment process (Berkman, 1996). It is especially crucial that staff who assist clients with HIV/AIDS work with the person in his or her system. In the case of people with HIV/AIDS, the client's system may include any or all of the following: family of origin, children, legal spouse, common law spouse, same-sex partner, friends, religious institutions, staff of community-based AIDS service organizations, and primary medical providers.

Germain (1981) and Germain and Gitterman (1996) discuss social work practice in terms of understanding and ability to intervene on both the ecological (or environmental) level and the individual level, with the client and his or her immediate system. Their perspective is easily generalized to all other mental health professions. Germain (1980) explains that "ecology seeks to understand the transactions that take place between environments and living systems and the consequence of these transactions for each" (p. 485). She then elaborates on how an ecological perspective is a useful lens through which to examine the social context of clinical social work and all psychotherapy. It is essential for workers to incorporate the ecological perspective into their clinical work with clients. This inclusion is particularly true for work with historically marginalized populations such as racial, ethnic, or sexual minorities, as information and resources have not always reached these groups equitably. By utilizing this broad systems perspective, a worker will be able to understand and correctly reflect back to clients how the biases and assumptions of the mainstream culture have affected them and contributed to their unique psychodynamic and psychosocial realities. This ecological approach informs the translational role to be of assistance to clients concerning medical decision making as it applies to protease inhibitors.

MENTAL HEALTH WORKERS' TRANSLATIONAL ROLES

An article published in the *New York Times Magazine* titled "When Plagues End: Notes on the Twilight of an Epidemic" (Sullivan, 1996), reflects some of the tensions that exist surrounding protease inhibitors. There is finally a reason to have hope that HIV disease may become a chronic and manageable illness for those individuals who can comply with the rigorous demands of dosage and who can tolerate a variety of difficult side effects of the combination therapies. Yet to proclaim that we are entering the "twilight of the epidemic" is overly optimistic, gives false hope, and is misleading. For one thing, there is neither clinical evidence about how long these drugs will prove to be effective nor proof that they work for every person with HIV and AIDS.

Protease inhibitors (saquinavir, ritonavir, indinavir, and nelfinavir) are among the newest antiretroviral weapons in the biomedical arsenal to combat HIV disease. These drugs operate to confuse the virus in its destructive replication pathway. Other classes of antiretrovirals include the nonnucleoside reverse transcriptase inhibitors (nevirapine) and the nucleoside analogues (AZT, 3TC, ddI, ddC, and d4T) (Overall Treatment Strategy, 1996). Although a complete discussion of the mechanisms by which these drugs operate is beyond the scope of this chapter, it is clear that a basic knowledge of these drugs and their effects and limitations is important for all professionals to provide optimal client support.

The protease inhibitors are very difficult drugs to take for a variety of reasons. They must be taken on exact schedules without any doses being missed. Three of them (saquinavir, ritonavir, and nelfinavir) must be taken with food, while a third (indinavir) must be taken either two hours after eating or one hour prior to eating to ensure the best level of absorption. If an individual is concurrently taking ddI, which also has to be taken either two hours after eating or one hour before eating but cannot be taken at the same time as indinavir, the scheduling of drug taking becomes a nightmare. When most PWAs have an extensive regimen of other drugs to take as well, the complexities of medication compliance is further compounded:

> "I was an attorney before I went out on medical disability," explained Bob, a client in private psychotherapy with one of the authors. "Managing my medical care and prescriptions, and monitoring when and how each needs to be taken has become my full-time job. I've put it all on my computer. There is simply no way else I could keep track of it all."

As this quote illustrates, even the most sophisticated consumer of medical care who has the capacity to organize his or her own life finds managing the required scheduling of anti-HIV drugs a daunting task. Thus, a single HIV-positive parent who relies on public assistance to care for her children, one or more of whom are also infected, has numerous realistic concerns about beginning protease inhibitor therapy. These concerns should discussed with an empathetic and knowledgeable professional who will not judge her (or him) for whatever decision she (or he) decides to make. In its simplest form, good mental health practice must have the capacity to begin where the client is at to allow empathy with all the issues that the client brings to his or her session.

BARRIERS TO SUCCESS
WITH PROTEASE INHIBITORS

As Strub (1997) notes, three factors highly relevant to successful combination therapy—compliance, absorption, and resistance—are only vaguely understood by the mass media, many people with HIV, and tragically, far too many physicians, psychologists, and social workers who work with HIV-infected clients. If a patient cannot comply with the strict and rigorous dosing, scheduling, and food requirements, the therapy is destined to fail because of the growth of insufficiently suppressed viral strains. Compliant patients unable to absorb the drug, due to diarrhea or gastrointestinal problems (including those caused by the drugs themselves), are also likely to fail therapy. Diarrhea can flush out the drugs before they are absorbed into the body and have the opportunity to suppress the virus. The age of protease inhibitor combination therapies is also the era of resistance-based treatment choices. In relation to triple combination therapy, resistance can develop to one drug, while the other two are temporarily repressing viral activity successfully (Protocols for the Primary Care of HIV/AIDS, 1995).

In addition to the difficulties inherent in the need for rigid adherence to scheduling, each of the protease inhibitors has side effects that can range from annoying to debilitating. Wright, Blackburn, and Taylor-Brown (1998) effectively summarize some of the difficulties in protease inhibitor therapy:

> Protease inhibitors in combination therapy carry the promise of prolonged health. This represents a major step toward transforming HIV from a life-threatening illness to a chronic illness resulting in reduced hospitalizations and enhanced quality of life. A barrier to the use of protease inhibitors is the need for life-long treatment. If protease inhibitors are not taken as prescribed, drug resistance occurs. For patients who are uncomfortable taking drugs, the need to take protease inhibitors forever will be a major barrier. What will happen as people do not take their protease inhibitors? They risk becoming drug resistant and providers will become frustrated with their noncompliance. Medication costs are another significant barrier. This complex information must be shared in a meaningful way. (pp. 59-60)

What we believe these authors mean by the need to share this information in a meaningful way is for workers to have the knowledge and skills necessary to translate medical issues into everyday language that patients can understand; patients can then communicate their feelings about whether to begin this therapy and, once begun, how to maintain such a rigorous medical regimen. In addition, professionals need to translate patients' concerns and reluctances to beginning this therapy to medical staff so that physicians, nurses, and physician's assistants will understand the various and complex reasons why certain patients decide that protease inhibitor therapy is not right for them.

As members of the treatment team, social workers, psychologists, and psychiatrists all play a vital role in translating patients' decisions concerning protease inhibitors to medical colleagues. They help the medical staff to not view these patients as noncompliant or self-destructive or as obstinate and simply refusing to do what is in their best interests.

Issues of compliance and adherence to medical regimens are not always an exact science. This is particularly so in nascent areas such as antiretroviral medications since it is still unclear as to what extent behavioral factors associated with medication adherence interact with biomedical advances to improve client outcomes (Epstein and Cluss, 1982). (Viral loads and T-cell counts are the current state of the art as biomedical markers for efficacy of antiretroviral therapy.) Clients' capacity to sustain long-term medication adherence has been shown to correlate with other life changes that affect quality of life and, ultimately, beliefs that one can make a difference in his or her health outcomes (Epstein and Cluss, 1982; Fincham and Wertheimer, 1985). Mental health workers are in a unique position to contribute to our understanding of this relationship and to ensure that patients who cannot, or choose not to, utilize protease inhibitors are respected as persons who have made a treatment decision which appears correct to them at the present time.

ADVOCACY AND EMPOWERMENT

As reported in *The New York Times* (March 2, 1997), some physicians are refusing to prescribe the new protease inhibitors to patients whom they believe will not be able to comply with the required rigid medication schedule. There are some doctors who maintain that poor compliance with the drug-taking regimen of protease inhibitor therapy could not only spell disaster for an individual patient but also create a potential public health risk through the spread of a virus resistant to many drugs (Sontag and Richardson, 1997). Some politicians rationalize that the high cost of these new drugs, combined with the limited funds available through ADAP (AIDS Drug Assistance Plans) or medicare, means that decisions have to be made about who gets the opportunity to benefit from the new drugs. This seems to be nothing more than old-fashioned American paternalism. Psychologists and social workers are actively engaging physicians to include the patients in the decision-making aspects of their care. "Doctors are making assumptions about who can handle this and who can't which inevitably brings a lot of prejudices to the surface" (Grossman, as quoted by Sontag and Richardson, 1997, p. 1). Bruce Agins, the New York State Health Department's chief AIDS doctor, said the state "was very concerned about people being denied access to the drugs in a wholesale way because they belong to a category of people like junkies" (Sontag and Richardson, 1997, p. 35). Social workers can be valuable patient advocates by working with physicians concerning realistically assessing an individual's likelihood of complying with treatment protocol.

It does not matter where mental health professionals practice, what their disciplines are, or what type of patients they treat; workers must first educate themselves about the intricacies pertaining to protease inhibitors to be prepared to work with clients. Whether a primary psychotherapist, drug counselor, medical social worker, or case manager workers must be conversant in the issues related to beginning and maintaining the difficult regimen of protease inhibitor therapy. We believe that the following tasks are necessary in work with people with HIV who are contemplating beginning protease inhibitor therapy:

1. Explain to patients that there now exists a new class of drugs that may help prolong their lives.
2. Translate for patients the realities of the difficulties regarding taking these new drugs, including that they have severe side effects and most probably must be taken for the rest of the patients' lives.
3. Using traditional social case work methodology, help them evaluate whether they feel that they want to begin this new treatment.
4. If they express an interest in beginning the new drugs, help them decide whether the rigorousness of the compliance issues makes these drugs a viable option for them.
5. If they do begin the new therapy and decide to discontinue the treatment, help them restructure the experience from one of failure and pathology to a self-empowering decision about their own health care.

In an article about African-American women with HIV disease, Wright, Blackburn, and Taylor-Brown (1998) explain some of the difficulties professionals may experience in achieving these tasks. "As social workers, one of our objectives is to provide an environment that will enhance clients' own skills and development, even if that means they reject what we believe might be best for them" (p. 57). These authors also state, "Once we have provided the information that they need to make informed choices, then we need to support them in their decision. Although admittedly, supporting a decision to refuse what we have to offer that would supposedly extend their lives is tricky for us" (p. 57).

Wright, Blackburn, and Taylor-Brown (1998) spell out specifically how mental health professionals can be helpful to clients considering protease inhibitors:

As social workers we need to assist our clients in evaluating whether to take this medication or not by:

- developing patient education materials that help women understand the medical and financial implications of the medications;
- provide opportunities to discuss their concerns with providers and
  other patients;
- working to maintain the relationship regardless of who the medical
  provider is or was—remembering that our client is of primary concern;
- need to assist the client in understanding past painful relationships
  or failures; and,
- by remembering to respect the right of the client to refuse treatment options. (p. 60)

Since its origins in Denver in 1983, the People with AIDS movement
has in fact been one contemporary example of a core principle of mental
health practice, insofar as it centers around self-empowerment for all
people living with HIV/AIDS. A key component of self-empowerment is
not to blindly trust one's health and well-being solely to any physician,
even a well respected and trusted one. Rather, patients should have a
healthy degree of distrust that becomes translated into each patient educating himself or herself about the illness and treatment options. Once educated, patients should decide, in partnership with the doctor, which treatments will be tried. All mental health professionals doing AIDS work need
to be aware of opportunities to remind clients of this fact.

Middle-class, well-educated clients who come from a position of privilege in this society, are more easily encouraged to be sophisticated and
demanding consumers of health care. Too often, poor and other marginalized clients have little experience in advocating for themselves with doctors,
nurses, and health care institutions and agencies. Thus, workers need to
instruct all clients on how to become self-empowered, self-advocating consumers of medical care without necessarily becoming adversarial. As professionals, "empowerment means that we strive to provide our consumers
with all the information we have at our disposal so that they can make
informed choices about their lives" (Wright, Blackburn, and Taylor-Brown,
1998, p. 60).

RACIAL AND CULTURAL BARRIERS
TO PROTEASE INHIBITOR TREATMENT

Many people of color in the United States have a significant distrust of
the traditionally white-dominated health care system. Western medical care

is underutilized by people of color. When people of color interact with Western health care systems, their cultural values related to health, illness, and help seeking are often at variance with the values of the dominant system (Dalton, 1991). The origins of this distrust are underscored in the legacy of the Tuskeegee syphilis experiments. For forty years, African-American men were viewed as specimens in an experiment and not as valuable human beings. These men believed that they were enrolled in a treatment study, when in reality they were denied treatment so that the effects of untreated syphilis could be observed under "natural" conditions through end stage—death. Trusting that they were being treated for the disease, they unknowingly infected their wives, lovers, and children. Given this historical context, it is understandable that African-American PWAs would be skeptical about the health care system (Wright, Blackburn, and Taylor-Brown, 1998). The legacy of the Tuskeegee travesty of health care understandably continues to exert a powerful influence on many African Americans regarding an unwillingness to trust the Establishment's existing medical system. Thus, since the development of the earliest antiretrovirals, many African Americans have not rushed to take these drugs, as they were being touted and pushed by the same Establishment (white) providers (Cargill, 1995). Health care professionals must not minimize these concerns or assume that a reluctance to use these new drugs is inherently pathological or indicative of emotional instability. "A major challenge in doing AIDS work is how do we communicate across cultures about medicines, illness, sickness and death, and how do you communicate new information in a way that is understandable and believable?" (Wright, Blackburn, and Taylor-Brown, 1998, p. 59).

WHEN PROTEASE INHIBITORS WORK

Therapists and counselors must not arrive at sessions with clients who are contemplating or taking protease inhibitors with any preconceived ideas of how clients should be feeling about this new development. This is a prime example of that old, but crucial, social work principle of always beginning where the client is at. Even just the potential to suddenly experience a change in health and outlook can be profoundly disorienting to some people. This is especially true if they have known they are HIV positive for many years, have been living with the knowledge, and have accepted that they have a life-threatening and probably terminal illness. One man explained some of his ambivalence about taking protease inhibitors:

There's a big tug of war going on inside me. Between the side that wants to live and the part that had already accepted that I was going to die. I had made peace with the probability that my life was going to be cut short. Now, I don't want to get my hopes up again. If they can restore my health with a pill, that will be far easier than trying to restore my shattered life.

Work with persons anticipating use, or questioning continued use, of protease inhibitors requires the provider to address issues of access, compliance, side effects, and maintenance early on and as frequently as necessary to facilitate the client's understanding of, and empowerment in, his or her health care (Soto, 1996).

The authors have spoken with many patients who are having attacks of anxiety and feelings of unreality, depression, suspicion, and anger in response to the improvement in their health. Usually they are confused by these reactions and often are ashamed to talk about them. As welcome as an improvement in their health may be, it is not a development that can yet be trusted to last, and because of this, the individual who is experiencing a dramatic resurgence of good health is often understandably reluctant to place much hope in this latest change. When an individual has invested considerable emotional energy and hope in previous possible medical breakthroughs, only to have his or her hopes shattered, it becomes increasingly more difficult to muster up the same optimism and hope as before. Experiencing periods of hope, coupled with letdowns and despair, can create powerful mood swings that lead in part to the well-documented emotional roller coaster of living with HIV and AIDS.

Therapists and counselors need to elicit each client's feelings about new treatment options and give him or her the opportunity to discuss and explore all of those feelings in depth. One client explained his feelings about beginning protease inhibitors in the following way:

It's a little like living on death row and getting a stay of execution. I had a date when I knew I was going to die, and now all of a sudden I'm going to be allowed to live for awhile longer. Who knows how much longer? Will I live to be an old queen? Will the virus mutate sometime in the future making the current treatments ineffective? Obviously I don't know. I do know that instead of being overjoyed, I feel like I'm being jerked around.

After finally deciding to begin taking the new drugs, and experiencing a remarkable drop in viral activity with a corresponding increase in his energy level, another patient concurred:

It's hard to put these feelings into words. I feel like I am simply supposed to be ecstatic that I am feeling better, and of course on some level I am. But this kind of about-face brings up multiple emotional issues. It's been impossible to say, "Hooray, all of my problems have disappeared."

Many individuals who are feeling better as a result of taking protease inhibitors feel guilty about their own good fortune, as they think about the friends, lovers, and children who have predeceased them, for whom these new treatments arrived too late. Numerous patients who are benefiting from the new combination therapies have described feeling renewed loneliness for the loved ones already lost to the disease. Again, therapists need to be alert to this dynamic and probe for any feelings that the client may have in this regard. After starting protease inhibitor therapy, one man gained weight and once again became robust at the same time that his best friend died. This juxtaposition of events greatly unnerved him and took away from the euphoria he was feeling about his own good luck. A common question is, "Why am I here to benefit from these treatments, when so many others whom I loved are already dead?"

Stabilized health as a result of the new treatments also has the potential to cause anxiety about financial matters. Some people with AIDS, believing that they only had a short time to live, cashed in life insurance policies and spent the money or applied for and got numerous credit cards and ran these up to the limits, thinking that their estates would be left to deal with the resultant debts. But now, as these individuals are living longer, they cannot afford to manage their current debt load and are extremely financially strapped. Others worry about how long various entitlement programs will continue to pay for their benefits. These benefits extend beyond cash resources. For clients who have moved out of their independent living situations into residences for persons with AIDS and other assisted-living arrangements, the benefits of biomedical sciences may jeopardize their status as a "worthy" recipient of continued support.

For patients whose health has improved so much that their physicians are questioning whether they can continue to justify a diagnosis of permanent disability, the good news is often accompanied by new worries. Although thrilled that they are once again feeling strong and healthy, they are frightened about the prospect of returning to work. People who believed that they were permanently retired due to having AIDS, and who have not worked for several years, have had no reason to keep up with current developments in their professional fields. They are worried about returning to work and not having the state-of-the-art expertise required to be competent. In addition, there are realistic concerns about what will happen to their insurance policies and other benefits if they do return to work. For clients with limited work histories, or who have been chemically dependent for much of their adult lives, the loss of social supports offered to PWAs can create a sense of dread and mean a return to a life with few options for stable income, medical supports, or housing. All mental health professions need to either research or develop relationships with experts in the area of returning to work and the effect this has on the client's benefits.

WHEN THE DRUGS DO NOT WORK

One scenario that is extremely painful and frightening for clients with HIV/AIDS, their significant others, and health care professionals treating these individuals and their loved ones is the reality that between 10 and 30 percent of those who take the grueling course of new AIDS medications fail to respond (Jacobs, 1997). Thus, it is clinically dangerous for professionals to allow their expectations and hopes for a dramatic improvement in the health of their clients to intrude into their daily interactions with these individuals. Clients who are debilitated by the severe side effects (which in the daily routine can be seen as *main effects*) of protease inhibitors sometimes feel poisoned by the new treatment. Clients who are unable to tolerate the side effects of the drugs often wrestle in sessions with "What good are the protease inhibitors if they are extending your life but destroying the quality?" These individuals need to be encouraged to discuss their feelings about the pressing issue of "At what price survival?" There are numerous patients who, after a very brief period of benefiting from the new drugs, become overwhelmed by the side effects and today are no doubt sicker than they were before they began the new wonder drugs. One client who has not been able to tolerate protease inhibitors stated:

> I don't like to whine, but it is really difficult hearing all the good news, and how these drugs have heralded the end of the plague. That has simply not been my experience. It's very lonely not being able to talk to other people about what it's like hearing all the good news and feeling totally left out. Even in my AIDS support group no one seems to understand how I feel.

"The perception that the plague is over has only compounded the misery of those who have failed on combination therapies" (Jacobs, 1997, p. 1). For people who have had their hopes dashed countless times, it is crushing to be left out of this so-called success story.

When an individual is unable to tolerate the numerous side effects, or is resistant to the new drugs, he or she is understandably disappointed and often angry that these drugs did not work for them. The patient previously quoted had to cease taking Crixivan because shortly after beginning it he began to experience suicidal thoughts in addition to bodily twitching and other symptoms of central nervous system disorders. On Norvir, he suffered even worse reactions, including hallucinations, severe nausea, diarrhea, and uncontrollable trembling. The side effects of delavirdine were also debilitating, and he had to stop taking it as well. He is currently hoping that new drugs enter the market soon, before it is too late. All nonmedical workers need to be knowledgeable about anticipated side effects and to inquire about what side effects, if any, the individual may be experiencing and how this is making him or her feel about this new regimen. In addition, patients need to be coached to request antinausea and antidiarrhea medications from their physicians. Providing clients with the information, encouraging proactive interactions with medical providers, and when necessary, advocating on their behalf are all examples of nontraditional mental health interventions that must be considered in work with clients faced with the critical decision of taking antiretroviral medications.

Jeffrey Karaban is deputy executive director of Body Positive, an AIDS organization in lower Manhattan. He sees a growing chasm between those who respond to combination therapy and those who do not. "A lot of old timers are feeling abandoned. They fear they'll become lepers, written off by drug companies who can't make a buck off of them" (Jacobs, 1997, p. 12). Karaban further explains how AIDS service organizations are developing specific services to meet the needs of both people who are benefiting from protease inhibitors and those who are not. Separate support groups are being formed at both Body Positive and at Gay Men's Health Crisis in New York City for clients who are successful on protease inhibitors and those long-term survivors who have had no luck with the drugs.

Most people who have improved as a result of taking protease inhibitors feel as if they are holding their breath, not allowing themselves to dare believe that their improvements will hold up in the long run. This uncertainty is not ill-founded and creates a very potent anxiety originating in the reality that, at the present time, the longest period for which protease inhibitors have been proven effective is eighteen months. It is very difficult to encourage people not to allow their dark thoughts about "what if's" to overpower them. During counseling sessions, they need to be reminded that we hope and want the benefits of all the new treatments to last for a long time. However, even if it is only for a year or two, their responsibility is to enjoy the improvements they are experiencing. Most patients who have shown improvement on protease inhibitors are confronting the paradox of now dealing with issues they thought they would never again face, such as work, feeling better, socializing, and even dating.

CONCLUSION

The AIDS plague is not over, and protease inhibitors have not ushered in the "twilight of the epidemic." They have become an additional and powerful weapon in our arsenal of treatments for HIV/AIDS. However, they have not even come close to solving many of the problems routinely experienced by people living with HIV/AIDS, problems for which they seek out mental health professionals for assistance. In fact, as this chapter demonstrates, the availability of protease inhibitors, while offering hope and improved health to many people, brings new and additional issues and dilemmas that make PWAs' plates just a bit fuller than they previously were. Incorporating the primary tenets of the ecological perspective with the translational role of psychosocial intervention allows the worker to join with the client system to enhance self-efficacy in making and sustaining difficult life choices associated with HIV disease. Nevertheless, as with all other facets of this illness, only by speaking up, ending the shame that accompanies silence, and facing the uncertainties and ambiguities honestly can each of us, provider and client, continue to refine what it means to be self-empowered, as we all live affected by HIV/AIDS.

Individuals who are infected with HIV but are lucky enough to have the money, time, and education to become treatment sophisticated now have a shot at surviving AIDS. Tragically, a growing majority of people with HIV do not have money, education, or even time to become as informed as they must to survive. This is where well informed and skilled mental health professionals can make an enormous difference in the lives of people living with HIV. All professionals must continue to advance the work with their clients to support treatment information and education, access to medications, maintenance of social supports as clients adjust to new medications and the prospects of returning to prior levels of functioning, lifelong adherence to medication regimens, and ultimately, the decision to take medications that may have limited effects.

"Accompanying the life-saving opportunity provided for the privileged by protease inhibitor therapy, there is also an enormous moral obligation" (Strub, 1997, p. 12). Social workers must mobilize to demand and deliver equitable and systemic access, trials, and real hope for everyone with HIV. The role of mental health professionals extends beyond the delivery of biomedical information and must encompass the capacity to work with the client system to translate information into useable terms. Professionals should then work with the client to actualize these options in a manner that optimizes health outcomes, self-worth, and personal dignity.

REFERENCES

AIDS Institute (1995). *Protocols for the primary care of HIV/AIDS in adults and adolescents*, Third Edition. New York State Department of Health.

Berkman, B. (1996). The emerging health care world: Implications for social work practice and education. *Social Work, 41*(5), 541-551.

Cargill, V. (1995). African Americans and AIDS. *HIV Newsline*, June, 38-40.

Centers for Disease Control and Prevention (1997). 1996 HIV/AIDS trends provide evidence of success in HIV prevention and Treatment: AIDS deaths decline for the first time. CDC Press Summary, February 28.

Dalton, H. (1991). AIDS in blackface. In N. McKenzie (Ed.), *The AIDS reader, social, political and ethical issues*. New York: Meridian, 205-227.

Epstein, L. H., and Cluss, P. A. (1982). A behavioral medicine perspective on adherence to long-term medical regimens. *Journal of Consulting Clinical Psychology, 50*(6), 950-971.

Fincham, J. E. and Wertheimer, A. I. (1985). The health belief model to predict initial drug therapy defaulting. *Social Science Medicine, 20*(1), 101-105.

Germain, C. B. (1980). Social context of clinical social work. *Social Work, 25*(6), 483-488.

Germain, C. B. (1981). The ecological approach to people-environment transactions. *Social Casework, 62*(6), 323-331.

Germain, C. B. and Gitterman, A. (1996). *The life model of social work practice*. New York: Columbia University Press.

Jacobs, A. (1997). The diagnosis: HIV-Positive. *The New York Times*, February 2, section 13, pp. 1-13.

James, J. (1996). The word from Vancouver. Being Alive. *AIDS Treatment News, 4*(10), 1-8.

Markowitz, M. (1996). *Protease inhibitors: A new family of drugs for the treatment of HIV infection*. Chicago, IL: The International Association of Physicians in AIDS Care.

Project Inform (1996, November). *Overall treatment strategy*. San Francisco, CA: Project Inform.

Sontag, D. and Richardson, L. (March 2, 1997). Doctors withhold HIV pill regimen from some. *The New York Times*, pp. 1, 35.

Soto, T. (1996). Psychosocial issues in protease inhibitor treatment. Presentation at the Center for Mental Health Services Mental Health Services Demonstration Program Steering Committee Meeting. Washington, DC.

Sullivan, A. (1996). When plagues end: Notes on the twilight of an epidemic. *The New York Times Magazine*, November 10, 52-84.

Strub, S. (1997). Treatment sophistication equals survival. *POZ,* April, p. 2.
Waldholz, M. (1996). New drug "cocktails" mark exciting turn in the war on AIDS. *The Wall Street Journal,* June 14, p. A1.
Wright, E., Blackburn, E., and Taylor-Brown, S. (1999). African-American women still remain invisible: Are mental health professionals doing enough? Clinical cultural competence issues. In Michael Shernoff (Ed.), *AIDS and mental health practice: Clinical and policy issues.* Binghamton, NY: The Haworth Press, pp. 235-248.

Chapter 2

Intrapsychic and Systemic Issues Concerning Returning to Work for People Living with HIV/AIDS

Michael Bettinger

Although some people with AIDS have continued to work throughout most of the course of their illness, others have retired because of complications related to HIV infection. With the success of combination therapies and protease inhibitors, many people with HIV disease have regained lost abilities, and a once-rare question has become common: "Should I return to work?" This prospect involves a host of practical questions, but it also raises psychological issues related to the meaning of work in a person's life, the changes in perspective that follow the adjustment to a life-threatening disease, a person's relationship to the future, and the difficult process of changing one's self-image; all are fertile areas for therapeutic exploration in counseling and therapy.

For most people, work is important for reasons beyond financial well-being. Along with gender, ethnicity, and sexual orientation, it is one of the primary ways people identify themselves. "What do you do (for a living)?" is almost always one of the first questions people ask one another in social situations, not simply because it is an easy way to break the ice and offer topics for continuing a conversation, but also because the answer provides a shorthand means for each person in the interaction to learn about the other. At the end of one's life, the obituary usually will note three things in the headline: the name of the deceased, his or her age, and what kind of work he or she did.

An earlier version of this chapter was published in *FOCUS: A Guide to AIDS Research Counseling*, *12*(8), July 1997, as "Regaining Lost Abilities: The Prospect of Returning to Work." *FOCUS* is a monthly newsletter published by the University of California, San Francisco, AIDS Health Project.

Work is central to self-image and self-esteem and is one of the basic marks—perhaps one of the defining conditions—of adulthood. For many people, especially those not directly involved in raising children, it is one of the things that gives their lives meaning. In the United States, with the exception of those over sixty-five and those raising children, adults are presumed to have jobs. And as the recent debate over welfare reform suggests, American society does not look kindly upon those who do not have jobs for which they get paid.

To be disabled is to be considered incapable or less able to work and therefore ineffective. Mental health professionals have long regarded work as a form of therapy for people with disabilities because working, even in a low-status profession, helps endow an individual with a sense of accomplishment and the feeling that he or she is not only a part of the greater adult community but also a productive member of society with an identity beyond that of "patient." Programs designed to help individuals with mental illness or developmental disabilities often incorporate a protected work environment as part of the overall program. The shift in identity from patient to worker often gives a person's life meaning, which results in enhanced self-esteem and often alleviates symptoms of depression.

DISABILITY AND THE RETURN TO WORK

For adults who find themselves unable to work due to the effects of HIV infection and for those who now have the opportunity to return to work, there are psychological and practical as well as financial consequences that blend with and reinforce one another. Most important, retirement because of disability removes a central focus in a person's life. This often creates an emptiness that has the potential to damage self-image and self-esteem, especially if it occurs at a time of life, in early to mid-adulthood, when a person would not have expected to face such limitations. While peers continue to be active and productive, a person disabled by HIV disease may not only lose the identity of a worker but also is at risk of seeing himself or herself as essentially defective because of the loss of that identity. A person with a long-term disability may take several years to grieve this loss and to mitigate potentially concurrent symptoms of depression before he or she adjusts to the circumstances, finds a new meaning in life, forms a new self-image, and bolsters self-esteem. Until recently, most people with HIV disease have not had the time to make psychological adjustments beyond confronting and accepting the possibility of debilitation and death and adjusting to the reality that "the future is now." For them, the world became organized around health care providers, medications, and HIV support groups, while they tried to cram a lifetime of activities into the present.

HIV-related disability has often meant putting a career on hold at a time when peers are advancing in their occupations. This can raise feelings of loss, anger, sadness, emptiness, and disorientation. But the idea of returning to work can also be emotionally traumatic. Looking for a job is, in any context, fraught with anxiety, as a person risks repeated rejection and the prospect of temporarily compromising goals. People with HIV disease reentering the job market may face these feelings and more—a sense of failure and regret, a fear of having lagged too far behind to catch up, grief at the loss of dreams and opportunities, anger at themselves for not trying harder to overcome disability, and psychological paralysis.

These feelings may be fueled by the practical challenges of dealing with résumés that are no longer so impressive and with professional skills that are no longer up to date. In addition, individuals reentering the job market at the same level they had been at when they stopped working may now be competing for jobs with younger people. America is an age-conscious society in which being older results not only in making an individual less employable but also raises anxieties about aging (something people with symptomatic HIV disease have up to now rarely considered). In this area at least, people with HIV disease share some of the challenges faced by women returning to the workforce after an absence for child rearing.

Being disabled can lead to severe economic problems and concerns about money that can only divert attention away from, or exacerbate, the psychological challenges of confronting the future as an able person. A person with HIV disease may have "spent down" life savings, cashed in retirement plans, maxed out credit cards and life insurance policies, and sold personal possessions. Being disabled and anticipating a shortened life span, a person with HIV disease may have adjusted to these conditions and to receiving financial support from government entitlements and/or private disability insurance.

However, when envisioning a normal life span, this financial instability can be frightening and can heighten anxiety about the decision to return to work and the process of job hunting. For some people, a "clean slate" may be inspiring, but for those who have let go of the means and form of a previous life it becomes unsettling in the context of extended life. Adding to this confusion is the uncertainty about whether health recovered by combination therapy will be permanent and by the understandable fear that working may mean disability income will be lost forever.

Finally, many people disabled by HIV disease have become used to a different way of life—a greater control over time; a slower pace and more adaptable schedule; a healthier balance of work and rest; the absence of the dysfunctional interpersonal "dramas" that arise in every work setting. For some, adjusting to disability, uncertainty, and a threat to life also nurtures clarity about what is important and what is unimportant, including a deeper understanding of the preciousness of life and a desire to live in the moment.

This change in perspective is often reflected in terms of work and career. It is not unusual to hear stories about a person with HIV who was a lawyer returning to school to become a therapist or for a businessperson to become an artist or for an artist to become a teacher. But recovering health, regaining ability, rejoining the workforce, and undertaking activities previously deferred may end this way of living, transporting a person with HIV disease back to where he or she was before becoming ill. Further, staying in, or returning to, the job a person previously held can, under these circumstances, lead to feeling trapped, frustrated, and disappointed.

ADAPTING TO CHANGE

Mental health providers can assist clients who are considering returning to work by seeking to help them understand the practical and emotional tasks they face and by helping them sort through the conflicts inherent in wrestling with these enormously complex and important issues. Part of this process is psychological, and part is practical. To deal with the practical aspects of resuming a career, or training for a new one, providers should refer clients for vocational counseling. To approach the psychological issues, clinicians should be aware of two sources of potential conflicts and ambivalence regarding returning to work or retraining— one intrapsychic, the other systemic.

To effectively address the myriad of intrapsychic issues, the clinician can begin by asking clients to explore the meaning of work and working (or not working) in their lives. The clinician should pay particular attention to how not working affects the person's self-image and self-esteem and the emotional issues that might make returning to work difficult. For clients who want to return to work, the psychological task is to move in a direction in which they will be able to redefine themselves as workers, acknowledging but disengaging from the image of themselves as being disabled. Intensively exploring the meaning of work with clients can help them locate internal emotional strengths and resources that they bring to this effort, which can be of assistance in keeping them on track during this often difficult period of change.

Intrapsychic homeostasis is powerful. Despite a natural capacity to adapt and readapt, some clients are likely to take comfort in the organization of their lives around HIV disease and to have difficulty changing this perspective. A similar phenomenon is seen among recently released prisoners who have a difficult time adapting to life outside of prison. Some commit other crimes or violate parole to be sent back to the familiar world of incarceration. In a similar fashion, some clients with HIV disease may find it difficult to readjust to a world defined beyond medical appointments, medication schedules, and other HIV-related activities. They may want to change their primary identity as a person living with a chronic and life-threatening illness, but they may not want to act or be different than they have learned to do to make healthy and necessary adaptations to living with HIV. Some clients struggling with returning to work experience difficulty letting go of what they have become used to, even when the familiar is a painful reminder of their health condition.

Any significant change in a person's life, including a positive one, has the potential to evoke feelings of loss and a need to grieve for what has been lost—in this case, a world organized around HIV disease and the self-image as a disabled person. To successfully grieve a loss involves forming a new relationship with what has been lost, whether this is a person who has died or, as in this case, an illness that is no longer what it was. This is often a confusing and baffling part of the intrapsychic journey of clients who are experiencing a renaissance of good health that is motivating them to contemplate returning to work.

In addition to the loss of viewing themselves as a disabled person faced with a shortened life span, clients may experience symptoms of depression combined with a variety of feelings about the improvements in their health. To make up for lost time, they may express a sense of urgency concerning deferred life activities. Feelings may resurface with a vengeance about the life partner a person never had, the forgotten sex life, the trips never taken, the house never purchased, the books never read, the family relationships never repaired. The mental health professional needs to inquire and elicit feelings about the toll HIV disease has taken on their lives, dreams, and expectations, even during this period of renewed vitality and optimism.

Also, since improvement in health rarely occurs without some setbacks, or the possibility of setbacks always haunting a person, clients who experience HIV-related symptoms or infections may emotionally regress to a "disabled" mentality for a period of time, when they become even mildly symptomatic after experiencing a period of consistent good health. They may find they have enough energy—be it physical or psychic—to be ambitious, but not enough energy to follow through on plans to pursue rejoining the workforce. Convalescence is difficult to manage both physically and emotionally and is often a bumpy road for the client, his or her support system, and the mental health professionals involved in caring for him or her. Finally, regaining strength and ability is likely to be complicated by survivor guilt, which may lead clients to act in ways that threaten, if not their survival, then at least their prospects for successfully returning to work. Throughout the process of discussing a possible return to work, clients may question the value of old ways of living, including ones with which they are about to reengage. The experiences gained during disability, of learning to live in the moment, for example, may help clients devise new (and perhaps unconventional) ways of living that are better suited to long-term adjustment.

For some clients, however, the process of looking at future possibilities may be a way of perseverating and of avoiding the difficult process of adjustment to new health and life. This is often true in clients who have a history of obsessiveness. Clinicians should heed such resistance, which may take many forms, and remain attuned to the pain clients express as they grieve the loss of a way of living and negotiate new lives. Counselors should also seek to help clients reestablish a balance between living in the present and planning for the future. This might involve helping clients understand and retain what they value about living in the moment, while defining long-term needs and strategies for satisfying them.

Systemic factors can also work in tandem with a client's intrapsychic issues to further complicate moving from an identity of a disabled person to contemplating a return to work. The other individuals in the person's life may be unconsciously invested in, or attached to, relating to the person with HIV or AIDS as permanently disabled. Members of the client's support system need to make their own psychological adjustments to accepting their loved one as a person with a chronic, life-threatening illness, and they may also be ill-prepared for the transition of their loved one into good health. Just as it is often difficult for a soldier to go from war to peace, caregivers can also find it difficult to go from illness to wellness. It is not unusual for partners, parents, or friends to want the familiar to remain familiar. Clinicians can help all people involved by providing a forum in which both systemic and intrapsychic issues can be openly discussed, by offering to see members of the client's support system along with him or her in family sessions that address these crucial changes that affect all of them and their social and emotional systems. The major goal of these sessions is to (hopefully) enlist the help of significant others in the process or, at least, to get them out of the way of the client's shedding his or her identity as a disabled person.

There are several possible approaches to dealing with systemic resistance regarding a client's need to move beyond an identity as a disabled person with HIV. The first is to help the client identify those resistances and understand that various people, possibly including himself or herself, will be pressuring him or her not to change. Identifying and understanding the sources of intrapsychic or interpersonal pressure concerning these potential life changes can be one useful place to begin intervention. Through dialogue with the therapist or counselor, it will provide the person contemplating such changes a way of understanding the reactions caused internally and in others.

Another strategy available to the clinician is to coach the client to recognize when significant others are creating obstacles to returning to work and to challenge those individuals expressing resistance. These individuals are often the very people who care most about the health and well-being of the potential worker. Depending upon a person's history and the dynamics of the relationship, including the levels of honesty and openness of communication, confronting loved ones with the obstacles they are creating to his or her efforts to redirect his or her life may be difficult. The clinician needs to employ techniques that include both problem solving and role-playing in an effort to empower the individual with HIV who is faced with the daunting task of discussing these issues with well-meaning loved ones.

Perhaps it is most important for the clinician to keep in mind that this time of change in health condition and possible readiness to return to work is exceedingly confusing for many people who are living with HIV disease. It is made more difficult by a society that is most comfortable with binary notions: one is either seropositive or seronegative; ill or well; with AIDS or without AIDS; able or disabled. However, these polar concepts are too limited for dealing with the new reality of HIV; there is a now a wider spectrum of illness and wellness than ever before. Clinicians need to take a psychoeducational approach and instruct clients that a broader range of possibilities exists. They must elicit clients' feelings about this evolving reality to validate the confusion many are experiencing, to help clients sort through all possibilities, enabling them to make informed decisions about returning to work and considering the future.

CASE STUDY

The following case study illustrates many of the factors described previously. In this particular case, the systemic forces created more of an obstacle for the client than did his own intrapsychic issues. Lawrence (not his real name) is a thirty-seven-year-old, gay, African-American male, from a working-class background. He graduated from a public college with a degree in electrical engineering but found he could not secure employment. Lawrence believed racism was the chief obstacle to his finding employment in his field so he joined the military, where he gained technical skills as an electrician. Upon discharge from the military, he worked for a major public utility as an electrician.

He seroconverted in 1987, as a result of an unsafe sexual contact; he and another a man were both using amphetamines, and the other man lied about his serostatus. He remained asymptomatic, although his CD-4 cells continued to decline, and he was eventually diagnosed with AIDS. At the same time, the utility for which he was working was downsizing and offering disability benefits to employees who were HIV positive, regardless of the actual state of their health. These disability benefits would, however, last for only five years. Lawrence took the offer and retired. At that time, his CD-4 cell count was almost zero. Since this was one of the lowest points of optimism in the medical battle against AIDS, he firmly believed there was no way he was going to outlive the disability benefits.

For the first three years on disability, Lawrence was quite satisfied with his life. He joined a gym and made considerable progress gaining muscle mass. These efforts at the gym also benefited him emotionally since he had been a skinny kid and had considerable shame about his body. During the time he was on disability, Lawrence began a romantic relationship with another man who was also disabled due to an AIDS-related condition whom he met while shopping in a supermarket. They eventually moved in together.

The presenting problem that initially brought Lawrence to therapy was depression. He had been urged to seek therapy by his AIDS support group, who had become concerned about a recent change in his mood and his reports that he was sad much of the time, had little interest in sex, and was having so much trouble sleeping that it was necessary for him to greatly increase his daily dose of prescribed sedatives. During the initial consultation, his affect was flat, and he related how he had become seropositive with the same affect used to describe how he met his partner and fell in love.

There were only two moments in the initial session when he was at all animated. The first of which was when he described the three great battles of his life: "racism, homophobia, and AIDS." The other time was when he proudly recounted being part of a team that had been sent throughout the state when storms knocked out the power supply, and he had to try to restore downed power lines, often while the storm was still in progress. He also proudly discussed his specialty of working with live power lines, a skill that required him to be extremely careful. Upon my questioning, he agreed that his steady and contained emotional nature aided him in these situations.

Soon after our work began, and just before protease inhibitors were approved for general use, he became eligible for protease inhibitors under a compassionate use program, as he had not responded to any of the other then available antiretroviral drugs. After several months of significant side effects from the first combination of drugs, his medical providers found a combination of a protease inhibitor and antiretrovirals which he could not only tolerate but which had a positive effect on his immune system. Soon his blood tests confirmed that his immune system was improving, and he also gained weight and regained strength.

Although this appeared to be good news, it initially led to considerable confusion on his part. He had been resigned to getting weaker and thinner and to dying soon. Now, for the first time since he had begun to decline, the process appeared to be reversed. After an initial period of hope and improving mood, his depression returned, and he agreed to begin treatment with antidepressant medication.

As treatment continued, Lawrence began to talk about how for most of his adult life he had identified with and invested in his work. After being African American, pride in his vocational skills was his strongest identification. In one session, he discussed how, while growing up, the adult men in his family would express pride that they would do the work that white people would not do, do it well, and work harder than whites would work. Discussing this memory had a profound effect on him. On one hand, it evoked feelings of sadness and loss, yet it also strengthened his resolve to try to return to work now that his strength was returning and his depression was abating.

As the end of the fifth year of disability approached, Lawrence became both fearful and elated. His fears revolved around financial realities since his private disability benefits would cease, leaving him with only Social Security Disability Income and Medicare, causing a considerable drop in his monthly income. Yet his elation was connected to beginning to view the loss of disability benefits as a potential opportunity to regain his independence by breaking free of his reliance upon government entitlements. As he explored his options about returning to work, he discovered that he could earn up to $500 per month without disturbing his SSDI or Medicare. He knew several contractors who would willingly hire him to do electrical installation work so finding work was not the problem.

In therapy, he successfully addressed the intrapsychic issues and worked through his various ambivalent feelings regarding returning to work. He was highly motivated to resume working by understanding the place work had always occupied in his life and identity. This caused him to recognize a deep belief that he needed something more in his life than he currently had. Some of his sadness stemmed from the reality that he was not contributing more to society. His improving health led him to realize that his personal values impelled him to work if he were able.

What surprised him most were the mixed messages he received from others regarding returning to work. The neighbor who depended upon him to be home in the mornings when the package delivery company arrived expressed regrets that Lawrence would no longer be there to receive packages. His partner expressed fear of being alone during the day and of Lawrence not being available to drive and accompany him to his medical appointments. Lawrence's mother strongly objected to the idea of him returning to work, expressing fears that he would overtax himself, causing him to become ill. She became hysterical several times when Lawrence said he probably would soon begin to work part-time. By discussing his mother's hysterical reaction to his plans for resuming work, he came to understand that much of his flat, unemotional style was an effort to be as unlike his mother as he could possibly be. Even members of his AIDS support group were not initially supportive of his desire to resume working; they told him that they were happy for him, but also that it would be difficult for them if he could not attend their daytime meetings because of work. The group said they saw him as an anchor, both emotionally and because of his success in avoiding opportunistic infections. The group members told Lawrence that they were worried the group would not survive without him.

Therapy sessions were very emotionally charged during this phase of treatment, as Lawrence grappled with increased insights and understandings about how he functioned in relation to the important people in his life. One major breakthrough occurred when Lawrence clearly understood how much he was affected by the expectations others had of him. This was a major revelation for him since he had always seen himself as an extremely independent person. This insight was but one example of the tremendous growth that Lawrence experienced through exploring all of his feelings and reactions pertaining to the role that work had historically played in his life before he became ill and his expectations for how returning to work would affect his identity, sense of self-esteem, and relationships. A combined intrapsychic and interpersonal examination of his relationship to working paved the way for Lawrence to begin to understand that much of his life had previously been dedicated to not acknowledging feelings. In sessions, he discussed both the meaning of work and the external pressures he was experiencing to remain on disability.

After discussing a variety of possible strategies in his sessions, Lawrence confronted both his partner and mother and was able to get them to stop actively resisting his efforts to resume working, though neither would ever actually become fully supportive of his transition back into the workforce. He began limited part-time work for a contractor who remodels houses, doing what Lawrence describes as simple work—running conduits, installing junction boxes, switches, and outlets. During our sessions, Lawrence was able to openly discuss feeling quite apprehensive about being back at work after a hiatus of almost five years. I also urged him to remember that he always maintained the option of deciding not to work if he found it too taxing, an idea he was reluctant to discuss in much depth. In a recent session, he was overjoyed to report that he had been able to tell someone he had met that he was no longer a person living on disability but was, once again, an "electrician."

CONCLUSION

Combination therapies including protease inhibitors are resulting in increased health for people with AIDS, who are now being presented with challenges previously unforeseen, including returning to work. Both work and being on disability have deep meanings for all people. Many clients who are on disability will now want to at least consider and discuss all the ramifications of possibly returning to work. To be most helpful to clients, clinicians need to engage clients in discussions that explore the historic meaning of work in their lives, as well as all the feelings accompanying the thoughts of reentering the workforce. When both the clinician and client have a fairly complete understanding of the complex relationship between the individual and his or her work history, only then can clinicians attempt to engage clients in an exploration of what the intrapsychic and systemic ramifications of returning to work may be. One important aspect of this exploration must be a realistic assessment of all the issues that have the potential to impede the person living with HIV from returning to work.

Chapter 3

An Exploration of Change:
The Influence of Combination Therapies
on PWA Support Groups

Mark Thomas

Since the early days of the identification of the acquired immunodeficiency virus, when the gay and medical communities struggled to understand terms such as AIDS-related complex (ARC) and gay-related immune deficiency (GRID), forums for people to share their concerns over AIDS-related issues have been widely utilized. These support group meetings have served to provide a safe space for people to explore their fears, reduce the isolation often associated with confusion and anxiety, share information, and provide support through illness and death.

In 1983, Gay Men's Health Crisis (GMHC) in New York City began providing supportive group services for people suffering from the enormous emotional consequences of witnessing life-threatening illnesses ravage the lives of friends, lovers, and often themselves. Unable to make sense of this insidious epidemic, the gay community rallied in an attempt to join forces, provide emotional and practical assistance to those in need, and be heard by a general population that appeared to be only minimally concerned with what was known as the "gay disease." These groups have evolved into the weekly, ninety-minute forums, run by volunteer mental health professionals at GMHC, that are provided for people living with AIDS, their loved ones, couples affected by HIV, and people in bereavement as a result of AIDS-related death(s).

People who suffer the physical and emotional consequences of having survived opportunistic infections resulting from HIV infection often feel burdensome to friends and family. This is true not only in relation to the need for practical assistance but also in the belief that their concerns may be overwhelming to people in their support system. People living with AIDS often describe being fearful of alienating those around them as a result of

WILLIAM F. RUSKA LIBRARY
BECKER COLLEGE

being a living reminder of those who have suffered and ultimately passed away. In the AIDS support group forum, the total experience of members' fears and feelings of confusion regarding the issues related to confronting mortality are validated by the other members and the support group leader. This often contrasts sharply with the often placating experience resulting from discussion with friends and family who may not be willing or equipped to manage the intensity of these issues, offering responses such as "Don't worry; you'll be fine," or "Try not to think about it." Through the utilization of a forum in which group members feel known and supported in the sharing of their triumphs, fears, and losses, support group participation often serves as the primary emotional outlet for people living with AIDS.

Throughout the history of AIDS-related support groups, the center of discussion has focused around an intense fear of sudden and debilitating illness, often greater than the fear of death itself. Members describe an anxiety regarding a pending succession of opportunistic infections, which are ultimately expected to lead to an inability to care for oneself and a loss of personal integrity related to a dependency on others for even the most basic needs. These fears become validated as group members witness the often painful illnesses and deaths of friends and fellow support group members as a result of AIDS-related complications. Group participants share common concerns regarding what their fate will be, who will be there to care for them as their illness progresses, and what steps may have the effect of postponing the inevitable. Further areas of support group exploration include the complex issues related to disclosure of HIV status to family, friends, romantic interests, and casual sex partners and the processing of the devastating feelings of being "contaminated" as a result of HIV infection. In addition, group members support one another in the mourning of many significant losses, which often include friends and lovers who have passed away, professional identity as a result of career abandonment due to illness, and financial security obliterated by the minimal income granted through state and federal benefit allowances.

Since the advent of recent medical interventions that have demonstrated some success in significantly lowering the concentration of virus for many seropositive individuals, there has been a distinct shift in the concerns of AIDS support group participants. Whether members have obtained the desired medical effects of combination therapies, have not experienced these beneficial effects, have been unable to tolerate the side effects, which vary significantly from one individual to another, or have opted not to begin treatment due to fear of toxicity, the emotive concerns for people affected by the AIDS epidemic have undergone dramatic change.

EFFECT OF COMBINATION THERAPIES
ON AIDS SUPPORT GROUP PARTICIPATION

National statistics have revealed that AIDS-related deaths have declined sharply since the advent of combination therapies to treat HIV infection (Centers for Disease Control and Prevention, 1997). This phenomenon is especially true in New York City, where, in 1997, deaths as a result of complications due to AIDS decreased significantly (New York City Department of Health, 1998). As expected, the same holds true for the number of participant deaths in PWA support groups. Although illness and death were an expected and not uncommon occurrence in support groups for people living with AIDS prior to the widespread use of combination therapies, the need to mourn the death of a fellow group member has become the exception. The consistent management of within-group crises has been replaced by a series of less immediate but equally significant concerns.

The Experience of Successful Medical Outcome
on Combination Therapy

For people who feel hopeful as a result of recent medical interventions, issues surrounding the mourning of friends and group members and the need to anticipate and tolerate unyielding personal crisis have been replaced by fears regarding a future that was previously not considered possible. A small survey conducted by the Group Services Unit at GMHC, in early 1996, assessed the most significant concerns for people who are experiencing the benefits of combination therapy, revealing that this population is most concerned about financial security. Although the thought of living on an extremely fixed income following years of preillness financial security appeared somehow tolerable when combined with the expectations of a limited life span, this issue becomes more daunting as life expectancy increases. It was not unusual for long-term AIDS survivors to have used their savings to live reasonably well in anticipation of a time when they would not be able to appreciate the world around them:

> Alberto, a forty-seven-year-old gay male, who for years has suffered through numerous opportunistic infections as a result of advanced symptoms of AIDS, was a successful employee of a major accounting firm until he was no longer able to work due to fatigue and illness. To maintain his modest apartment, unaffordable on his now extremely limited income, Alberto made the decision to cash in his retirement accounts. This decision seemed logical given Alberto's certainty that he would not survive long enough to use them for the purposes that he had originally intended.

For the past eighteen months, Alberto has had an undetectable viral load and a dramatic increase in T-cell count as a result of his adherence to combination treatment. His energy has returned, he has regained the twenty pounds lost as a result of illness, and (for the first time in many years) he experiences himself as a healthy man. Alberto's excitement and optimism about the potential for a life span greater than what had been expected is coupled with an overwhelming fear regarding his ability to financially provide for himself in the event that he lives significantly longer. He is certain that his Social Security will be minimal since, as a result of his illness, he paid into the system only until he was forty years old. When considering a return to work, he questions who will hire a middle-aged accountant that has been out of the workforce for seven years. In addition, Alberto is concerned that by returning to work, he may be compromising the benefits that, although minimal, he has come to rely on and will sometime need again.

Alberto's practical and emotional struggle to find answers to these questions is a long and often overwhelming process that requires support and guidance. Support group members who are experiencing beneficial effects of combination treatment are able to share their concerns regarding a desire to return to work, which is combined with the fear of being unable or unprepared to do so. As Alberto's plight illustrates, the questions that arise include, "What if I give up my benefits, and am not able to maintain my health for the long term?" "How can I reenter the workforce when I have been out of the work arena for a number of years, and my professional knowledge has become obsolete?" "Who will hire me with this gaping hole in my résumé?" The emotional concerns of these issues are shared and explored in the context of GMHC support groups designed specifically for this purpose: at the time of this writing, the practical solutions remain unanswerable, as state and federal agencies scramble to provide workable answers regarding benefit options and opportunities for retraining people living with AIDS.

Individuals with HIV who are experiencing the often dramatic benefits of combination treatments describe feelings of "cautious optimism" and cannot help but consider themselves human guinea pigs. As with any new medications known to have a high degree of toxicity, many questions arise regarding the efficacy of these treatments. Currently, data regarding the effects of protease inhibitors used in combination with other classes of HIV medications date back approximately two years. Little is known about the long-term effects of these powerful chemicals on the human body or how long these medications will continue to be effective. A feeling of being in a type of "holding pattern" regarding the need to make a plan for the future often results, as illustrated by the following case example:

> Cynthia is a thirty-four-year-old woman who discovered that she was HIV positive shortly after her marriage to Robert (who is HIV negative) six years ago. Although the couple had originally planned on having children, this plan was abandoned to avoid the risk of putting the child through a short, potentially painful experience. Cynthia and Robert considered adoption, but Robert's hectic work schedule (which often forces him to be out of town), coupled with the expectation that Cynthia's illness would continue to progress, thus leaving her unable to care for the child, put an end to these plans. Both Cynthia and Robert missed the presence of children in their lives, and knew that, given the opportunity, they would be good and loving parents.
>
> Cynthia began a combination treatment regimen approximately one year ago. Since that time, her viral load has become undetectable, and her T cells have approached the low end of the normal range. As a result of their strong desire to have children, the couple again began to consider adoption. Although Cynthia and Robert feel enormously fortunate to experience a decreased threat of AIDS-related illness for the very immediate future, planning for the distant future seems premature. Will Cynthia become resistant to the medications that appear to be prolonging her life? Would the couple be able to afford child care if Cynthia were unable to care for the adopted child? Although the couple acknowledges that no one has a guarantee of a long and healthy life span, the odds against this expectation appear to be heavily weighted, given Cynthia's uncertain condition.

As a result of Cynthia's HIV status, and the uncertainty of the long-term effects of combination therapy, the couple is experiencing confusion regarding how to plan their lives together. The argument that "no one is guaranteed to have a tomorrow" has allowed the couple to make many decisions affecting the quality of their relationship but is less helpful to Cynthia and Robert as they are confronted with matters as important and life altering as taking full-time responsibility for a baby. Cynthia shared these concerns in her women with HIV support group, in which she was able to reveal that a large part of her struggles centered around feelings of inadequacy as a spouse and a parent as a result of her HIV infection. She was relieved to find that a number of group members identified with these frustrations. Within group, the benefits and risks of parenthood are openly discussed and considered without the guilt that often accompanies this dialogue with a partner and co-parent.

Another major concern for people with AIDS who are benefiting from their use of combination therapy is the prospect of living significantly longer with irreversible disabilities resulting from opportunistic infections. This concern is often voiced in the support group at GMHC for visually impaired people living with AIDS. Group members are legally and, in some cases, completely blind as a result of a variety of illnesses resulting from a compromised immune system:

> Tom became completely blind at the age of twenty-three, when he discovered that he had AIDS, and suffered from meningitis that resulted in the severing of his optic nerves. Although Tom was told that he would not live through the night, days turned into weeks, and weeks into years. He began to feel physically healthy and slowly developed the realization that his death was not as immediate as had been expected. He started to make short-term plans for his life.
>
> Tom worked to reinstate a quality to his life that would allow him to feel productive and comfortable. He learned to independently walk with a cane, joined a gym to regain his weight, developed a relationship, and worked to build a support group for people who are visually impaired as a consequence of having AIDS. Due to Tom's complete blindness and his determination to enjoy his life, he became a role model for other members of the support group, most of whom anticipated the progressive loss of the little vision that remained for them. Members openly expressed being inspired by Tom's ability to take control of his life.
>
> Tom emotionally shared with the group his conflicting feelings regarding the potential for an extended life span as a result of combination therapy. He admitted that a large part of his motivation to reassemble his life following his blindness was the thought that his time was limited. Tom confessed to the group that, for him, the thought of becoming old as a blind man was very difficult and sometimes overwhelming. Other group members identified with his struggle.

Tom was inspired to enjoy his life, despite his handicap, due to the "now or never" perspective that resulted from his expectation of a shortened life span. His description of fears regarding growing old without vision inspired a group discussion about the ability to tolerate and adapt, in the short term, to the physical limitations resulting from having a severely compromised immune system. Group members indicated that living with these dramatic limitations (vision loss, fatigue, etc.) becomes increasingly daunting with the anticipation of having to manage them for what could be a number of decades.

The case examples presented here illustrate the emotional conflict that is experienced by many people who have attained promising medical benefits from medications used to control HIV. Individuals describe both a feeling of excitement at the thought of having potentially escaped the death sentence once invariably linked to an AIDS diagnosis and concern regarding the need to be prepared, both practically and emotionally, for what may be an unexpected future. Support group participation to investigate the joys and anxieties resulting from this experience, in a forum that feels safe and understanding, is often an invaluable experience, as people living with AIDS struggle to make plans for their lives.

The Experience of Medication Failure

A variety of circumstances, some currently understood by medical science and others not, have resulted in a population within the community of people living with AIDS who are not having a drastic reduction in viral load nor an increase in T-cell count as a result of the use of protease inhibitors. For many, the side effects of these toxic medications are so detrimental to any existing quality of life that individuals discontinue treatment. For others, these medications are tolerable but ineffective. Still others have difficulty maintaining the stringent medication/meal schedule necessary for these drugs to be effective; this is especially true for people who may not be able to plan their next meal, due to a reliance on others for food, and for people who have experienced a degree of dementia as a result of their diagnosis and who are therefore unable to accurately keep track of the rigorous schedule demanded by these medications.

Support group participation has revealed that people for whom the medications have failed have, to a large degree, lost the feeling that they are a part of a large, vocal, and determined community of people living with AIDS; they believe instead that they have become a more invisible minority within the HIV-infected community. A fear exists regarding a sense of being defeated and forgotten regarding treatment development. As a result, many people have become increasingly isolated, socializing less with friends who are uninfected or who have had more successful treatment outcomes to avoid the feeling of being a reminder of the realities of AIDS. Group members have indicated that their tendency to isolate becomes most pronounced as they become increasingly ill and when the need for support is most great.

Support groups to address these issues provide a forum for the exploration of these concerns in a world that has become increasingly weary of hearing about them. Ironically, the standard efforts used to recruit group members have proven virtually ineffective for groups that focus on medication failure, in large part due to a reluctance to be identified with this newly formed, at-risk population.

> Marc, a thirty-seven-year-old gay male who has experienced severe illnesses as a result of long-term HIV infection, began combination therapy approximately eighteen months ago. As a result, Marc experienced a minimal decrease in his extremely high viral load and an increase in T cells from single digits to approximately sixty.
>
> Members of Marc's PWA support group have had a variety of outcomes as a result of beginning combination therapy. Marc identifies more strongly with the group members who are having a successful outcome than with those who feel that the medications do not offer them the promise of an extended, healthier life span.

Marc illustrates the tendency to avoid ruling out the effectiveness of combination treatment, despite strong evidence that its utility is severely limited. Although Marc's hopefulness should not be discouraged, and may be useful in increasing his day-to-day quality of life, it is difficult to imagine that it represents the full spectrum of his feelings regarding his experience with protease inhibitors.

The sense of denial exemplified by Marc's reluctance to confront the efficacy of combination treatment can be understood from variety of perspectives: Marc has a strong investment in believing that he will continue to enjoy his life indefinitely and is resistant to the thought of becoming ill in a world in which AIDS-related illness and death have declined significantly. In addition, Marc has had a long history of affiliation with the gay AIDS community, many of whom are experiencing beneficial treatment outcomes. His need to identify with the larger community of people living with AIDS requires a minimization of the degree to which his health remains at risk. Finally, Marc's long history of surviving life-threatening illness has provided him with the status of being enormously fortunate and almost blessed—a position that has been a large part of Marc's self-image. This image becomes threatened as Marc witnesses improved health for those around him, while not including himself in this more fortunate cohort.

A feeling of undefined guilt often accompanies the experience of an unsuccessful outcome on combination therapy. People for whom combination treatment is ineffective often feel that they have failed the medication rather than having the perception that the medications have failed them. Although this may not be a rational view, people in this circumstance often blame themselves for the limitations of the medications used to treat their HIV infection. In an attempt to make sense of an often unexplainable situation, people wonder, "What did I do wrong that other people have done right?" This guilt becomes compounded as individuals are forced to explain to family members, friends, and partners that the apparent "good news" regarding the treatment of HIV does not apply to them. This increases the feeling of being a source of concern and burden to loved ones. This irrational sense of guilt and failure intensifies feelings of anxiety, depression, and isolation.

To provide the support and knowledge needed to encourage feelings of hope and inclusiveness for people who are disappointed with the effects of combination treatment, support group models now offer psychoeducational information regarding the use of holistic, alternative treatments that have long been considered vital in the maintenance of mind/body health for people living with AIDS. These "wellness groups" have been effective in recruiting people who continue to have health concerns and who are reluctant to identify with a cohort that has ruled out the usefulness of medical treatments which include the use of protease inhibitors. Using this model, group members are able to look beyond combination therapy for treatment of their HIV and gain some control in the maintenance of their health.

THE INTEGRATION OF SUPPORT GROUP EXPERIENCE AND THE SOCIAL WORLD

The definition of what it means to be a person living with AIDS has undergone as many changes as has the ability to treat opportunistic infections. At the beginning of the epidemic, a diagnosis of AIDS almost certainly meant rapid and painful physical deterioration that would ultimately lead to death. Now, the possibility for individuals to survive for longer periods of time, and in some cases indefinitely, has resulted in a wide range of AIDS-related experiences regarding the maintenance of health and quality of life. Never has this been more true than with the advent of combination therapies to treat HIV infection.

Long-term support groups for people living with AIDS have provided an arena for people to more fully understand the joys, anxieties, and fears specific to an array of HIV-treatment outcomes. Within these forums, which often include long-term supportive group relationships concerning the experience of having AIDS, participants gain a sense of trust and affiliation as a result of their often dramatic history as a group. This history includes the shared experiences of hope, loss, and mourning. Over time, group members are able to develop an understanding of one another and appreciate the emotional ramifications of one anothers' experiences. Recently, these understandings have included the variety of physical and emotional effects that have resulted from the availability of combination therapies.

The range of experiences described by support group participants often reflects the experiences within the social circle of group members. As a result, increased understandings of group participants' feelings as they relate their histories with combination therapy become generalized to their social interactions. In this way, the abilities of group members to deal more sensitively with friends and acquaintances who may be struggling with health-related issues become enhanced. As a result, relationships within and outside of the group become strengthened, feelings of isolation are reduced, and the perception of being a single community that continues to struggle with the fight against AIDS is promoted.

IMPLICATIONS FOR THE PWA SUPPORT GROUP LEADER

The nature of discussion in PWA support groups has become less crisis driven since the advent of a number of medical interventions used to ward off the insidious effects of HIV. Participants continue to struggle with issues central to the maintenance of their emotional and physical well-being. These struggles remain directly linked to the intensity of the experience of living with a potentially life-threatening illness. Currently, however, many members are working through the less immediate process of evaluating how to proceed with their lives, given the hopefulness and ambiguity of their present situation.

The seasoned PWA support group leader, accustomed to managing the immediacy of fears regarding death and illness, may feel less useful as group dynamics become less crisis driven and move toward a focus on life planning and the potentially long-term management of uncertainty.

> Helen, a forty-eight-year-old clinical social worker who has led a PWA support group as a volunteer for seven years, shared with her supervisor that recently she has been having difficulty coming in to run her group. She indicated that she does not look forward to the experience the way she once did. Helen reported that while she used to leave her group with the feeling that she had accomplished something important, her more recent experience feels somewhat different and less rewarding. Helen was encouraged to bring this issue to

her supervision group—the resulting discussion revealed that a number of her colleagues identified with her experience.

Helen had a history of becoming energized by the PWA support group that she facilitated, and she missed the feeling of effectively managing the chaos that was often a part of the forum. This example illustrates the necessity of group leaders' recognition of their own ego needs as they facilitate AIDS-related support groups. This becomes especially significant as the needs of the group participants change. As crisis transforms into the exploration of more long-term issues in PWA support groups, the dynamic of the group changes drastically. This change may prove to be difficult for some group members and must be investigated within the context of the group as a process issue. Similarly, this change in group dynamic may become intolerable for the group leaders, who must explore this issue with colleagues and/or supervisors to minimize the risk of instilling in the group the feeling that the leader has become less invested in the life of the group.

The investigation of group dynamics is further necessary as the facilitator helps the participants manage the range of individual outcomes to combination therapy. The goal of the group leader must be to promote the feeling that all members are welcomed and encouraged to share their varied experiences. It is common for group participants who are having favorable treatment outcomes to minimize their feelings of hopefulness in an attempt to protect those members of the group for whom the medications have been less effective. Conversely, group members that have not experienced a beneficial reaction to combination treatments are likely to minimize their experiences of fear and increased hopelessness to avoid the perception that they have somehow failed or to protect other participants from the awareness that illness and death may continue to be a part of the group's experience. Ironically, this tendency for the group to protect itself from the experiences of its own members results in decreased feelings of group safety and affiliation. The careful processing of each member's history with protease inhibitors will promote further understanding of the emotional reactions of people who have experienced a variety of treatment outcomes. In addition, such dialogue will minimize the destructive risk of unexpressed shame and potential anger within the group, relieve the discomfort associated with secrecy, and promote the feeling that no one experience is more valid than another.

The process of investigating group dynamics is a fundamental tenet of group facilitation. The exploration of defense mechanisms in the provision of AIDS-related therapeutic support, however, has historically been a complex issue. It seems clear that certain defenses are useful in the maintenance of the emotional health of people living with life-threatening illness. In the example presented earlier, Marc had a history of exaggerating the beneficial effects he experienced as a result of combination therapy. In more therapeutically oriented groups, these defenses may be challenged within the context of the group meeting. In this case, the group leader has the responsibility of ensuring that the confrontation is done as gently as possible to ascertain from the group member a fuller array of feelings regarding his or her medical condition. Issues of hopefulness must be encouraged and combined with the experience of confusion, anger, and despair, which are inevitably a part of the emotional experiences of all group members regardless of medical treatment outcome (Gushue, 1997).

SUMMARY

The advent of recent medical interventions designed to significantly decrease the viral load of people living with HIV has dramatically changed the content of AIDS-related support groups. Commonly, the primary issues of these groups have become less crisis driven, moving away from the management of members' fears regarding illness and death and the experience of having these fears become realized. Support group discussion centers more on the anxiety and confusion arising from the potential for some group members to have an unplanned, extended life span and for others to feel excluded from the advances that medical science has achieved in the fight against AIDS. Support group facilitators must be aware of the ways in which the group members react to this shift in content, especially in relation to the group's ability to process the varied outcomes of these treatments for individual members. In addition, facilitators must carefully investigate the ways in which this dynamic shift effects them in the provision of supportive group services for people living with and affected by AIDS.

REFERENCES

Centers for Disease Control and Prevention (1997). *HIV/AIDS Surveillance Report* (year-end edition) 9(1). Atlanta, GA: Author.
Gushue, George V. (1997). Beyond Science: Miracles, Miracle Cures, and AIDS—The Role of the Therapist. In L.A. Wicks (Ed.), *Psychotherapy and AIDS: The Human Dimension.* Washington, DC: Taylor and Francis.
New York City Department of Health (1998). *AIDS New York City: AIDS Surveillance Update.* New York: Benjamin Mojica.

Chapter 4

Telephone Support Groups
for HIV-Positive Bereaved Mothers
of Young Children

Lori Weiner

INTRODUCTION

The telephone was first used as a method of outreach in 1953 by the Samaritans for suicide prevention (Grimed, 1979). Since this time, telephone support has been utilized for crisis intervention (Hornblow and Sloan, 1980), outreach for physically disabled people (Evans et al., 1984; Evans and Jaureguy, 1985), ongoing psychotherapy (Shepard, 1987), elderly individuals with visual impairments (Evans and Jaureguy, 1982), and for HIV-infected persons living in rural communities (Rounds, Galinsky, and Stevens, 1991).

In 1990 to 1992, I, along with several of my colleagues, conducted a study on the effectiveness of telephone support groups (Wiener et al., 1993). We ran telephone support groups for HIV-infected children and healthy children living in families with AIDS. We also ran these groups for HIV-infected and non-HIV-infected mothers, HIV-infected and non-HIV-infected fathers, adoptive and foster parents, grandmothers and grandfathers. The telephone support groups were a creative and therapeutic way to help HIV-infected children and their family members, who either did not have access or did not feel comfortable attending a face-to-face group, cope with the impact of this disease on their lives. The groups provided a sense of confidentiality not afforded in a face-to-face group and helped create a climate of acceptance and support for individuals who were often isolated because of the stigma associated with HIV/AIDS and the lack of adequate support networks in their communities.

Our telephone support groups were short-term, meeting once a week for one hour and fifteen minutes and lasting four to six weeks in duration.

The leader provided basic structure for the group by opening the first session with an explanation of the group's purpose and then asking the members to introduce themselves. In each subsequent group session, the leader began by summarizing the prior group session and then opening the discussion up to group members. For the last group session, the members were asked to prepare a story, poem, or prayer that had been a comfort to them. The leader remained an active participant by sharing a poem as well. During the last group, the members were also invited to discuss their feelings concerning the group experience. In each group conducted for the study, as well as the many telephone groups conducted since the study was completed, members chose to share their names and telephone numbers either during or at this final group session.

In the midst of the HIV epidemic, one of the greatest social work challenges is finding the time, energy, and skills to help the bereaved. In a medical setting, we often find ourselves immersed in a multitude of medical, social, financial, and emotional crises. When a moment is found in which we can take a deep breath (no one is standing at our office door, the phone is not ringing, and the list of phone calls to return is manageable), we cherish that moment. But for me, that moment has frequently been filled with guilt. The reason is that the people who often need me the most are the parents of those whose children who have died. They are no longer surrounded by their child's medical emergencies but often wish they were. As horrific as the child's course of illness might have been, most report wanting to go back to those days, even just for one day, to hold their child once more. Due to the flurry of activity and complex care which often precedes the child's death, the quietness that follows can be deafening. Parents frequently report feeling abandoned by the medical staff. As one parent stated, "I know that people need to go on helping the living, but what about me? How can they go from being here all the time, to not even calling?" This is just one more loss that parents need to adjust to and mourn.

Being acutely aware of this sense of isolation, I try to keep in touch with bereaved parents weekly for at least the first few months. However, between 1994 and 1995, it seemed that 25 percent of my days was spent on the phone with bereaved parents. Soon after a child's death, most parents find it helpful to review over and over again the days and moments prior to the death. Real grief work is essential as well as emotionally exhausting. I was finding it increasingly difficult to balance those calls during the day with my day-to-day responsibilities—providing comprehensive psychosocial support to children and families living with HIV. It began to take longer for me to transition emotionally from getting off the phone to "being there" with the child who came to my office for his or her session full of life and hope for the future. I then found myself "putting off" making those calls and leaving each day feeling as if I left many things unfinished. Due to a need to provide support to parents grieving the loss of their child, my own need to have a specific time to provide such support, and the success of the previous telephone support groups, I decided to form a similar group for bereaved parents.

As a result of the success of the previously conducted telephone support groups, I used the same format for the bereaved parents groups. However, the groups were held monthly instead of weekly and over a period of one year. This enabled members to experience many "firsts" without their child, such as the first Christmas, Easter, Halloween; the first day back to school; their child's birthday; as well as the first anniversary of his or her death.

Jenny Kander (1990) writes in great length about the needs, tasks, and challenges of the bereaved. Her premise is that to have experienced a loss does not have to leave the survivor a "helpless victim," unless he or she chooses that style of being. She outlines responsibilities in grieving as in every other aspect of life. The responsibilities she includes were chosen as the shared goals of this group:

- Physiologically counterbalance the impact of grief
- Confront the reality of the death
- Bring feelings and thoughts into the open
- Make use of available resources
- Manage one's own health care needs
- Complete that which remains unfinished
- Find release from guilt and regrets through forgiveness
- Regain and maintain some sense of inner integration
- Redefine the self
- Keep communication channels open within the family
- Assist children in the family with the grief
- Grant permission to cease grieving

GROUP MEMBERSHIP

The only criterion for entry into this support group was having lost a child to HIV who was treated at the NIH four or fewer months prior to the group starting date. Five women fit the criterion. All five women were contacted by phone to ask if they would be interested in participating, and each of them was. They ranged in age from twenty-five to forty-two, and their deceased children ranged from three to ten years of age at the time of death. Two of the members' children died within minutes of each other on the same day. Two died at NIH; two died in their home hospitals; one child died at home. For two of the group members, their deceased child was their only child. One of the members had another HIV-positive child who, at the time of the group, was relatively asymptomatic. One of the group members was single and living with her mother. The others were either married or involved in a committed, cohabitation relationship. Two of the members had acquired HIV through IV drug use. At the time of the group, both had been clean for many years. The other three groups members acquired HIV through sexual contact.

Geographically, the members represented three states on the East Coast and one in the Midwest. Some of the members had met in the clinic while their children were receiving treatment, but none of the members knew one another well. The group began when we agreed on a time during the day that would work best for the telephone conference call. At the members' request, I audiotaped each group, due to a concern that there might be times when one or more members might not be physically well enough to participate. Except when noted, all members were available for most of the group sessions. If a member did miss part of a group due to a conflicting appointment, the tape of that particular group was offered to her. No member requested a tape, either while the group was run or since the group was completed. The remainder of this chapter will review the group as it progressed from the first session until it was completed one year later.

SESSION ONE

I began by introducing the goals of the group and then asked each member to introduce herself. Each member described in detail not the course of her child's illness but the days and moments prior to and following her child's death. Each member reviewed the last words she had said to her child. Most believed that the death occurred only after they personally gave the child permission to die. For example, one mother reported, "I told my daughter that she did not have to stay here any longer for me . . . that I would be all right . . . that we would be together again. Then I asked her if she was ready to go with Jesus. She said, 'No.' A few moments later I asked her again. This time she said, 'Yes.' She died in my arms only seconds later." All of the group members described their child's funeral as a "celebration of life" and a very fulfilling memory. A few of the members talked about looking for a "sign from God" to know that their child was okay.

Along with filling the void in their lives, the struggle to find an identity other than that of an effective advocate for their HIV-infected child was a theme that permeated throughout all the groups. The women were enormously supportive of one another and of the group process. They shared telephone numbers at the end of the session. Of note, although all of the group members were also receiving treatment for their own HIV infection, not one of them addressed her own health status during this initial group session.

SESSIONS TWO AND THREE

I began the next group session, as I did all the sessions that followed, with a summary of the prior group. I outlined the issues raised and the needs identified by the group as well as by individual group members. I discussed adaptive and maladaptive coping styles, using their own experiences as examples. During the second and third group sessions, some members felt the need to again review the moments prior to their child's death. It was clear that most of the members were experiencing physical as well as emotional exhaustion due to a poor sleep pattern than had emerged as a result of the unstable nature of their child's health for weeks prior to his or her death. This pattern was not reversed following the child's death. Each member described herself as having difficulty falling and staying asleep and experiencing early morning rising. They described in detail how painful early mornings and late evenings were—a time when they found themselves alone with their thoughts. Therefore, as reflected in our first goal, we discussed ways to physiologically counterbalance the impact of grief. This led to full discussion of their own health care needs, and members encouraged one another to visit their physicians. They did, and there was much discussion in the following groups about the results of their blood studies and different treatment options.

The emotional impact of grief became stronger by the third session. As one member stated, "I've been up, down, inside out, and around. I thought I was doing so well. It took three months to realize she was finally gone." What became increasingly clear was that the issues of each member's own identity were clearly intertwined with strong, unresolved feelings of guilt. Two of the members began drinking. One of them had tremendous insight into this behavior as a way of trying to survive, as the following dialogue illustrates: "After crying for the past few weeks, I went to AA and made a ninety-day commitment. It was because I realized that any life I knew as a sober individual was with my daughter. She was my sobriety. I don't know how to live for myself." A second member added, "The question that continues to come up for me is—'Why am I still alive and her dead? I am struggling with myself and I am struggling with God.'" A third member responded with, "I know exactly what you're saying. I feel like I need a 'moral inventory' because guilt has really set in. I asked God to forgive me for what I did in my past and to let me forget. I was able to while my son was alive, but now, the only way I can go on is to go back and forgive myself for giving him this disease which he didn't deserve. But I'm not ready to forgive myself yet." A fourth member added, "I do not feel the same degree of guilt. But I felt much more important when my daughter was alive. The doctors and nurses cared what I said. I was important. My daughter needed me. I don't like surviving. Not without her." The fifth member remained quiet until I asked her if she would like to share her thoughts. Her response was, "My son made my life so complete. I never felt the anger or the 'Why me?' phases. What was most important was the love we had for each other and how strong that love was."

Survival, finding comfort in remembering the love between mother and child, renewing spiritual faith, strengthening one's identity, and the reduction of guilt became the stated goals of the next several sessions. I had asked the members to give thought to a different issue at the end of each session that reflected the group theme. For example, at the end of the third session, one member mentioned the word "gift." So I asked each person to either write down or to just think about the different "gifts" her child gave her. During the next session, after my introductory summary of the previous group, we would review what the members had prepared. The group reported finding this helpful, as other members always seemed to raise issues of which they had lost sight.

SESSIONS FOUR, FIVE, AND SIX

The frank and open discussions that guided our previous groups continued. Some of the members discussed the realization that they did not feel comfortable in the "outside world," that is, the world outside the AIDS community. Some began making plans to volunteer, others to become a foster parent. Another member came to terms with her partner having forced them to live in secrecy about the HIV diagnosis and that she could no longer comfortably do so. She ended this relationship and began a new one shortly afterward. Relationships and members' own emotional and sexual needs were honestly discussed. Speaking out and a feeling of empowerment was heightened when one group member agreed to be interviewed on national television. Yet others still struggled to find a way to "contribute" and/or find a place where they felt they best "belonged."

The reality of the child's death became clear to each of the group members, though in different ways. Some relied on their child to remind them to take their own medication. Others had a schedule that was difficult to change or habits that were hard to break, such as waking up at a certain hour to give medicines, reminding their child to do homework, or even learning not to look each week for the toys on sale in the Sunday newspaper. September was a very difficult month for those group members whose children were in school. Shopping for new clothes for the school year was always an exciting time. Watching neighborhood children walk onto the bus was just one more painful reminder of their child's death. These losses needed to be grieved, and the members brought their own losses to the group to be worked through.

While guilt, forgiveness, and acceptance of one's self remained important themes, existential beliefs and death also became a topic of discussion. One group member stated, "No one could have told me that there was such a thing as a 'good death'—not possible, no way, no how. Don't even TALK to me about dying. Well, I've turned about 180 degrees on that subject." This led to a discussion about each member's childhood thoughts, fears, and fantasies about death. At the end of the sixth group, they came to the conclusion that, although they do not welcome death, people have a lot of control over how and where they die. As one member summed it up, "We don't always have a choice, but we do believe that the end of this life is not the end of the road." Interestingly, the members later reported this particular session to be one of the best.

SESSIONS SEVEN, EIGHT, NINE, AND TEN

During the seventh session, one of the members was hospitalized with *Pneumocystis carinii* pneumonia (PCP). As this member was having too much respiratory difficulty to remain on the telephone, her mom joined the conference call for a few moments. Not surprisingly, there emerged much discussion among members about the fragility of life as well as a review of their children's illnesses. The members, in general, were feeling more positive about themselves and increasingly at peace with life without their children. They were able to look with more investment into the needs of the well children in their homes and into ways to strengthen those relationships. Halloween and Christmas were difficult holidays to get through and calls to one another took place frequently during these times. The course of bereavement was best described by the group members as a "horrible roller-coaster ride," and little events that "pulled them down" were often discussed. For example, one member who thought she was doing great became quite depressed with the first snowfall: "I always needed to protect my daughter . . . how can I just leave her out there in the cold?" For one member, survivor guilt was heightened significantly when her doctor informed her that she was in a small group of what were called "slow progressors or long-term survivors." "I feel guilty about being well. My son isn't even here to share this with me. I feel bad even telling you or other friends who are not doing well. Why me anyway? People think that I'm a nothing. I used to use drugs and they think 'she shouldn't be living.' " The rest of the group responded with support for these feelings, along with some spiritual guidance: "There is a reason you are here. There is something important for you to do. It's up to you to figure out what that is and not get absorbed in self-pity."

By the ninth session, most members reported feeling as if a different phase of grief had begun. New relationships outside of the group were forming. A few of the members who had long-standing problems with their parents gave one another the courage to address these issues and to make visits back home. For the most part, these visits did not go well. One parent was reported to have said, "If it wasn't for you, our grandchild would still be with us." Another group member returned from her visit to her parents and stated, "Well now my child dumped me and my parents dumped me. If I had a legitimate disease such as leukemia, I bet my mom would be by my side. But I don't. I have an illegitimate disease. AIDS is an illegitimate disease." It was inspirational how the members were able to support one another with tremendous insight throughout these difficult times of awareness and to share in one another's hurt, disappointment, and need to "move on." As one member said, "Just let go of it; they're never going to change. My parents are the same way. I'm angry with them but I am also worried about them because when I die, they're going to go on a terrible guilt trip and I won't be there to help them."

The member who had been previously diagnosed with PCP continued in poor health, which greatly affected group dynamics. CMV retinitis resulted in loss of sight in one eye and a new life of continual infusions of IV medications. She was often either too ill to join the group or only able to stay on the telephone for a short period of time. When she did join the group, it was usually from a hospital room. In her last group session, she commented, "I'm glorified that God gave me my child and I cherish my days." Three weeks later, on the day that her mother called to say that her daughter had died, I received a beautiful card and picture from her in the mail. The card read, "Dear Friends, God Bless You All." The picture was of her holding her child just moments after her child's death. On the back it read, "Homeward Bound, I Love You All."

SESSIONS ELEVEN AND TWELVE

The eleventh session began by sharing with the group the news of their friend's death. I read the note I received from her as well as the inscription written on the back. They talked about how "ready" this group member seemed to be and the peace she felt about dying. Each member was asked to think about what it would take for her to feel a similar peace. Since two of the other members had been hospitalized the previous month, the conversation was very real for them. They talked at great length about feeling "blessed" that they were able to live long enough to care for their HIV-infected children, as "no one could do as good a job as the child's mother." As our group was coming to an end, there was considerable discussion about separations and losses each had experienced in her life. Each member was helped to refocus on living and the goals she had for herself.

In this session, it seemed that the members felt as if they needed permission to say good-bye to some of their grief. For example, one member was planning on getting married and did not know how to "bring her child along." As part of their "end of group exercise," as well as our final goal to "grant permission to cease grieving," I asked each member to write or do something in an attempt to say good-bye to her child. Two members were able to write their child a letter, which they shared with the group during the last session. Another went to the cemetery and spoke at great length to her child. One group member felt the need to go back to the room in the hospital where her child died, following which she reported to the group, "It was just a room. Every tile on the floor had an echo and a story of its own and I needed to hear them all. And I did. I heard her laugh and I heard her cry. I saw the pajamas she wore and I saw me for the first time from the outside and how I sat in that chair. I had to take a step back. Then I realized, I really realized that that was then and this is now."

During this "last group," each talked openly about how much they appreciated having the group and one another. They asked if they could have a "reunion group" in a few months, and one was scheduled for two months later. Three members were present. Although they reported some very difficult days, the gains they felt they had made in their lives and in the group continued. They reported feeling ready to end the group "for now." As one member so eloquently stated, "I can really say now that my child lives on in my heart. So do all of you. I can honestly say that I've learned who I am through my child's life and through my child's death. What a trip this has been."

CONCLUSION

Identification and universality have been described by several authors as key elements to support groups (Yalom, 1981; Lieberman, 1983). Lieberman (1983), in his study of widow support groups, indicated that the members attached a new social meaning to the loss through normalization, a process of perceiving that one's thoughts, feelings, and behavior are not aberrant or unusual but are common to those undergoing the same experience. In this group, the members not only felt ostracized by society and often within their own families because of the death of their child but also because they are HIV infected as well. The descriptive data presented here support the theory that they developed a sense of community and normality as a result of being part of the telephone bereavement group.

The stated goals of the group were met. The group members made tremendous strides in the enormous challenges that faced them. They began taking better care of themselves while confronting the reality of their children's deaths; they openly discussed their fears, anxieties, disappointments, and hopes for the future with other group members, and most important, allowed themselves to recall, remember, and feel. They individually and collectively struggled with releasing themselves from their guilt and regrets in an attempt to maintain and regain some sense of inner integration. All members still had more work to do, as grief is an evolving process. Most of this work will entail continuing to make sense of the loss of their children while establishing a new relationship with those children—not the physical relationship that they had while their children were alive but a new way of relating (Kander, 1990). I believe most of the group members will be able to allow their deceased children to be a creative force in their lives. They were a creative force in mine. That is not to say that in some of these groups I did not find myself eating a pound of M&M's. I did. There was hardly a group during which I, along with the group members, did not shed tears. I, too, knew and had my own special bond with their children as well as with the group member who died. The monthly calls allowed us all to grieve, to say good-bye, and to say hello all over again. The month I asked them to share the gift that their child had given them, I spoke about the gift of being their facilitator during this process. I learned as much, or more, than I gave. We often feel we "know" what the grieving process is like for our clients, but it was a privilege and a gift for me to experience the year with them. I truly believe that I helped them tremendously during a time when so many people abandoned them in both their personal and professional lives.

In summary, I strongly recommend this psychotherapeutic modality to all social workers involved in the HIV epidemic. It is a practical, cost-effective and therapeutically sound means of reaching people who may not be geographically able or emotionally ready to attend face-to-face groups. Telephone support can also allow the social worker to reach a population of clients whose connection to an agency is often terminated following the death of a family member. The group members of this particular group reported the experience to be an invaluable resource during the intense bereavement period. Group cohesiveness, self-understanding, and the sharing of both wisdom and hope was clearly evident throughout each of the sessions. During the last group, one parent eloquently reflected on the group experience:

> I could never have imagined anything lonelier than losing my daughter. I felt empty, raped, with no reason to keep on living. This group gave me a sense of belonging, and it made me feel needed and understood again. I don't know how long each of us may be on this earth but we need to make the most of each day we have. We have a reason to live. We owe that to our kids, and we now owe that to each other.

REFERENCES

Evans, R. L., Fox, H. R., Pritzl, D. O., and Halar, E. M. (1984). Group treatment of physically disabled adults by telephone. *Social Work in Health Care, 9*(3), 77-84.

Evans, R. L. and Jaureguy, B. M. (1982). Phone therapy outreach for blind elderly. *The Gerontologist, 22*(1), 32-35.

Evans, R. L. and Jaureguy, B. M. (1985). Cognitive therapy to achieve personal results: Results of telephone group counseling with disabled adults. *Archives of Physical Medicine and Rehabilitation, 66,* 693-696.

Grimed, G. W. (1979). Telephone therapy: A review and case report. *American Journal of Orthopsychiatry, 49*(4), 574-584.

Hornblow, A. R. and Sloane, H. R. (1980). Evaluating the effectiveness of a telephone counseling service. *British Journal of Psychiatry, 137,* 337-338.

Kander, J. (1990) *So Will I Comfort You . . .* Goodwood, Capetown, South Africa: National Book Printers.

Lieberman, M. (1983). Comparative analyses of change mechanisms in groups. In R. Dies and K. MacKenzie (Eds.), *Monograph I: Advances in Group Psychotherapy: Integrating Research and Practice* (pp. 191-208). Madison, CT: International Universities Press.

Rounds, K. A., Galinsky, M. J., and Stevens, L. S. (1991). Linking persons with AIDS in rural communities: The telephone support group. *Social Work, 36*(1), 13-18.

Shepard, P. (1987). Telephone therapy: An alternative to isolation. *Clinical Social Work Journal, 15*(1), 6-65.

Wiener, L. S., Spencer, E. D., Davidson, R., and Fair, C. (1993). National telephone support groups: A new avenue toward psychosocial support for HIV-infected children and their families. *Social Work with Groups, 16*(3), 55-71.

Yalom, I. D. (1981). *Existential Psychotherapy.* New York: Basic Books.

Chapter 5

HIV Prevention, Women, and the Kitchen Sink Model

Annette "Chi" Hughes

As we approach a time in the history of HIV disease when optimism often outweighs cynicism and hope replaces hopelessness, we are still confronted with the staggering statistics pointing to an increase in the incidence of HIV infection in women. Sadly, this has been the reality since the late 1980s. This is coupled with an increase in the death rate of women with HIV, while their male counterparts are experiencing a longer life expectancy and improved quality of life. The mass media and others on the periphery of the epidemic appear perplexed by this phenomenon; however, a review of the course of the disease and this country's response will elucidate the many reasons, including denial, fear, and distrust, for the current state of affairs. Concomitant problems of sexism (leading to the traditional exclusion of women from medical research studies and drug trials), racism, and homophobia, which are indelibly woven into the very fabric of the United States, also contribute to the different effects of HIV disease for women and men. These very issues will continue to cause a disparity, one fatal to women, in the availability of care, treatment, and social support, if not confronted directly through services and programs designed by and for women. I have had the distinct experience of working in the field of HIV/AIDS since 1984, the defining experience of being African American and female for forty years, and the exhilarating experience of being lesbian for who really knows how long. It is through these lenses of experience that I present this chapter.

AIDS IS NOT A GAY DISEASE—OR IS IT?

Gay-related immune deficiency (GRID), one of the first names in the nomenclature for HIV disease, suggested to Americans that there was a disease that was capable of choosing its host body based upon sexual orientation. Had this been true, it would have been the first time in the history of the United States that such a thing occurred. For some heterosexists, the perceived absurdity of homosexuality in and of itself confirmed the existence of GRID. In addition, there was emerging medical data to support the reality of GRID. Convinced of its existence (evidenced through the mounting number of men becoming ill), gay men (mostly white) launched what was perhaps their greatest collective humanitarian effort to date. Garnering expansive resources and using its networks of bars, social groups, political organizations, etc., the gay community became the harbinger: "Our semen may be lethal; something intrinsic to who we are and what we do may be making us ill. Protect yourselves and your sexual partners!"

Nowhere in this message was there any mention of women, not even gay women or lesbians, possibly being at risk of GRID. (The first female case of AIDS in the United States was reported in 1981.) It appeared that gay men of color were also let off the hook. However, within a few years, other "risk" groups were identified: intravenous/injection drug users, Haitians (men and women), and hemophiliacs. This still left the majority of Americans free from the worry of contracting HIV, with the exception of those who irrationally feared contagion through handshakes, sneezes, tears, and toilet seats. Five years into the epidemic, with cases of HIV infection identified in women, prevention messages still were targeted to "risk" groups to change certain "risk" behaviors. With the fear of infection minimized for most Americans, the country took a "business as usual" stance. What was even more curious was the unwillingness of many to show compassion to those who were infected with was being called a fatal disease. Health care providers refused to care for people with AIDS, many members of the clergy preached condemnation, and family members turned away. Yet the gay community forged ahead in the areas of advocacy, education and prevention, treatment, and compassionate care.

The first people I met on the front lines of HIV efforts were gay men and women (lesbians) responding to the call from their community. In my community of Washington, DC, it was lesbians who raised the issue of women becoming infected with HIV. While other parts of the world, particularly Africa, showed equal rates of HIV infection in both men and women (with no particular reference to sexual orientation), the United States continued to see the disease as the sole purview of a few small risk groups. Five years into the epidemic, HIV/AIDS still was considered a gay disease.

The first woman I met with HIV disease was an African-American woman in Washington, DC, in 1985. She had made her way to the gay clinic because that was where she had heard she could get help. In a voice barely audible through her shame and fear, she explained that she was a recovering heroin addict, clean and sober for three years. As far as she could discern, she had not had sex with a gay man. Since becoming sober, she had not been sexual. In 1985, there was very little information available about HIV and women, and very few, if any, prevention campaigns targeted women who were not injection drug users or sexual partners of men who used injection drugs.

Lesbians were thought to be at the lowest risk for HIV infection, regardless of the fact that some lesbians were injecting drugs and having unprotected sex, both with men and women. Smug in the belief that "we're not plagued with frequent STDs," and with no proven cases of woman-to-woman transmission of the virus, most lesbians minimized the possibility of HIV risk for most of the first decade. Subscribing to the adage "we teach what we need to know," a small group of lesbians, with assistance from a local foundation that provided a small grant, launched the first forum on Women and HIV in the District of Columbia in 1985. By this time, I had attended countless forums, conferences, and meetings concerning gay men and HIV. Communities, other than those of white gay men, have played catch-up since the beginning of the epidemic in terms of developing strategies for preventing transmission of HIV.

In the early and mid-1980s, many members of the African-American community intentionally distanced themselves from AIDS, especially as the disease was speculated to have originated in Africa. Blacks were unwilling to assume yet another stigmatizing association. Theories of genocide surfaced in pockets of the black community, including suspicions about the possible clandestine role of the federal government in spreading the disease in communities of color. Although there was recognition that AIDS was affecting the African-American community, a hands-off approach and denial became the first line of defense. Anti-AIDS sentiments, coupled with racism and homophobia, drove black men and women with HIV, as well as those at risk for HIV, further into their respective closets.

Finally, when women were targeted for HIV-prevention efforts, it was largely due to their identification as "vectors" of the disease through sex work and perinatal transmission. Blamed for infecting their johns, female sex workers became scapegoats. Castigated for infecting innocent babies, women with HIV were frequently counseled to terminate pregnancies. Yet another closet door swung shut.

Some familiarity with the history of AIDS assists in understanding why we are where we are in 1998. From an emotionally detached perspective, I can say that AIDS has afforded many burgeoning professionals and concerned lay people an opportunity to study the etiology of an epidemic as it becomes a pandemic. This process has required the understanding of bodies of information, from the intricacies of the immune system to the inequities in access and provision of health care. It has also required the unlearning of information and practices. Prevention and education strategies purported to work for white gay men did not work for black gay men, women, or women of color. In the early 1990s, AZT therapy was thought to be harmful to men of color due to their higher death rate from the disease and shorter life expectancy after diagnosis. These outcomes were erroneously linked to the use of AZT and later attributed to African-American men entering the health care system later in the course of the disease than white gay men.

Today, the same holds true for women. Late entry into care has been linked to a shorter life expectancy for HIV-infected women. The suspicion surrounding AZT as well as other medications, still persists in some communities. I have spoken to women who participated in studies who admitted to not taking the doses as prescribed for study participation, fearing harmful effects. Women have confided in me that even after filling prescriptions they would leave full bottles of antiretrovirals to collect dust in a cabinet. As recently as 1997, women were significantly underrepresented in AIDS clinical trials due to lackluster recruitment of women and mistrust and lack of information on the part of infected women.

HIV PREVENTION AND WOMEN: THE KITCHEN SINK MODEL

Many women at high risk of HIV infection, or living with HIV disease, experience multiple vulnerabilities, i.e., substance abuse, mental illness, domestic violence, and poverty. When these issues are addressed it is often separately, leading to a fragmentation in service delivery. For some the fragmentation is another stressor or barrier to services. One-stop shopping for social services, or the settlement house model, is the one most requested by clients. In the absence of much-needed qualitative research to understand what produces better outcomes for women at risk, the Kitchen Sink model was designed to address as many of these vulnerabilities as practical. The model appears to address the most salient needs of the women served.

Since 1990, I have been able to work exclusively for and with women at high risk for HIV infection, and I have also worked with women with HIV disease through PROTOTYPES, A Center for Innovation in Health, Mental Health, and Social Services. This work has taken me to San Juan, Puerto Rico; Juarez, Mexico; San Diego and Los Angeles, California; and Boston, Massachusetts, to work on a project titled the WHEEL. The WHEEL, an acronym for Women Helping to Empower and Enhance Lives, is a comprehensive pilot test of an HIV-prevention intervention that targets women at risk for HIV infection. Initially funded by the National Institute on Drug Abuse, the WHEEL targeted women who are sexual partners of injection drug users. Because of the universality of some of the needs expressed by this population of women, the model has been replicated and adapted for other populations of women at risk. The WHEEL intervention can be used as an addition to an existing program or as a freestanding health education/ behavior change program. Two types of WHEEL interventions were developed—group and individual. A brief description of each will follow later in this chapter.

Study participants ranged from twelve to seventy-three years of age. A total of 2,792 females were recruited for the study from the cities mentioned previously. These cities were chosen because of the high incidence of substance abuse and HIV infection. Developing prevention interventions for culturally diverse groups of women could have been an impossible feat, given the differing belief systems, cultural norms, and behaviors of the targeted populations. Some of the women did not acknowledge their risk (78.6 percent of the total sample believed they had a 25 percent or lower chance of contracting HIV); others believed they were unable to change the circumstances that placed them at risk (abusive relationships, economic dependence); still others felt that the risk of abandonment and/ or rejection by a partner far outweighed the elusive risk of HIV infection. Women described numerous reasons for continuing to engage in HIV-risk behaviors, including not knowing or understanding what behaviors constituted "risk."

One factor leading to the adaptability of the WHEEL to diverse cultures was allowing women at risk to design their own interventions and then making the interventions as accessible as possible. Believing that any intervention targeting women would have to have a component of personal empowerment, a multidisciplinary and multicultural team of women came together to design the intervention. The team included community activists, former drug addicts, survivors of domestic violence, psychologists, AIDS advocates, and researchers. Integral to the first discussions about the intervention was the identification of our (program staff) own risk for HIV infection, with the focus being on behaviors. This led to an acknowledgment of the difficulty of changing our own behaviors as well as our partners' behaviors. The other focus of the work group was a review of our own roads to personal empowerment. We identified things which we thought were important to us in achieving our current station in life or simply the opportunity to sit at this table designing an intervention. Each person's path was different but consisted of similar components: personal growth, spiritual growth, networking, economic survival, advocacy, learning skills, relationships, health, self-knowledge, planning and decision making, social activities, and self-actualization. How, if appropriate, would these elements be woven into a prevention intervention that simultaneously addressed cultural differences and varying literacy levels?

The next step was to conduct focus groups at each of the study sites. Participants were asked to discuss issues that were important to them, including topics on which more information was sought. It was no surprise when focus group participants identified issues and topics of interest similar to those identified by the work group. Priorities identified by women participating in focus groups were safety, relationships, sexuality, health, addiction, and survival. One theme consistent among many of the women at risk is, "AIDS is not the most important thing in my life." AIDS simply had to wait its turn, and since HIV posed no immediate threat to life or limb, it could wait indefinitely. The challenge here was to weave HIV information into their self-defined priorities. Curricula for educational groups were developed on all of the issues identified by the women. Once the intervention began, it became clear that a group on parenting was needed. This curriculum was designed and added to the intervention. Curricula were designed in consideration of various cultures, cultural norms and beliefs, and literacy levels. In each group curriculum, HIV-prevention information was taught and related skills were practiced. For instance, the curriculum on parenting includes a discussion on developmental milestones for children and infants, options for disciplining children, and ways to talk to children about sex and HIV.

It would not have mattered how inclusive, creative, or effective the WHEEL would have been if we had not been able to recruit participants for the intervention. I will never forget a woman I saw in San Diego, on a popular sex work strip, whom outreach workers had identified to be at high risk due to her frequent exposure to STDs. When the outreach staff approached her, she greeted them warmly with a hug. After a brief assessment, they began their appeal to transport her to an STD clinic and then to a safer location off the streets. Standing aside, attempting to blend into the bustle of the strip, I heard her plead, through lips covered with sores, "Pray for me; please, just pray for me." Within seconds, she had rushed past me and faded in with the countless others, many as vulnerable as she. Feelings of inadequacy and hopelessness engulfed me. We had not, at that time, developed a prayer intervention.

Although sustained behavior change is the crux of any HIV-prevention effort, there is significant groundwork that must be laid before behavior change can be adopted and maintained. There are some intervention strategies that have been successful for the women with whom I have worked. By "successful," I mean intervention programs that have educated women about their risks, provided opportunities to share what they learned with significant others, afforded them a chance to experience self-efficacy, given them skills to reduce their risks and opportunities to practice those skills, connected them to much-needed resources in their community, and provided a forum for them to define their own needs. These were some of the outcomes of the WHEEL. In addition, using univariate measures indicated that the intervention effected significant behavior change between baseline and follow-up for sex risk, drug use, and trading sex.

INVENTING THE WHEEL

The success of the WHEEL comes from the wellspring of experience and wisdom inherent in the community. Frontline staff for all these programs have been members of the communities targeted for interventions. Typical staff members included women who were peers, such as former sex workers, former inmates, single mothers, lesbians, social workers, young women, women with HIV, recovering addicts, hair braiders, and a wife of a preacher. Life experience, leading to empathy and sound judgment, proved to be the salient qualification of each of these staff. Most had a desire to share something life sustaining with their community, having had firsthand experience of the ravages of HIV disease. There is the risk of the staff overidentifying with clients, which leads to the blurring of appropriate boundaries. The sensitive nature of the topics discussed (violence and victimization, substance abuse, sexual abuse, corporal punishment) in the interventions may bring up issues for the staff as well as the clients. Also, it is recommended that staff in recovery have at least two years of abstinence from drugs before being hired to this work professionally. Trained as HIV pre- and posttest counselors and phlebotomists, staff receive periodic instruction in professional growth and development. Social workers were used to provide crisis counseling and to assist with group facilitation and conduct needs and HIV/AIDS risk assessments.

Extensive community mapping and networking preceded the implementation of the participant intervention. WHEEL staff interviewed staff of other community-based organizations (CBOs) to identify available resources, screen for woman-friendly services, and develop networks for referrals to and from the WHEEL project. A resource directory was developed from the community networking process to assist staff in referrals and to distribute information to clients. Outreach staff were the project's ears and eyes to the community, providing valuable feedback on the success and problems of the project.

Individual Intervention (One to Three Sessions)

The individual intervention provided one-on-one sessions throughout the course of the intervention. Session one was a needs assessment and HIV/AIDS risk assessment, conducted by a counselor using two forms designed specifically for the WHEEL. In addition to questions about drug use behavior, the HIV/AIDS risk assessment asks about the potential for domestic violence in relationships. If the woman requests help for an abusive relationship, she is referred to the mental health clinician. Through these assessments, staff are able to determine each woman's ownership of risk as well as what resources she needs that the program might be able to provide, either directly or through referrals.

Following the needs assessment and risk assessment, the counselor administers what is called "enhanced HIV pretest counseling." It is called "enhanced" because it incorporates a more extensive risk assessment than the one used earlier and helps a woman identify the pros and cons of HIV testing. An integral part of this session is a condom use demonstration and drug works cleaning demonstration, when appropriate. If the participant requests HIV-antibody testing she is referred either within or outside of the group. Testing is session two, and session three is HIV-antibody posttest counseling. For women who test negative, prevention is reinforced. For women who test positive, the goal is to assess for coping ability and refer to health services.

Group Intervention

Women participating in the group intervention receive all the components of the individual intervention plus participation in three group sessions. Recommended for women who are able to make a longer-term commitment to the program, group sessions consist of the delivery of structured modules, teachback opportunities, and a graduation ceremony.

Teachback sessions allow a woman to teach what she has learned in the WHEEL group sessions to whomever she pleases. Literally she "teaches back" something of import she wants to share. Teachbacks have been given to daughters, girlfriends, and neighbors in a variety of settings. However, in preparation for teachbacks in the community, a participant is given the opportunity to practice teaching others (her peers in the group sessions) before she completes the enhanced intervention. Here she gains confidence, practices techniques, fields questions, and receives feedback from other participants. Upon completion she is ready to take her knowledge to the community and has the chance to give something back to the people she cares about.

Sessions average two hours each and are conducted over a period of several weeks. The first two group sessions are topical (parenting, survival, relationships, sexuality, keeping yourself safe, health, and addiction). The topics chosen most often were parenting, survival, addiction, and safety. For participants with children, the parenting module was the most popular. It is highly informative and interactional and includes practical responses to some of the difficult issues of parenting. Session three allows for a teachback of the information learned in the previous two sessions. It ends with a graduation ceremony and the presentation of graduation certificates to the participants. This ceremony is open to family members and friends of the participants and is often the highlight of the intervention. Many women, upon completion, admitted that the graduation represented the first time they had been acknowledged for completing anything.

Every effort is made to "meet women where they are at," psychologically, emotionally, educationally, and otherwise. Educational groups are held in participants' living rooms, recreational centers in housing projects, churches, and drop-in centers. Chemically dependent women who attend meetings "high" are allowed to participate in group sessions as long as they are not disruptive and do not bring drugs on site. The harm reduction model has proven to be an essential tool for developing trust with chemically dependent women and homeless women who visit program drop-in centers on a regular basis. If a woman identifies herself as being in an abusive relationship and requests information or assistance, crisis counseling is available. Certificates of completion for the intervention help some women meet requirements for probation and the Department of Children and Family Services. Participants who are required by the Department of Children and Family Services to attend parenting groups are able to meet part of this requirement by attending the parenting group session. Group facilitators/counselors can write letters attesting to the participant's involvement when release of information forms are completed. Similarly, women required to attend domestic violence groups and/or receive domestic violence counseling are able to meet a partial requirement by participating in the WHEEL group and individual counseling sessions.

Language in the curricula acknowledges same-sex relationships and any composition of family identified by the participants. Cutouts and pictures are used to aid women who are preliterate or prefer storytelling as a means of learning and teaching. Women are taught to "teach others" in the way most comfortable for them, thus fostering a sense of self-efficacy. Teaching tools are made available at no cost and a number of participants have taught their daughters, girlfriends, and partners or simply brought them to groups.

HIV-prevention intervention groups are presented as "health education" groups in the community, making it safer for battered women to attend and to remove the stigma associated with HIV. The health module includes information on HIV transmission and on mental health and spiritual well-being. It also includes a section on "What prevents me from getting my health needs met?" Module three, sexuality, asks such questions as, "Why do women have sex?" and "What if your partner won't wear a condom?" Through role-playing, women are shown how to problem solve if confronted with this dilemma. "Keeping yourself safe," the module on violence and victimization, addresses violence in communities as well as in the home.

The women most at risk for HIV infection are the women most at risk for poverty, substance abuse, inadequate health care, violence, and marginalization by virtue of their "minority" status. It simply is not enough to address HIV/AIDS prevention exclusively, when a woman cannot prevent poverty, read above the fifth-grade level, protect herself from an abusive partner, or refuse just one last hit off the pipe. Interventions that improve the overall quality of life for women will likely be well-received and even welcomed into communities.

Women assume numerous complex roles that define their importance within their family structure, their communities, and their personal lives. HIV-prevention interventions must address as many roles as possible (spouse, partner, mother, daughter, single parent, employee, and provider). The relational nature of women—or the ability to view one's self as an integral part of another human being's life—provides an open door for those of us seeking to understand some risk behaviors of women. Strategies must derive their focus from the definition of the problem as articulated by the population targeted for the intervention. Help-seeking practices, health locus of control, and other theories used to understand health-related behavior should be used as informational guides. However, women are quite capable of speaking on behalf of themselves and conveying their needs, if given an opportunity.

LOOKING TO THE FUTURE
WITH THE PAST ALONGSIDE

In a society that has relegated women to second-class status, it does take everything, including the kitchen sink, to elevate women to first-class status, yet it does not require taking the finite resources away from men. However, it does require an acknowledgment of the mistakes made in the first decade of the AIDS epidemic and a sincere willingness to correct them. Efficiency in program design (integrated services), efficacy in outcome, and equal and fair access to health care and other resources will close the widening gap currently experienced by women at risk for and living with HIV.

Now it is old news that women (along with teens) are one of the fastest growing groups of people with HIV in the United States—a distinction that possibly could have been avoided. Lessons of the past must inform the future of HIV-prevention (primary and secondary) programs for women. Mandatory testing of pregnant women, as stipulated in the CARE Act Reauthorization, is reminiscent of the "woman as vector" syndrome and may serve to scare women away from prenatal care. Names reporting at a time when the number of women with AIDS is increasing may prevent women from seeking care. These two issues alone present an ambiguous picture for women and AIDS policy.

Services are changing (traditional AIDS service organizations are attempting to provide more programming for women) and improving to meet the needs of women at risk and women with HIV disease. Unfortunately, this is happening at a time when conventional AIDS funding sources are appearing to decrease. As clinical trials prove the efficacy of even more drugs, threatening to command a larger percentage of current available funds, social service providers are clamoring for their share. Where will services for women fall? Other funding available for welfare reform and vocational training and job placement must be tapped to supplement programs targeting women at risk and women with HIV. Women are concerned about their survival. Once again, the kitchen sink approach may be helpful. Service provision for women with HIV will parallel services for men in some areas, but when the paths diverge, women and their advocates must make sure women are at the table having their say.

Most reasonable people are clear that AIDS is not a gay disease. One year to the millennium, and one year to the third decade of this pandemic hold promise for some and uncertainty for others. AIDS, with its challenges and triumphs, is a stern teacher and unrelenting reminder of the vulnerability of the human condition. It also supports the adage that necessity is the mother of "intervention."

Chapter 6

Losing Lawrence:
The Death of a Child
in a Residential Child Welfare Facility

Gerald P. Mallon

HIV and AIDS have changed the way that many human service professionals view death. Those working with populations affected by HIV have
learned that death no longer predominantly occurs for the very old, those
at the end of the life cycle. Even with that sad reality firmly entrenched in
our professional collective consciousness, those of us who work with
adolescents still believe that teenagers are not supposed to die. When they
do, their deaths send out shock waves that reverberate to anyone who has
ever come in contact with them, especially the organizations that have
worked with them. Every organization has its own culture, and it is within
the context of that culture that each organization also deals with loss.

After watching friends die for more than a decade, I have, unfortunately, become an expert at recognizing the face of AIDS. I saw the expression
of that illness come through the door of our group home two years ago,
when a sweet young man named Lawrence* was admitted to our program
in New York City. Although his medical report identified him as "a
healthy adolescent," anyone who saw him would know immediately that
he was not well. Lawrence was in fact skeletal. He was stooped and small,
vulnerable and shriveled, appearing to be more like an old man than a
seventeen-year-old. His skin was blotched and discolored; his hair was
sparse; his eyes were sunk deep into his head. His skin was stretched
across his skull, pulled so tight that there was a visible tautness at the
temples. This was not how one normally expected a seventeen-year-old to
look.

---

*To protect this young person's confidentiality, his name has been changed.

Green Chimneys Children's Services is a voluntary nonprofit child welfare agency that contracts with the New York City Administration of Children's Services (ACS) and other local social services' districts. The agency is licensed by the New York State Department of Social Services to provide residential care, including independent-living skills programming or life skills for adolescents preparing for discharge on or before their twenty-first birthday. The agency provides a continuum of services for adolescents including two independent-living programs based in New York City, the Gramercy Life Skills Residence and the Supervised Independent Living Apartment Programs (SILP).

The Gramercy Residence, where Lawrence lived, is a group residence located in the East Midtown section of Manhattan in an upscale community known as Gramercy Park. The residence houses twenty-five adolescent males between the ages of sixteen and twenty years old, all of whom are at the older end of the age range continuum in the foster care system. Residents are expected to complete high school, attend college, gain work experience, learn to manage their financial resources, and demonstrate their ability to manage other life skills that are critical for living independently. Green Chimneys' residents live in, and access services from, the agency until their twenty-first birthday, at which point they are discharged to live in the community. The expectation is that they will live independently and self- sufficiently without relying on the benefits of public assistance. Referrals, based on the needs of the residents, are made to our program by the New York City Administration for Children's Services.

Both staff and residents who live in our group residence at Green Chimneys knew that the day would eventually come when a client with AIDS entered our facility. In fact, I do not think that a day has gone by in the ten years that I have worked with Green Chimneys that I have not thought about HIV or AIDS striking one of our clients. Although we have cared for many clients diagnosed as HIV positive, we had been anxiously awaiting the day when one of our clients would become symptomatic with HIV disease. Over the years, our staff had participated in numerous training programs and had developed a relationship with a competent medical facility nearby, but nothing prepared us for the devastating reality of AIDS, especially when we were forced to confront it in a seventeen-year-old.

Lawrence was sent to live at Green Chimneys by the New York City Administration for Children's Services. He came to our program as a planned placement, which meant that we received and reviewed some material about his history and his needs before we accepted him for admission into our program. We would have accepted Lawrence as a client had the referring agency informed us that he had AIDS, but the Administration of Children's Services (ACS) completely omitted any mention of his HIV status, though they assuredly were aware of it. This meant that we were not prepared when he was admitted to plan for his unique social, psychological, and medical needs. ACS's refusal to share this important information had profound implications for our program.

As a follow-up regarding the referring agency's failure to inform us that Lawrence had AIDS, we contacted ACS to explore with them why they had not shared with us this critical information. They admitted that they had known Lawrence was HIV positive but decided not to reveal this information because they feared that no agency would accept him if they knew of his HIV-positive status. New York City has several programs that address the needs of pediatric AIDS cases, but they did not then, nor do they now to my knowledge, have policies that speak to the needs of adolescents whose lives are affected by HIV. In response to our call, during which we expressed our concern about not being notified of Lawrence's HIV status and health needs, the representatives of ACS said, "So I guess you'll want us to find him another placement." They were shocked when we said absolutely not. After having Lawrence in our program for only a few days, we realized that moving Lawrence would be a mistake. He was fragile, scared, and in need of physical and emotional care and nurturing. We believed our program would provide an environment in which his needs could be met.

Since Green Chimneys has always worked with a large population of gay, bisexual, and transgendered young people, we have earned a reputation for working with those whom other agencies might perceive as being "different" or "difficult," but Lawrence was our first youth who had symptomatic HIV. Lawrence was not gay or bisexual, nor was he a hemophiliac or an IV drug user; he was born HIV positive. Lawrence's case was of extreme interest to the medical community, as he was one of the oldest individuals to survive an HIV-positive birth. Lawrence was admitted to our residence on the Friday evening of a holiday weekend, so he was not introduced to many of the staff until the following Tuesday. When the staff met him, everyone commented on his thin appearance, skin discoloration, and weakened physical condition. After the initial medical assessment, our nurse immediately brought him to the hospital where he was examined and had blood samples taken. After analyzing the results, the hospital admitted him. They confirmed what we already knew: that Lawrence had full-blown AIDS.

The hospital was not a new place for Lawrence; he had spent many of his younger days there. Although he was new to our program and was hospitalized almost immediately after he arrived, both staff and fellow residents quickly developed a special bond with Lawrence and began to visit him on a daily basis. During this first hospitalization following his admission to Green Chimneys, Lawrence spent several days in the hospital before being discharged back to our care. After his third or fourth hospitalization, however, the staff began to express some concern about whether we were the appropriate facility for him, given his serious medical needs. We knew our program was not a medical program that was equipped to meet his intensive health care needs; we were in fact a life skills residence (an irony which we did not realize at the time), designed to prepare young people to live independently. Despite this, we believed that we could care for his emotional needs, and we would devise a plan with the hospital's assistance to manage his medical needs.

Lawrence begged us many times not to send him to a hospice or other health care program. He asserted very clearly, "I feel comfortable at Green Chimneys." After discussing it, also involving Lawrence in these important decisions about his own life, our treatment team determined that, unless ACS could find a better place for him (and we did not think that place existed), and since he was often clear that his relationship with peers and the staff sustained him, it was best that he remain at Green Chimneys. All of our residents (who, due to confidentiality issues, were not told by staff that Lawrence had AIDS) had extended themselves emotionally and physically to be extra kind and generous to Lawrence. They sensed, without anybody telling them, that Lawrence was very ill. Many of our residents had lost family members and friends to AIDS so they were familiar with how people with AIDS look. However, Lawrence's having AIDS never deterred the majority of residents from showing compassion for him. Their ability to reach outside of their own concerns and worries to be available to a peer who was dying was a very moving testimony to their humanity. Their concern for Lawrence shaped their reactions to his eventual death. One resident summed up his feelings this way:

> I knew he had AIDS; no one ever told me that because they are not supposed to tell you and that information is confidential, but I knew just by looking at him. I had an uncle who died from AIDS, so I know that look. But it didn't really matter what Lawrence had—all that mattered was that he was a nice guy and he was sick—so we visited him. I know that if I was as sick as he was, I would have wanted people to visit me.

Having a resident with end-stage AIDS was very emotionally difficult for both staff and residents, and at times, it seemed that the strain of caring for a client with AIDS was wearing everyone down. As unsettling as Lawrence's illness was for staff, clients, and for Lawrence's family, no one ever lost sight of how difficult it was for him. One afternoon while visiting Lawrence during his final hospitalization, we brought with us a video of an action movie that he had requested. As we all sat together silently watching the film's beginning screen credits, Lawrence turned to us with an exasperated expression on his face and exclaimed in an annoyed tone, "Could we please fast-forward this part? I don't have much time you know!" Embarrassed, we jumped up quickly and fast-forwarded the film to the start of the action. This was but one example of how, at times, Lawrence demonstrated less denial about his condition than did staff.

Lawrence celebrated his eighteenth birthday in the hospital. He had many visitors that day, receiving many gifts and lots of attention. Everyone knew this would be his last birthday, although this thought remained unvoiced by the staff and other Green Chimneys residents who shared the day with him. In the midst of celebrating his birth, we were all very much aware of the inevitable reality that we would soon be dealing with the opposite extreme of life—his death. The death of a young person hits a special nerve within all of us because young people are simply not supposed to die. The reality that we were helpless in the face of death left most staff members feeling frustrated and vulnerable. Each of us handled these feelings in different ways.

In staff meetings, we prepared for the consequences of this stressful event. We had, during many meetings, discussed the potential for emotional fallout on many fronts, but with the exception of the following incident, to our surprise, both staff and residents responded in a consistently compassionate and caring manner to the stress of Lawrence's illness. There were literally no incidents of residents acting out feelings that arose as a result of Lawrence's deterioration. The following incident was as close as a staff member came to acting out his own feelings related to Lawrence's condition. One day, I noticed that Lawrence's social worker was at the residence when he would normally have been visiting Lawrence. When I inquired about why he was not at the hospital, he remarked in an agitated tone that Lawrence was not his only case and he had other work to do. I gave him one of those glaring supervisory looks that nonverbally says, "Now tell me why you're really not going to the hospital."

At this point, the worker, a forty-five-year-old MSW, acknowledged that he was having a difficult time with Lawrence's illness. His remarks conveyed his distress:

> I have never known anyone personally who has died. I know that it's crazy given that I am forty-five years old, but I have never personally

dealt with death before. And it's just so unfair that this eighteen-year-old boy should be in the hospital dying. I find myself feeling helpless when I visit him. What can I say? What can I do for him? I mean, there's nothing that I can do to stop him from dying. It's just so sad. It's even affecting my sleep. I feel really sad and depressed about it.

We spoke for a long while that day about loss, about issues pertaining to death and dying, and about the seeming unfairness of it all. I acknowledged that it was difficult for this worker to deal with illness and death and supported the normalcy of what he was feeling. I also pointed out ways in which he could be "present" for Lawrence. I suggested they could watch a video together, he could bring Lawrence a favorite food or beverage, read to him, play a game with him, and sometimes, I noted, it did not matter what he did with Lawrence—it only mattered that he was present to sit with him, even in uncomfortable silence. I also offered to go with him to visit Lawrence, suggesting that going together would give us an opportunity to support each other after the visit. We went together many times to visit Lawrence and also paired up other staff and residents to visit as a model for processing and supporting each other after spending time with him. This strategy was particularly useful when Lawrence's condition deteriorated.

During the course of Lawrence's illness both the staff and residents who lived in the Green Chimneys program needed support and opportunities to vent their sadness and their anger about his infirmity. Due to confidentiality issues, we were never able to openly discuss Lawrence's illness with the other residents, though many of them guessed that he was terminally ill. Residents were encouraged to visit Lawrence in the hospital and to spend time with him, and many did visit, especially if they were accompanied by a staff member. Others did not visit, sending their regards with those who did. As a means of assisting the young people with their own bereavement issues, we were very conscious of the need to provide both formal and informal opportunities for them to process their feelings of loss. Weekly groups that focused on issues of attachment and loss were conducted by our social work staff. These sessions provided residents with opportunities to talk about Lawrence's illness, to share feelings of loss that they had experienced in other parts of their lives, and to voice their own fears about HIV and AIDS. Individual sessions were held informally and conducted on an as-needed basis, especially with those residents who had developed a significant bond with Lawrence. The importance of these sessions is reflected in the comments of one of the residents who knew Lawrence:

Lawrence was a cool guy. Even though he was sick and all, he had a good sense of humor and he was fun. When he got sicker I visited him a lot in the hospital—it was scary to see him that sick. He was the same age as I was—it's hard to see someone who is your own age just lying there like that. When he died I went to his funeral—it was really sad. The staff here did a lot of things that helped to make people feel better—they had groups and whenever we wanted to talk privately we could. It didn't bring Lawrence back—but it made his passing easier to deal with. I still miss him—his picture is on the wall in my bedroom—every now and then I look at it and think about him.

Staff members in the program were also encouraged to visit, and like the residents, some went frequently; others did not. As Lawrence's illness progressed and when it became apparent that his death was imminent, some of the staff who had visited the most and been the closest asked for opportunities to process their own pain. Although the staff discussed their feelings during individual supervisory sessions with me, I thought it was important that all of us had an opportunity to process our feelings with professionals who were not so intimately involved in Lawrence's case. Arrangements were made for two skilled professionals—both clinical psychologists with many years of experience in working with HIV illness and bereavement issues—to come to the agency to conduct a five-session grief/bereavement group for any staff who wished to participate. The agency's administration agreed to fund these sessions. This was one concrete example of how administration supported staff during this crisis by recognizing and responding to the debilitating consequences of dealing with the terminal illness of a child. The staff members who participated reported that these sessions, which were opportunities to cry, grieve, and process their own fears about illness and death, were critical for them. Recalling this experience, now almost two years later, one staff member's sentiments vividly illustrate the complexity of these feelings:

The group was very useful for me. As a social worker with adolescents, I had never had the experience of having a client die. It was painful to watch Lawrence. I would be lying if I didn't say that it affected my work with the other guys. Sometimes when some of the guys would complain about what I thought of as petty things, not getting their allowance, having an argument with another resident—I wanted to scream, "What are you complaining about? I have to go in ten minutes to visit a seventeen-year-old who's in the hospital dying."

I knew as a professional that their issues were important to them, but somehow their complaints paled in comparison. There were times when I was just so sad that I could hardly speak, but when that happened, I somehow managed to talk about it and of course, I always felt better. I think that in some sense it showed the other guys how much we cared about all of them.

As the administrator of this program, the most difficult time for me was when Lawrence took a turn for the worse. As I sat in his room where Lawrence lay curled up in a fetal position with the covers pulled up to his head, I recall thinking, "Could this get any worse?" As impossible as it seemed, he was even skinnier than he had previously been. His hair was matted from lying on his pillow, and you could see his pulse beating in the vein on the side of his head; his breathing was shallow, and it was apparent he was nearing the end. He was scared—you could see it in his eyes, and most of us felt powerless over what was happening—there was little we could do except to be there. We held his hand, we watched TV with him, we combed his hair, and we sat and waited as he slept. His doctor said he could die that night or in two weeks. Instead, he clung to life for almost three more weeks.

During this last phase of his illness, the staff members grew more and more fatigued. The stress inherent in caring for a dying person was felt by everyone in the program—both staff and residents. The residents, except for two young men who were his closest friends, no longer visited Lawrence. Staff members, especially our two social workers, were saying— and feeling very guilty about it—that they wished Lawrence would die. I realized they needed a different kind of support. Staff needed to know it was all right to experience these feelings and to express them. The grief and bereavement group helped a great deal, but they needed more individual supervisory time to process their feelings, and sometimes, they just needed an opportunity to cry.

On Sunday, February eighteenth, at 8:20 p.m., with both of his social workers present, Lawrence took one last deep breath and let go of life. Both social workers said they felt it was important that they were there with Lawrence. In being present at the time of Lawrence's death, they supported each other, sharing both their overwhelming sense of loss and their profound relief.

Planning for Lawrence's funeral arrangements preoccupied most of our attention the next several days. Our residents and staff were at the funeral home in Brooklyn to mourn with his family. Our agency contributed a substantial sum of money to help his family with the expenses, and we gathered together for both nights of the wake at the funeral home. We came together one final time to pay tribute to Lawrence in the chapel on the day he was laid to rest. Staff members silently hoped this would be the last time we would have to face the dismal task of burying one of our residents whose life was taken by the terrible plague of AIDS. The impact Lawrence's death had on our organization was significant. For many weeks, the staff and Green Chimneys residents were in a bereaved state—numb. Staff members and young people grieved individually and collectively in different ways. Several of us posted photos of Lawrence in our offices, and residents put pictures of him in their rooms. Others placed the program from his "Going Home" service on their walls or doors—it was a durable reminder for us of who he was. Almost two years after Lawrence's death, those mementos still hang as a remembrance of the lost life of a young man.

It is an unfortunate reality of child welfare that even in death there is paperwork, but it was in this process that I found what could perhaps be the lesson in this sad story. When I called the New York State Department of Social Services office to inform them of Lawrence's death, I spoke to a supervisor, one who has never been known to give out complements, and she said, "Well, Lawrence may not have come to your program in the right way, but it sounds like he came to the right place."

Epilogue

In writing this chapter, one thing became clear to me. Initially, we were unprepared for the crisis that ensued when we were asked to care for a very ill child with HIV illness. That our agency's administration provided us with unqualified support enabled the staff to feel taken care of, and thus, we were then able to be nurturing and supportive of the residents and one another. The expression of grieving, sadness, and other "nonprofessional" feelings were encouraged in both the staff and residents. My assessment is that because staff were given numerous opportunities to grieve, they were able to engage in a parallel process with the residents and facilitate the appropriate expression of the residents' feelings of sadness and loss. I believe this was probably the single reason why there was virtually no acting out by the adolescents who were residents of Green Chimneys during the time of Lawrence's deterioration, death, and the period of grieving that followed. The lesson for other agencies is that when support and care is provided in a consistent and unambiguous way, from the highest levels of administration through middle management and supervisory staff to line workers, the manifest humanity of the organization becomes the cultural norm for all the clients and professional staff. This contributes to professional staff being emotionally available to work effectively with the clients during a period of crisis for the entire therapeutic community. This support and tolerance for a broad variety of emotional expression enables the clients to sense that they are cared for, and consequently, they are able to respond appropriately.

In some ways, I believe many of us think Lawrence prepared us for the future. That feeling was confirmed just recently when three of the young people from Green Chimneys went to the doctor to obtain the results of their HIV tests. Although one staff member accompanied them to obtain the test results (at their request), the remainder of us staff who were at the residence waiting for them to return, held our collective breath and said silent prayers. As soon as they returned, we met individually with the boys and then as a group to discuss their status. Two of them informed us that they were positive, while one remained negative. I could not help but remember Lawrence when these young men told us that they were infected with HIV. They are only seventeen years old. This is not supposed to happen to teenagers—and so the story and our work continues.

Chapter 7

A Question of Survival: Issues in Counseling Homeless Persons with HIV

Ken Howard

INTRODUCTION

When considering the combined issues of HIV and homelessness, there immediately arises a "chicken or the egg" situation: Are people with HIV at risk for becoming homeless, or are people who are homeless at risk for being exposed to HIV? The answer is a little of both. Presented here are some of the issues that arise when social workers provide individual counseling to people who are dealing with the combined issues of HIV and homelessness.

At the time this chapter was written, I was the HIV mental health counselor for Foundation House Transitional Group (FHTG) (formerly the West Hollywood Homeless Organization) in West Hollywood, California—a nonprofit, multiservice program for homeless men and women over age twenty-one. FHTG operates several homeless services community outreach teams, a storefront, multiservice, drop-in facility called the Hollywood Access Center, and a sixty-bed shelter and transitional living facility called Foundation House. FHTG serves many people who are facing the multiple stressors of homelessness and HIV, along with diagnoses of substance abuse, psychiatric disability, or post-traumatic stress disorder. Sorting these issues out and prioritizing them in developing a treatment plan requires special considerations during assessment.

This article was originally presented at HIV/AIDS '96: The Social Work Response, the Eighth Annual Conference on Social Work and HIV/AIDS, May 29-June 1, 1996, Omni Hotel at CNN Center, Atlanta, Georgia.

Although the rate of HIV infection in the general population of the United States is estimated to be about 1 percent, among homeless people nationwide, estimates range from 5.5 percent to 45 percent (St. Lawrence and Bayfield, 1995). In some subgroups, such as IV drug users, it can be as high as 40 to 80 percent (Fetter and Larson, 1990). At Foundation House, the overall HIV rate hovers around 50 percent (Paradise, 1996). This elevated rate in the shelter, as compared to others in the Los Angeles area, is believed to be due to the combined high rate of IV drug use and the large gay population in the city of West Hollywood (currently estimated at 30 to 42 percent of city residents) (Economic Roundtable Team, 1994).

Foundation House also attempts to create an atmosphere of safety and comfort that is particularly welcoming for people living with HIV. This is accomplished by giving priority admittance to clients who are referred by AIDS service organizations for housing and counseling services (as required by funding sources such as HOPWA and the Ryan White CARE Act) and by in-house practices, such as having a weekly HIV support/education group, literature on bulletin boards from local AIDS service organizations, support for modified diets, consideration of physical abilities in the assignment of house chores, and mandatory, monthly HIV education and prevention classes. There is also strong enforcement of rules for residents and staff against the use of slurs and discriminatory statements to harass another resident on the basis of any individual difference, including sexual orientation and HIV status.

CITY OF WEST HOLLYWOOD PROFILE

Foundation House's home, the City of West Hollywood, was incorporated as a separate city in 1985 and carries as its motto, "The Creative City." It has a strikingly high proportion of white-collar workers in the entertainment industry and is described in city profile documents as comprised largely of "white single adults living alone in apartments, with notably strong concentrations of gay men, seniors (particularly women), and recent immigrants from Russia" (Economic Roundtable Team, 1994). Obviously, this is a somewhat unusual profile compared to many American cities. Although education and employment rates are high, so too are housing costs, which contributes to the problem of homelessness. It is not unusual to find nonluxury one-bedroom apartments ranging from $700 to $900 a month.

It is estimated that 7 percent of West Hollywood's population are people living with HIV, again higher than the estimated national average of 1 percent (Paradise, 1996). Los Angeles County in general differs from the nationwide picture of HIV and AIDS in several ways. More of the L.A. County cases are male (92 percent versus the national 82 percent), more are believed to be caused by male-to-male sex (71 percent versus 41 percent), and far fewer are believed to be the result of injection drug use (8 percent versus 27 percent) (Being Alive, 1996). Awareness of regional demographic differences helps to highlight where community education and prevention efforts should be directed, and it also underscores the necessity of HIV services tailored to the needs of local populations.

HIV COUNSELING NEEDS ASSESSMENT

Given this context of Los Angeles County, the City of West Hollywood, and Foundation House, there are issues in counseling the multiply diagnosed resident. With the multiple stressors such clients face, the age-old social work ethic of "start where the client is at" is particularly relevant here in discovering what needs the client has and which ones to address first.

Maslow describes the five basic needs of humans for psychological health as (1) physiological, (2) safety, (3) belongingness, (4) esteem, and (5) self-actualization (Lester et al., 1983). The clients of Foundation House also follow this hierarchy in the issues that they present in individual sessions, in the same order that Maslow describes, from the most basic to the most esoteric. Although these clients are dealing with HIV, very often HIV is not the "presenting issue," as it often is with clients in other settings, such as AIDS service organizations or community mental health clinics. For the homeless person with HIV, there is panic, but the panic is not, "What do I do with my life now that I have HIV?" or "What happens if I get sick?" or "How on earth do I tell my boyfriend/girlfriend/mother/roommate?" It is, "How do I survive *today*?"

There is a tendency in these clients to avoid HIV-related issues altogether and to focus instead on issues of immediate gratification. These are directly in line with Maslow's theory that physiological needs, such as food, clothing, shelter, and basic subsistence/survival money, take precedence over processing issues, such as life purpose following HIV diagnosis, HIV-related losses, self-care for HIV, and abstract or existential issues, such as fears of death and dying. It is a kind of denial, but less a denial than it is a subjugation of one crisis to deal with another, more pressing one.

Most homeless people, regardless of HIV status, are focused on issues of daily survival, and it is difficult to redirect them to think about the future, whether it is related to vocational training/planning, long-term health management, or substance abuse recovery, because of the immediacy of basic needs (Fetter and Larson, 1990). One study of homeless people with mental illness found that they "tend to place a high priority on meeting their basic subsistence needs first, before addressing their mental health needs, whereas mental health professionals often place a higher priority on providing traditional mental health treatment, underscoring a need for comprehensive systems of care that can include housing, health, mental health, and other social welfare needs" (Levine and Rog, 1990, p. 964). This can also be applied to homelessness and HIV, a situation in which we often want to rush in and help the client deal with HIV before they are ready to do so.

HOMELESSNESS AS A PHENOMENON

The primary crisis of homelessness is a multilayered phenomenon. A recent survey characterized it as "a symptom of underlying societal and community problems, such as inadequate or unaffordable housing, poverty, illiteracy, and substance abuse" (Fetter and Larson, 1990, p. 381). Another contributing factor to homelessness is mental disability. One study found that 90 percent of homeless people had diagnosable mental disorders, while another study found that 82 percent reported multiple disabilities (Grunberg and Eagle, 1990, p. 521).

Homelessness is described not only as "lacking a place to live," but also includes the concept of "disaffiliation," which is defined as "the absence of affiliative bonds to family and community, characterized by social, familial, psychological, and interpersonal disarray" (Grunberg and Eagle, 1990, p. 521). Add HIV to this, and the disarray becomes traumatic.

People with HIV experience a loss of housing for a variety of reasons, including (1) loss of income due to lost employment, (2) difficulty receiving financial assistance, (3) discrimination, (4) inability of caregivers to continue care, (5) decline in health that makes current living arrangements impractical, and (6) living on the economic margin before HIV diagnosis (McDonnell et al., 1993).

Homeless people who live in a shelter have their own set of characteristics. "Shelterization" has been described as "a process of acculturation . . . characterized by a decrease in interpersonal responsiveness, a neglect of personal hygiene, increasing passivity, and an increasing dependency on others" (Grunberg and Eagle, 1990, p. 524). All too often, community-based support systems such as family and friends are lacking or inadequate, which reinforces isolation and contributes to low self-esteem, loss of will/hope, lack of interest in self-improvement, and a sense that the shelter resident has no control over his or her life (Grunberg and Eagle, 1990). It is important to note that these characteristics were describing homeless people living in shelters and did not necessarily include the additional issue of HIV, which would certainly exacerbate these feelings. Conversely, people with HIV who are already experiencing depression, anxiety, and lowered self-worth would experience a compounding of this if faced with homelessness and an increased loss of autonomy and identity (McDonnell et al., 1993).

Although some of these "shelterization" characteristics are evident at Foundation House, the "neglect of personal hygiene" is not seen due to a shelter requirement for daily showers. Foundation House is unique among area homeless shelters in providing an atmosphere of safety for residents of all sexual orientations as exemplified by the fact that some gay men occasionally can be seen giving each other new haircuts or experimenting with color. This phenomenon illustrates that when a supportive, nondiscriminatory environment is provided to these clients, they form a community among themselves. They create bonds that allow for this playfulness that is generally not found in shelters where clients have a sense of guardedness or fear because of their sexual orientation, HIV status, or gender status that "has to" be hidden for self-preservation from either fellow residents or even program staff.

TREATMENT CONSIDERATIONS

It has been noted that the psychosocial difficulties concerning HIV often emerge long before physical symptoms develop, including loss of work, social isolation, financial problems, and the illness/death of members of the social support network (Lutgendorf et al., 1994). These are in addition to emotional responses, such as a diminished sense of self-efficacy, despair, anxiety, depression, and maladaptive coping mechanisms, such as denial, avoidance, substance abuse, and unprotected sex (Lutgendorf et al., 1994). In the chaos that can accompany homelessness, there is even more opportunity for substance abuse, anonymous sex, and avoidance of self-care. These psychological stressors can affect the physical course of illness: studies on myocardial infarction patients showed that quality of life factors such as mental and emotional well-being influenced disease course and symptoms, even at long-term follow-up, and similar studies regarding HIV have shown the positive correlation between mental health and immune function (Lutgendorf et al., 1994).

Lutgendorf and colleagues (1994) describe the primary tasks people with HIV face, including (1) taking control of one's health and making treatment decisions, (2) dealing with the threat of an early death and a sense of urgency to attain life goals, and (3) facing the stigma of HIV and notifying others of one's status. The social worker can assist the client with all of these tasks in the treatment plan, and in our Foundation House program, "taking control of one's health" and "dealing with a sense of urgency" can apply also to securing stable housing and a reliable source of income to maintain it. Facing the stigma of HIV is also heightened in the shelter setting, since the scrutiny of society at large exists in a microcosm in the atmosphere of group living, even in a shelter that is gay- and HIV-friendly.

Lutgendorf and colleagues (1994) also describe how the reaction to HIV, as with any traumatic event, shatters an individual's basic assumptions about the world and requires the construction of a new meaning. This happens at the time of a seropositivite diagnosis and in the transition from asymptomatic to symptomatic AIDS (but less so, ironically, from symptomatic to full-blown AIDS). Constructing this new meaning, or adjusting one's identity as a person living with HIV, is similar to the person who is homeless establishing a new identity in the community. Old work roles and former residences no longer apply, so the overall task in counseling and in case management in the homeless rehabilitative program is to assist the client with adapting to this new identity and forming new coping skills.

The task of forming these new coping skills is important for not only practical issues such as securing housing but to address psychological issues as well. Lutgendorf and colleagues (1994) found that maladaptive coping strategies such as denial and disengagement were associated with greater depression, while active coping such as planning and positive reappraisal were related to less depression and higher CD-4 cell counts. Support groups and individual counseling play a role in this also, since maladaptive coping is related to HIV-related deaths of loved ones and the anticipation of one's own death. Without an opportunity to process such feelings, clients are at risk because "carrying undisclosed emotionally laden information may have negative health and immune consequences" (Lutgendorf et al., 1994, p. 229).

Sally Jue has described the characteristics and coping skills of long-term survivors of HIV/AIDS. She found that although beliefs vary, long-term survivors have an active and flexible coping style that includes the importance of forming supportive, close relationships with others; active, usually traditional medical treatment in an equal and collaborative partnership with their medical provider; acceptance of HIV as a part of their lives; and luck. In contrast, they rarely use denial and tend to confront problems directly (Jue, 1994). She also describes the characteristic of forming specific, realistic long- and short-term goals. Certainly, social workers can assist in these tasks, but Jue warns that "therapy is most effective when it is approached from a client-empowerment perspective . . . as equal partners with the therapist in determining the direction of therapy and forming treatment goals and plans . . . in a way that supports their right to self-determination and their ability to manage their lives responsibly" (Jue, 1994, p. 331).

CONCLUSION

Part of the work that we do as mental health professionals is to recognize the client as our partner in assessment and to allow him or her to decide where on the pyramid of the hierarchy of needs he or she wishes to begin treatment. The challenge for the social worker, then, is to focus on the "start where the client is at" approach, address the resistance of the client that arises from his or her anxiety (Rosser and Ross, 1991), and explore his or her immediate needs before addressing the level of traumatic response to HIV. Afterward, other aspects of the treatment contract can begin, such as assisting the client in managing his or her response to HIV, substance abuse recovery, and processing past trauma. This requires the worker to focus first on empowering the homeless HIV client by being tolerant of him or her as he or she works through defenses, allowing the client to determine the pace of his or her highly individualized rehabilitational program. This emphasis on the client's pacing allows him or her to lower defenses and to increase active coping skills when faced with multiple stressors, when even HIV is second or third on the list.

Since the voices of homeless persons with HIV are too often kept far from public forum, presented here (with kind permission) is a poem from a resident of Foundation House, "S," who was diagnosed with HIV in March, 1996, titled, "Time":

> Time—
> What does the future bring?
> Anything you like it to be
> Be careful what you ask
> It may not be what you want
> Expect the unexpected
> If you don't like it,
>   change it for the better
> We live only once
> Time—we need to use it to our advantage . . .

REFERENCES

Being Alive (1996). *Being Alive Newsletter.* Los Angeles, CA: Being Alive/ People with HIV/AIDS Action Coalition.

Economic Roundtable Team (1994). West Hollywood Community Needs Assessment, March. Los Angeles, CA: Economic Roundtable.

Fetter, M. S. and Larson, E. (1990). Preventing and treating human immunodeficiency virus infection in the homeless. *Archives of Psychiatric Nursing, 4*(6), 379-383.

Grunberg, J. and Eagle, P. F. (1990). Shelterization: How the homeless adapt to shelter living. *Hospital and Community Psychiatry, 41*(5), 521-525.

Jue, S. (1994). Psychosocial issues of AIDS long-term survivors. *Families in Society: The Journal of Contemporary Human Services, 75*(6), 324-332.

Lester, D., Hvezda, J., Sullivan, S., and Plourde, R. (1983). Maslow's hierarchy of needs and psychological health. *The Journal of General Psychology, 109*, 83-85.

Levine, I. S. and Rog, D. J. (1990). Mental health services for homeless mentally ill persons. *American Psychologist, 43*(8), 963-968.

Lutgendorf, S., Antoni, M. H., Schneiderman, N., and Fletcher, M. A. (1994). Psychosocial counseling to improve quality of life in HIV infection. *Patient Education and Counseling, 24*, 217-235.

McDonnell, J. R., Persse, L., Valentine, L., and Priebe, R. (1993). HIV/AIDS and homelessness. *Journal of Social Distress and the Homeless, 2*(3), 159-175.

Paradise, F. (April, 1996). Executive director of Foundation House transitional group. Personal communication.

Rosser, B. R. S. and Ross, M. W. (1991). Psychological resistance and HIV counseling. *Journal of Gay and Lesbian Psychotherapy, 1*(4), 93-114.

St. Lawrence, J. and Bayfield, T. L. (1995). HIV risk behavior among homeless adults. *AIDS Education and Prevention, 7*(1), 22-31.

Chapter 8

Support Groups
for HIV-Negative Gay Men

Steven Ball

In recent years, an increasing consensus among AIDS educators indicates that education and information have not been enough to stem the growing tide of new seroconversions among previously uninfected gay men. Prevention professionals have begun to acknowledge an ever-increasing need for primary prevention and counseling targeted specifically to HIV-negative gay men. HIV-negative support groups that address more than safer-sex issues, including the "whole" person within his environment, have developed independently and have been integrated into already existing HIV-prevention programs.

One example of the operationalizing of this understanding can be found within Gay Men's Health Crisis (GMHC). First in the substance use, counseling, and education department (SUCE) and more recently in the prevention department, the organization has offered multiple workshops and groups that have proved to be a healing antidote to the ongoing stressors of staying HIV negative. In an environment in which the link between sex and survival has been turned upside down, groups for HIV-negative gay men offer invaluable forums for normalizing fears, clarifying values, disseminating information, and building a community of concern to mitigate overwhelming feelings of loss and isolation that might otherwise lead to self-destructive behaviors.

Social group work seems to be a necessary next step in prevention efforts because it acknowledges and clarifies the needs of uninfected gay men, while at the same time it induces more community validation for a group that, until recently, was seldom targeted. For those of us working in prevention, the ongoing psychological toll of AIDS on the uninfected became like an elephant in our living room: everyone knew it was an issue but no one knew how, or felt entitled, to broach it.

No one could have predicted the extent of the damage that AIDS would continue to wreak in this decade. Who would have predicted that reactions to HIV testing would divide gay men into positives—those who were infected—and negatives—gay men who escaped the fate of infection but found themselves in a wasteland of death, illness, suffering, sadness, and seemingly endless tragedy? Nonetheless, openly gay men continued to adapt to their new world, and others continued to come out. As all of these men proceeded with their normal human strivings for connection, testing became an important right of passage in gay male development. It has affected every permutation of interpersonal relating, from friendships to early dating to committed partnership.

The growing invisibility of uninfected gay men whose needs were scarcely recognized by medical and mental health providers served to expose many of these men to an acute mental health crisis that often exacerbated behaviors and thought patterns which put them at risk for contracting HIV. Some of the HIV-negative gay clients whom I saw in my private psychotherapy practice walked through their days like zombies, burdened by unattended grief for too many losses. Inhibited and intimidated by the more obvious need of HIV-positive men and those who have full-blown AIDS, many HIV-negative men felt guilty about expressing their particular concerns and needs. By the late 1980s, many gay men unconsciously accepted the general public's equation of a gay identity with an AIDS identity. The implicit organization of a gay identity around HIV seemed to limit the roles of HIV-negative men to those of caregiver or outsider.

AN INTEGRATED MODEL

There came a point at which I felt both personally and professionally compelled to argue against this narrow, false definition of what it is to be an HIV-negative gay man. I was exhausted from feeling angry and helpless as I watched gay men die of AIDS, while I witnessed healthy gay men unable to feel joy or pleasure in life. Most agencies, at the time, were still not ready to take on what was seen as a controversial use of limited resources. I found it less restrictive and more expedient to set up groups in my private practice so I could experiment without the confines of the economic, administrative, and time restraints of social or AIDS service organizations. At the time of this writing, I continue to offer two long-term HIV-negative therapy groups in my private practice. The interactional/existential model used in these groups primarily focuses on interpersonal learning, illuminating members' limited views of themselves and their world, as their growing need for interaction and intimacy helps them to improve and expand their relationships outside of the group. It has been the effectiveness of these long-term groups in helping members understand the difficulties of being HIV negative that motivated me to start experimenting with a time-limited group model for these men.

Based on a combination of my private practice groups, as well as experiences with various brief treatment models, I began developing a model that could be integrated into larger prevention programs. The basic assumptions that underlie the use of this brief model are (1) large numbers of men should have access to the service; (2) multiple groups can provide a link among the members of different groups and the various segments of the gay community, thereby stimulating the environment to further respond to their needs; and (3) more volunteer facilitators would be likely to take on group leadership with a proscribed investment of their time. As of March 1996, GMHC has offered ten, ten-week groups that have been co-led by various HIV-negative gay professionals and trained peer facilitators. Almost 200 HIV-negative gay men have interviewed for the groups thus far, and approximately one hundred have participated.

These mutual aid groups have developed out of a long tradition of social group work that utilizes a remediation model, which is already used to address a broad range of social issues that affects individuals. Additionally, the HIV-negative groups draw on a synthesis of other theoretical perspectives, most notably, existential group therapy (Yalom, 1985) and narrative therapy (White and Epston, 1990). All of these influences are client centered and supportive. Rather than a professional treating pathology, the leader is an informed participant in a network of reciprocal relationships. This moves away from a more traditional problem-focused approach to group work, in which the therapist is the expert who holds the answer and the group is primarily a context in which to change the individual. Clinical skills are useful, but the ability to picture a rich and varied life for HIV-negative gay men is essential. This faith offers some promise of healing.

Of particular importance in this model are stage-specific interventions that use an adult developmental perspective of relationship building. While the definitions of group stages vary slightly among the numerous authors who have described models of long- and short-term group work, all seem to incorporate at least three stages into their understanding of group development: the beginning stage of engagement, the middle phase of differentiation, and the final stage of termination. In all groups, regardless of the stated theme, members struggle with the generic themes of affiliation, defining the rules for power and control, creating boundaries among members and between members and the outside world, and ultimately dealing with separation and grief issues as dramatized by the inevitable ending of the group experience.

General themes of being HIV negative coincide with specific stages. During the first stage of engagement, members focus on their ambivalent connection to the AIDS community and are generally asking for the answers to help them stay uninfected. As they move into the middle phase of differentiation, members often wrestle with the discomfort of feeling closer to the other members of the group and with their desire for connection. In the final phase of termination, members investigate ways to continue to appreciate and enjoy their lives, while gathering their inner resources to deal with the pain and loss that is still to come. The themes that emerge in each particular stage are integrated into the group leaders' understanding of group development to help leaders recognize predictable group behaviors during specific stages and to relate these behaviors to the difficulties of being HIV-negative gay men. This knowledge helps leaders direct the group experience and prevent it from getting sidetracked on issues unrelated to the goals of the group.

The interactional model of group development merges with an understanding of the use of narrative therapy both as a concept and as it relates to the role of the facilitator in a group. Narrative treatment emphasizes the telling of personal stories, but unlike more traditional therapy that might focus on what went wrong, narrative treatment searches for the emotional health, the heroic measures that cause people to fight back and survive. Narrative therapy maintains a strengths perspective. Additionally, since we are just beginning to adopt a vocabulary for the realities of uninfected men, there are few true experts. The inclusion of a narrative viewpoint gives the fullest freedom for both members and leaders to be important sources for information and for reconfiguring their present life stories.

Group leaders help members to recognize and normalize AIDS-related trauma that members may not have connected previously to the impact of AIDS. Often, for example, there is an initial sense of taboo about admitting to guilt or shame related to being HIV negative. For many, this seems like melodramatic whining. However, as members begin to identify with one another's struggles, they hear their own experiences reflected back to them in a myriad of different situations, both within and outside of the group. Through externalization—a central intervention strategy in narrative therapy that defines the problem as external to the individual—members are able to acknowledge the oppressive impact of AIDS phobia, homophobia, and years of stigmatization. The struggle is no longer an internal one rooted in the past—in a "pathology-saturated" character—but instead it is an external and current battle against the communal tragedy of living in the era of AIDS. This reformulation of hard-earned heroism can become the foundation for more adaptable life stories that evoke members' speculations about what kind of futures they can have if they continue to see themselves as strong, competent, and supported.

MEMBER PROFILES

The current climate of change in HIV prevention has begun to incorporate and validate the issues faced by HIV-negative men. After almost a year of offering HIV-negative groups at GMHC, what we encounter from new prospective members in the pregroup interview process is an acceptance of the idea that HIV-negative gay men *do* have a unique set of cultural and psychological issues. Yet confusion remains regarding how these issues specifically affect their lives and behaviors. They are intrigued by the group flyer that lists "identity, life expectations, dating, unsafe sex, isolation, ongoing losses, and the future" and then states that "the aim of the group is to explore and get support in dealing with these important personal issues. Through the group experience, members will learn coping skills while gaining a renewed self-acceptance and commitment." It seems most men who interview are experiencing some developmental discomfort as their old beliefs, attitudes, and coping mechanisms wear thin.

Many younger men who came out post-HIV report that their social, recreational, or sexual patterns are less pleasurable than they anticipated they would be and that they either no longer have, or never really had, a sense of belonging to a gay community. Feeling once again like an outsider creates a regression that reactivates old developmental issues and childhood wounds. As when one first acknowledges one's homosexuality, being HIV negative unconsciously replays being stuck in a circumstance beyond one's control and feeling unacknowledged while anticipating great losses. Since early in their childhood, most of these men have struggled to find a world that is kind to them, a world they can trust. They are still looking for something more substantial. They sense that they have to grow, but they do not have a strong vision of what they are growing into.

Older men, such as myself, who were out pre-AIDS are often exhausted by the subject of AIDS, but more important, we are still looking for a new sense of belonging and control in our lives that can be translated into our sexual and romantic encounters. We want to counteract the learned helplessness that causes many men to retreat into a global ("It affects all I do") or stable ("It will *always* be this way") vision of their relationships and their immediate community. With members' impaired sense of a future orientation, it becomes necessary to expand their frames of reference away from the helpless tunnel vision of safer-sex discussions, which characterize most prevention workshops and groups, and toward a focus of empowerment based on interpersonal relating and individual behaviors.

MEMBER SELECTION

Similar to most groups, the face-to-face pregroup interview is not only diagnostic but also an orientation process that obtains an agreement from the potential members to work cooperatively within the short-term format. The interviewer looks at individuals' interpersonal patterns and roles in "natural" groups in their lives to date, including their family of origin or family of friends. People are excluded if they are in an acute risk stage, including a crisis of pathology (eruption of psychotic process, suicidality, homicidality, or extraordinary, severe anxiety) or a situational crisis, such as the recent death of a loved one. Clients excluded from joining a group are referred to the appropriate mental health support or, in the case of acute bereavement, perhaps into a grief group. They are encouraged to return for a group in the future, after more immediate concerns have been addressed.

The importance of the process of selecting and preparing the members for group cannot be emphasized enough and is one of many areas that warrants further study and experimentation. Group construction includes the traditional complexity of composing a group, with a balance between homogeneous and heterogeneous elements. It is true that heterogeneous factors, such as age and experience differences, initially can create a baseline tension. However, when correctly facilitated, these differences can be used to build interpersonal curiosity that accelerates the pace of the group. Of course, group composition also needs some homogeneity of ego strengths so as not to set up one or more members as a scapegoat or an outsider. For instance, a member at the very beginning of his coming-out process would probably be better served in a coming-out group, if others were not at the same stage in this process. In the groups at GMHC, as we continue to experiment with the effect of group composition, we are presently working to balance different ages, experiences, relationship statuses and developmental levels within one group.

Although an acknowledgment of the similarities in experience of being HIV-negative defines the beginning efforts of group cohesion, the members inevitably end the ten weeks with a sensitivity to each member's right to be different. Certain themes related to individuality, separateness, and autonomy, clearly lacking in the general safer-sex guidelines of past prevention campaigns, can be derived directly from the differences, not the similarities, among group participants. The interpersonal and experiential variety of members captures the essence of membership within a community, and as a result, the groups more effectively reflect their outside environments.

THE STAGES DESCRIBED

Roy MacKenzie (1990), a leader in the subject of time-limited group psychotherapy, thoroughly describes a six-part system that incorporates effectively the developmental stages of a group into a therapeutic "road map." The group initially deals with the issue of affiliation of each member as they "size up" and seek approval and acceptance from the other members of the group. In the first group, the leader is active in providing structure and often asks members to share the goals that they determined in the pregroup interview. Commonly, men start by acknowledging their general anxiety and fear about having sex or dating, in general, and express concerns about how this group and how these particular men could be helpful. Some men discuss their concerns about safer sex. Others might talk about recent relationships with HIV-positive men and how these connections are complicated by issues of safety and disclosure. All of the men seem to grapple with how to articulate clearly their particular concerns about being HIV negative.

After leaders reiterate the ground rules shared in the pregroup interview, they clarify the general consensus of the work to be done, which is to establish a safe place where members not only share one another's personal accounts of living as urban gay men, but also focus on interpersonal learning that will help them feel more connected to their world outside of group. Toward the end of the first group, the ten members separate into pairs; each partner interviews the other for five minutes and gathers information that includes a glimpse of each person's past, present state, and envisioned future. Members are then reintroduced by their partner to the group. This is one of the only structured exercises done in every group's process. Leaders are constantly encouraged to bring new ideas to the process and to share the effectiveness of those ideas in the weekly supervision group.

Group leaders often ask members, as a home assignment, to notice how the first group affected their daily lives. One set of group leaders experimented with having the members fill out a weekly card; the members could then reflect on the group during the week and note issues and concerns they have difficulty sharing in group. At the beginning of the next group, members hand the cards back to the leaders. The leaders read the cards after group and usually respond by encouraging the members to raise their concerns in group. These weekly cards help leaders monitor individual concerns that might not be appropriate to the agreed-upon goals of the group and to monitor potential group dropouts. Other leaders have written a weekly letter to the group in an effort to enhance continuity, their observations of the group life, and the bridging of the group into the outside world.

Throughout the initial phase of the group, leaders encourage members to tell their specific narratives without the powerful social forces of what is politically or socially correct. In the first three groups, men tend to talk about themselves in connection to those who are HIV positive or have AIDS, minimizing their own needs. It seems as if it is safer to talk about grieving and loss because these ideas are more socially acceptable then talking about their desire to stay negative or to make meaningful connections. These beginning groups are described to the members as a first date. This metaphor of dating is often invoked throughout the group process to mirror the developmental stages in building a relationship, normalizing the members' conflict between getting closer to one another and running away from emotional connection.

By the third group, the stage of differentiation develops and is exemplified by the recognition of individual uniqueness that includes physical, sexual, and spiritual differences that exist among members. The group has moved out of childhood, so to speak, and is moving into adolescence, when subgroups emerge, conflict and power struggles are explored, and sex becomes the pervasive topic. Although anxiety remains high during this stage, it is acknowledged more readily. Interestingly, confrontation frequently focuses on how the different members choose to interact socially and sexually with HIV-positive men. As the therapist reinforces productive interactions that focus less on content and more on how they are dealing with one another interpersonally, these men begin to realize how their feelings and emotions affect their behaviors both within and outside of group.

When men begin to reveal ambivalence regarding safer-sex practices, it often signals the beginning of the third phase of individuation. Safety has been tentatively established, and members begin to disclose their personal concerns. Sex remains one of the most common areas of discussion. In some groups, a battle may develop between "sex positives" and "sex police." In some groups, members express frustration about continuing to deny themselves pleasure. Most groups find themselves locked in a heated debate over the condom question and oral sex. Members may believe that the leaders are privileged to the latest safer-sex information and are intentionally withholding answers from the group. After the leaders explore the source of these feelings and fantasies, they can then attempt to emphasize that there are no magical answers to safe sexual encounters. Members then begin to consciously realize that they have to struggle with finding out what is individually acceptable for them.

As members continue to acknowledge their mutual conflicts, they move tentatively into the stage of intimacy. As the group becomes more consciously familial, the content of the group sessions concerns interpersonal acceptance, rejection, and realistic expectations of one another. If the groups work harmoniously, this stage quickly intertwines with the phase of mutuality, in which members experience how moments of altruism and reciprocity can exist while still holding on to their own distinctive needs, wants, and desires. In one group, a poignant moment occurred one evening during the ninth group, when members started fantasizing about what it would be like if they all lived together, going into great detail about how it would be to come home to one another, even discussing whether or not the leader would be there. They joked about how each one would take care of the others and how it would feel to be surrounded by men with whom they could share their true feelings about the day, about last night's date or sex, and about their relationships. They still had doubts that they could even create this sense of closeness and trust with friends outside of the group— but the success of the group was to know it was possible.

As is the case in all brief groups, the final phase of separation and termination concludes with many members experiencing a desire for the group to continue to avoid confronting the loss. Throughout the group process, the methodical countdown to termination enables the men to use the group as an emotional laboratory in which they can explore and experiment with issues of anticipatory loss similar to those that many were experiencing and might experience in their daily relationships. As members process the loss of the group identity, a final task is for leaders to assist members in identifying triggers for feelings of isolation to help members resist returning to a place of obscurity once the group is terminated.

Many men express a desire for another group experience, and some have gone on to other groups. Some are training to become peer facilitators in future groups. For many of these HIV-negative men, the ten-week support group offered the first safe place where they could openly explore their emotional response to the AIDS epidemic, while gaining a sense of membership, acceptance, and approval in a community setting. One favorite closing exercise is to have the men write a letter to themselves that they would like to receive one month after their group terminates, which reminds them of their group experience and helps them stay connected to whatever they found most helpful. Co-leaders collect these letters in the final group and mail them one month later. Hopefully, this helps integrate the story of the group into the narrative reality of their life. Keeping these men healthy and HIV negative requires helping them find hope for their future, confidence in their ability to make significant, meaningful connections with one another, and faith that they can find a way to appreciate life, even while they gather the inner resources to deal with the pain and loss that is still to come.

Although the response from focus groups suggests that these groups have proven important and effective resources for many participants, they are by no means a panacea to seroconversion. Nonetheless, the time has come to expand prevention campaigns at both the individual and community levels to reach out to those who are less able to access the social services they both need and deserve. These men would benefit from group interventions to strengthen their capacity and motivation to believe in a future for all gay men and to provide an integrated understanding of their guilt about survival.

REFERENCES

MacKenzie, K. R. (1990). *Introduction to time-limited group psychotherapy.* Washington, DC: American Psychiatric Press.

White, M. and Epston, D. (1990). *Narrative means to therapeutic ends.* New York: W. W. Norton and Company.

Yalom, I. D. (1985). *The theory and practice of group psychotherapy,* Third Edition. New York: Basic Books.

Chapter 9

Finding Their Voices in Group: HIV-Negative Gay Men Speak

Carl Locke

The Titanic syndrome is some are prepared with life vests, some accidentally survive, some come to their senses but are too late to be saved, and others refuse to admit their peril and go down dancing.

"Rick," a fifty-one-year-old gay white man
stating his view on gay men
and how they are dealing with HIV

In the foreword to William I. Johnston's book, *HIV Negative: How the Uninfected Are Affected by AIDS* (1995), Eric Rofes writes, "Testimony is crucial for survivors of any disaster. Amid the earthquake detritus and hollowed-out shells of buildings at the battlefront, men and women emerge compelled to bear witness to horror and atrocity" (p. v). The concept of *bearing witness* is perhaps most often associated with the Holocaust but has been applied to many communal tragedies, including AIDS (Kayal, 1993). Bearing witness serves many functions, including making note of the event(s), recording it, sustaining the memory of the event and its consequences/lessons, telling of personal stories for individual growth as well as for larger change, and organizing affected communities politically.

I heard the quote at the introduction to this chapter from a member of a support group for HIV-negative gay men that I was conducting, and it is an example of bearing witness. The analogy to the Titanic serves as a provocative introduction to the struggles faced by gay men who are not infected with HIV. Prior to the HIV-antibody test, there was no distinction between the infected and uninfected. It was thought or assumed all gay men were or could be infected. Today, many gay men know their HIV status or assume knowledge of it. HIV status, as well as its psychosocial implications, has become integrated into the identities of gay men (Ball, 1996; Johnston, 1995; Odets, 1995). For uninfected gay men, the impact of the identification with HIV and AIDS, experiencing the pervasive trauma and loss associated with this epidemic, and testing HIV negative deserves much attention, especially if they are to remain uninfected. Many gay men experience very complicated feelings about testing HIV negative. If one's identity as a gay man is intertwined with HIV, discovering he does not have HIV often causes great anxiety, conflict, and confusion rather than relief.

Complicating this further is the fact that testing HIV negative does not mean one can never become infected. The status of being HIV negative is not irreversible. Rofes (1996) writes, "I believe gay men will pay dearly if we do not begin addressing HIV-negative issues directly. Not only will we see increased rates of new infection among HIV-negative gay men . . . but . . . 'the silent epidemic' . . . will continue to damage our physical, emotional, and spiritual health" (p. 6). Ball (1999), writing in this volume, provides an overview of how group work can be an effective modality for meeting the unaddressed needs of HIV-negative gay men. Using quotes from participants in support groups for HIV-negative gay men, this chapter gives voice to numerous concerns expressed by uninfected gay men who participated in two different ten-week groups run at Gay Men's Health Crisis from 1994 until 1995, and serves to illustrate the psychosocial issues and dynamics faced by men who remain uninfected.

COMPOSITION OF GROUPS

The two groups examined in this chapter began with ten and nine members respectively, and each group had one participant dropout. The groups were cofacilitated by myself and another social work colleague.* The ages of the men in the groups ranged from twenty-eight to fifty-three. The men were in various stages of coming out in terms of their identification as gay, some having come out prior to the onset of the AIDS epidemic and others afterward. Relationship status varied among members. The majority of the men were single. Some were in relationships with HIV-negative men, and others were in relationships with HIV-positive men.

---

*I would like to acknowledge Scott Whipple, CSW, who cofacilitated the two groups described in this chapter. All the work was a collaboration, and his insight, support, and skills were invaluable to the success of this endeavor.

Some of the relationships were monogamous and others were nonmonogamous. One member was divorced from a woman after a long heterosexual marriage. A few of the single men were widowers, as their lovers had died from AIDS-related illnesses.

SPECIFIC TECHNIQUES UTILIZED

An adaptation of the diary concept was adopted as a central technique used by the facilitators in running these groups. Instead of requiring each member to record thoughts and feelings in a journal, the idea was broken down into smaller, isolated tasks. The men were given a blank index card at the end of every session (starting with session two) and were instructed to use the card in any way they wanted. However, it was suggested that the members write down thoughts, feelings, or reactions about the group that came up during the week, write something specifically to the facilitators, or use the cards as a type of diary. The men were asked to turn in the cards to the facilitators at the beginning of each session. Group members were given the opportunity to discuss anything they had written on the cards with the group. The original goal was that, by the end of the ten weeks, the men would have a journal of the group process without having to think of it as such. The cards were also an invaluable tool for the facilitators to receive immediate feedback from group members about how each was experiencing the group and what issues were shared as opposed to individual concerns. The information obtained on the cards helped the leaders provide structure for group discussions based directly on feedback from the members. Eventually, responses were written on the cards by the facilitators before the cards were returned to members the following week. The facilitators' comments mainly encouraged members to bring up the topics in group and provided positive reinforcement and validation for expressed feelings.

THE BEGINNING PHASE OF THE GROUPS:
FINDING A PLACE

Many, and perhaps most, gay men who are not infected with HIV do not incorporate being uninfected by HIV into their concept of self. This is in marked contrast to most HIV-positive men, for whom HIV status is an integral component of their identity. The uninfected gay men who participated in the groups discussed in this chapter identified strongly with AIDS and with HIV-positive men, even while intellectually knowing that they were HIV negative. An example of the confusion that arises out of this fusion of identities was often expressed on the cards turned in to the facilitators. Early in the group process, Shaun, a thirty-four-year-old gay man, wrote:

> Joining this HIV-negative group, while the payoff is yet to be seen, was my personal statement of just how plugged in I am to the plight of HIV-positive people specifically, and gay people generally.

For Shaun, joining an HIV-negative gay men's group was about his identification first with *HIV-positive* gay men and second with the gay community at large, and nowhere does he mention the plight of men, such as himself, who are HIV negative. Although something drew him to participate in the groups, he was unsure just what that was at the beginning of the group experience. His stating "the payoff is yet to be seen" provides a vague hope that there will be personal benefits to him from coming to this group. Unsure of what the group had to offer and why he felt he needed to be there, he resorted to the common "solidarity" he felt with HIV-positive men. Not only did Shaun come to the group because of his connection to men with HIV, but also because it proved his connection to the gay community at large. The blending of HIV and the gay community are evident in Shaun's reasons for participating in the group. He felt torn between feeling connected to HIV-positive gay men and to the gay community, but at the same time, he did not really feel as connected to either as he would like. What eventually emerged during group discussions was that his lack of feeling connected to the gay community was directly related to his being HIV negative, which he viewed as extremely different from being HIV positive.

The men in the group often discussed how the focus of the gay community had been primarily on AIDS for over a decade. This was specifically a condition Shaun did not share "with the gay community." Group members often expressed feelings of not belonging to the gay community because they were HIV negative. Exploration of these feelings revealed that they often stemmed from the entanglement of interests, purposes, and identities between being gay and being gay with AIDS in the gay community. This process has been termed "the homosexualization of AIDS" (Odets, 1995). Shaun's comment illustrated that one way of not feeling disenfranchised from a community overidentified with AIDS was to not identify as different from HIV-positive men.

Another example of how this disenfranchisement is experienced was seen in the following story, shared with the group by Dan, a forty-three-year-old man:

> I was attending ACT UP for a while in the beginning. I remember people assuming you had to be sick if you were involved. One day, this guy I had met at the previous week's meeting came over to me. I was excited because I thought he was hot. He started asking me if I was taking supplements or vitamins, and I said "No." He handed me a bag full of vitamins and liquid supplements, saying he could no longer use them and that I should try them. I didn't know what to say. I just took the bag.

In this example, Dan illustrated the assumption that all gay men are HIV positive or should act as if they are. After this incident, he reported feeling uneasy and like "a spy" in ACT UP meetings. He felt as if there was no place for him in ACT UP since he was HIV negative, and he only went to a few more meetings before dropping out. Both Dan and Shaun related feeling alienated from HIV-positive gay men and indirectly from the gay community. How they dealt with this feeling was somewhat different. Whereas Shaun refused to identify as different, Dan could not rid himself of the feeling and began to feel unwanted and like "a spy."

It cannot be overstated that this "homosexualization" of AIDS is experienced by all HIV-negative gay men and is dealt with in some manner. Much of the beginning process of these groups focused on uncovering the ways in which group members identified with, and simultaneously felt alienated from, HIV-positive men, while helping them shift their focus from thinking and talking about HIV-positive men and their issues to thinking about HIV-negative gay men and personalizing these issues as immediately relevant to themselves. We attempted to reduce the group members' focus on men with HIV/AIDS by asking them about their feelings and experiences pertaining to the epidemic and reframing what they shared into a context of not being infected, yet still being affected, by the presence of AIDS in their lives and community.

Lack of Support

The feeling of not having a place in the gay community because they were HIV negative was not limited to men attending these groups. It was often echoed by friends, colleagues, and even the institutions within the gay community. James, a thirty-four-year-old man, after discussing with a friend his participation in the group, heard the following reaction:

Is this what it has come to—groups for men who are not sick?

Another member related a similar reaction to telling someone about being in this group:

> My friend was almost angry about it. He said he couldn't understand what there would be to talk about. If you don't have the virus, you should be happy about it. Why would a group be necessary? He said it was probably just a bunch of whiney men getting together and couldn't believe I was a part of it. He also felt it was a misuse of funds for GMHC to sponsor such a thing.

Another example of this awareness was the following, shared on a card:

> It seems it's easier and more acceptable to talk about being HIV positive than it is to talk about being HIV negative.

The feelings of not belonging to the gay community and resistance to supporting the space to express such feelings also came from uninfected men themselves. James related the following story:

> I feel I need to pull back at times when talking with HIV-positive men. At work I heard a rumor, which turned out to be true, about a fellow employee who had AIDS. He was at the end of the lunch table when I heard others talking about him. I felt like I peered into his closet or personal life and did not want to or need to know his status. It just so happens that he was on my subway car later and I was on my way here. He asked where I was going, and I told him about the group and then just shut down. I felt very guilty and then angry that I knew this man's status and that I felt like I needed to hide where I was going because of it.

Many members of the group echoed feeling the need to "pull back" when talking about their own experiences of being HIV negative with HIV-positive gay men. In pursuing this further in the group, most men felt the urgency and crisis faced by men infected with HIV had to take priority over their issues as uninfected men: "After all, it's a life-threatening illness." Several men commented that discussing feeling depressed, lonely, or afraid could not compare to the intensity of these feelings for HIV-positive men. Because of this self-imposed, and community-sanctioned, prioritization of HIV-positive gay men's issues, the group members had imposed a "not so significant" label on their own struggles and problems. By downplaying the very real reactions, challenges, and problems they faced, they participated in minimizing the validity of their concerns. By declaring their problems "as not so bad," they expressed an ambiguity and discomfort with creating a place to address issues faced by HIV-negative gay men. As group leaders, we spent time validating the feelings of men who experienced confusion, difficulty, and struggle concerning having a place in the gay community as uninfected gay men. By identifying and sharing just how difficult it was to be an HIV-negative gay man, the men began to feel less isolated with these feelings and consequently began to grow more accepting of their right to have a place within the gay community where they could receive much-deserved attention.

No Place to Escape

One recurring theme expressed by group members was that testing HIV negative was not a permanent condition. This was evidenced by sentiments such as, "I don't feel like it's *if* I am going to be infected, but a matter of *when* I will be infected." Illustrating the concerns about the possibility of becoming infected, one group member shared the following:

> Sun(day)—Low key—nice—napped, shopped, met a friend of a friend who was positive and he told me he was positive. I wonder— how long before it hits me? Can I escape it?

All of the men in these groups expressed similar feelings, although in varying degrees.

James wrote:

> After seeing *RENT* over the weekend, I thought, "There is *no* place to escape from HIV and AIDS." [Three of the characters in the play are infected.]

Tom, in his forties and in a long-term relationship with a man diagnosed with AIDS, related a story after seeing the Broadway play *The Heidi Chronicles*. He felt he could not get away from AIDS. He wrote:

> My lover returned to NYC after a two-week vacation with his relatives. While I was happy he was back, I noticed a definite rise in my overall anxiety level. I realized that the two weeks he was gone, I hadn't had to worry about his health.

The group members often spoke explicitly about feeling disenfranchised, the inevitability of becoming infected, and a lack of control over their lives.

These experiences translated into feelings of being lonely, isolated, guilty, angry, and overwhelmed, which they began to relate to their not being infected with HIV. These issues, although initially difficult to talk about, became increasingly clear as the group matured. The subject easier to talk about in the early phase of the group was sex.

Sex

Both groups began with members discussing sex by rigidly regurgitating safer-sex messages ingrained into contemporary gay culture by a generation of prevention efforts. Discussion of "non–politically correct" desires, thoughts, behaviors, and even feelings was very uncomfortable and frequently policed by other members. Paul, a thirty-eight-year-old man, in a brave first-session statement, exclaimed, "I just want to get fucked without a condom!" He had never had anal sex without using condoms, as he had not been comfortable with anal sex in his twenties. He felt that the epidemic had lasted longer than he expected, and he wanted to know how much longer until he could "do it" without a condom. Immediately, Mark, a forty-three-year-old member, responded with as much energy as Paul had used to express his desire for unprotected anal intercourse, "I think that is a very dangerous thought."

The comment came very early in the group process when trust had not yet been established and risk taking was premature for most members. As facilitators, we acknowledged the risk Paul took and validated his expressed desire and obvious frustration with safer sex. Mark was encouraged to elaborate on how Paul's expressing desire was dangerous *for him*. We attempted to have him own the feeling that it was dangerous for him to hear other people express a desire for unsafe sex by having him restate his reaction. Mark's comment was an example of attempting to suppress the sexual desires of HIV-negative gay men. In response to Mark's comment and in a continuing effort to establish a safe place for members to express anything they felt, the leaders reminded the group that feelings were not good or bad and that understanding desires was the first step in beginning to negotiate how to fulfill them in a safe and emotionally satisfying way. Another example of the group feeling the need to give the correct "party line" was illustrated by the men's responses when asked if they had difficulty using condoms. In the beginning, most members denied problems, but discussions during later sessions revealed that most men expressed varying degrees of difficulty using condoms.

In early group sessions, sexual discussions followed a very rational approach that was framed in terms of gathering the latest information and looking for external, socially approved guidelines. A universal question concerned oral sex and its safety level. Although the facilitators attempted to frame sexual behavior choices as part of each man's assessment and decision-making processes, the members wanted instruction on the risk of unprotected oral sex. In his third group session, James wrote:

> I would really like to talk about the "nitty-gritty" of HIV transmission. I know "the rules," but not everyone agrees on them. What do we really know? I would like to discuss sexual practices that are considered "possible safe". . . . My latest guide from GMHC is dated 1991. Has it changed?

Both groups asked the facilitators for GMHC's "latest" on safer-sex guidelines and, specifically, GMHC's stance on oral sex. GMHC had recently developed a brochure on oral sex, which was given out during one group. The brochure summarized by stating oral sex is a low risk for HIV infection. It then advised the reader, "It is up to you what risk you are willing to take, and up to you to decide what you put in your mouth." After reading this, Rick responded, "I thought you were offering a passport to pleasure, but this is not it."

Nick, a thirty-year-old group member who recently had come out as gay, discussed his struggle with wanting to sexually experiment but being afraid this would cause him to become infected. He had never had anal sex and wanted to try it. In addition, he had never tasted semen. He said he knew he "could not taste cum," but he wondered how risky anal sex is even with a condom. The following two questions, which Nick wrote on his card one week, indicated that it was highly likely that he was having even deeper struggles and confusion regarding sex, guilt, fear, and intimacy:

1. Anonymous sex: If you are used to a lot of anonymous sex, does it affect your ability to get into relationships?
2. Sexual compulsion: What is it? How do you know that you may be compulsive? What to do about it?

Indications of compulsive sexual behavior were not reported by Nick. He did, however, raise the aforementioned issue of wanting to explore his "sexual self" and of being afraid that if he did, he would become infected with HIV. The leaders felt that it was likely that his normal desire to explore sex as he matured was in conflict with the AIDS-prevention messages he had absorbed. He was eventually able to understand that his fear of infection was merged with a fear of, and guilt about, sex. Wondering if his sexual desires were compulsive were in part his way of coping with the confusion and anxiety that accompanied his sexual desires. If he was to define himself as sexually compulsive, he would then be able to get support from within the gay community to not act on his sexual desires. What became clear during the course of the group was that Nick's conflicts about his sexual desires ran very deep, and addressing them was beyond the scope of these groups.

Two group members, Turner (a thirty-six-year-old, gay white man) and Ralph (a fifty-two-year-old, gay white man), were sexually abstinent and explained that abstinence was a way to cope with the anxiety regarding AIDS in their lives. Turner was in recovery from alcohol abuse, in therapy, and taking Zoloft for depression. It was with much discomfort that he shared this information with the group. In a discussion of anxiety experienced after having sex, he shared the following:

> Well, here we are, all sitting around talking about difficult and painful feelings that are a part of being negative. We retest and never believe our results. People are living with HIV for ten-plus years now. Would it be so awful to just become infected and have it over with and live a somewhat normal life span? HIV may become a chronic disease, not a fatal one.

This statement reflected disenfranchisement from those infected but also the desire (conscious or unconscious) to be HIV positive and the feeling of not being able to remain HIV negative. To remain uninfected appeared to cause suffering that Turner felt would be worse than being HIV positive. In this case, his only way to manage remaining uninfected was through complete sexual abstinence for three years. It was again important to highlight that Turner's experience of living as an uninfected gay man was so difficult that he felt becoming infected would decrease his anxiety and be an *improvement* in his life. Many of the men in these groups experienced this feeling on and off in varying degrees.

THE MIDDLE PHASE OF THE GROUPS: ANGER

Anger was expressed by group members in various ways and was targeted at HIV itself, infected men, AIDS service organizations, the larger gay and mainstream cultures, media, and at themselves. Shaun wrote:

> Court TV began this week covering the case of a Brooklyn boy who, in 1984, contracted the HIV virus from a blood transfusion during surgery. By virtue of the fact that at the beginning the case covers

what we knew and didn't know in the early 1980s, I found myself flashing back to the early 1980s and the intense fear I felt about the disease and what to do when the HIV tests would become available. I also, while watching the case, have felt intense anger at our government for not caring, because it was mostly affecting gays, and letting this disease get totally out of hand.

He continued this theme on a different card, after another session:

Angry at press for how OJ trial was handled and related it to the lack of sensitivity to gay male plight. Also related anger at how press covers gay issues (Pride Parade) and AIDS (recent lack of news coverage).

Nick, the man struggling with his desire to experiment sexually, wrote:

Resentful that heterosexuals my age are not sitting around discussing death and that's what we're doing. That is what makes me resentful.

Joe, a forty-seven-year-old gay man who explained he came to group because he was afraid of HIV and wanted to discover what he really was afraid of, stated in his fifth group session:

I feel anger and resentment at the resources and energy spent toward people who are sick, and to be honest, sometimes at sick people themselves.

Joe explained his comment as stemming from his frustrations that the only focus of the gay community seemed to be AIDS, when at least half of gay men in New York City were not infected with HIV. These uninfected men were men such as himself. He wanted to be included and legitimized in his struggle. Another member responded, "I feel like the positives have taken over."

Self-Directed Anger

Many times, anger surfaced in ways that appeared to be homophobic, resulting in important discussions about the ability to express difficult feelings without becoming destructive. Shaun raised the issue when he shared the following story with the group:

I was in the grocery store and in the fruit and vegetable section. I saw this queeny guy there and I started to feel uncomfortable. I was uncomfortable with this feminine guy and it stuck with me. The more I thought about it, the more I wondered; why should this guy being himself and out shopping make me feel so uncomfortable?

When the group discussed Shaun's experience, Shaun was able to admit feeling afraid people would identify him with this other effeminate man. He further acknowledged that he was afraid he himself identified with the effeminate man and did not like the association. The group was able to relate his experience to his discomfort, on some level, with being gay.

Shaun, in a later session, shared another experience, in which he was at a classical music concert and saw two men sitting a few rows in front of him. He described an "obvious" air of physical closeness between the two. At times, they casually touched each other, and it appeared to Shaun that they wanted to put their arms around each other but resisted. He was angry that they didn't. He said he was angry that the world was such that "even at a classical music concert where there must have been other gay men" this couple was not able to show their affection for each other. He was able to share feeling envious of what he was viewing as an ideal of a gay relationship. What is significant about Shaun's second story is that it further fleshed out the homophobia with which he was struggling. His first story demonstrated his fear of "being like" the "queeny guy," while the latter showed his fear of not being like the two other men. In both cases, he projected aspects of himself onto others and judged them harshly, thus judging himself. Psychoanalysis terms this projective identification. Simply put, it is an unconscious process of projecting aspects of yourself that you do not claim onto others, resulting in an attraction-repulsion "tug of war." Projective identification is very much a part of homophobia. Homophobia, whether resolved or unresolved, can resurface in HIV-negative gay men because the feelings of isolation, fear, the need to hide (their status as uninfected men), social unacceptance, and anger are feelings experienced by every gay man during his coming-out process.

Coming-out references were often made during the group process and were referred to by the facilitators as something all of the men had in common. Group members related current feelings of isolation and depression about being HIV negative to the same feelings they experienced when coming out. Having to tell people you are HIV negative was also related to having to tell people you were gay. For men who felt they fought the battle of internalized homophobia, it was disconcerting and overwhelming to realize how HIV resurfaced or exacerbated this struggle.

Jim shared how growing up Catholic instilled in him guilt and strong negative self-judgement. He was conflicted because he also found himself drawn back to the Church at this time in his life. He wrote:

> It's easy to make the leap from gay men dying to a moral stance of deserving it. I know it's part of my own homophobia and want to keep it in check.

Ralph wrote in his journal:

> A friend and I were talking about an acquaintance of his who dresses very outrageously and I said, "He takes the subway like that?" Was my comment a type of homophobia? I felt it was more a concern for his safety.

After discussing this with the group, Ralph felt his initial reaction was complex, and homophobia may have been a part of it, although he was genuinely concerned for this man's safety as well. On his card, Ralph wrote:

> I've always prided myself in being very liberal. In matters of sexuality, I suddenly (or maybe not so suddenly) find that I am not only conservative but reactionary. I'm not happy with this turn of events.

DEPRESSION AND FEELING OVERWHELMED

Symptoms of depression were expressed by most men in the groups. Members reported crying spells, overwhelming feelings of grief and loss, and previous consultations with mental health providers. One group member was currently taking the antidepressant medication Zoloft. Tim, a forty-two-year-old gay man in a relationship with a symptomatic HIV-infected man, wrote:

> The only thing that came up this week relates to last week's loss issue. While watching *The Heidi Chronicles*, the speech delivered by the gay doctor about being at another memorial service brought me to tears. Despite knowing the speech from the play, despite our talking about it in last week's group, I got two sentences into the speech and was in tears. It is things like this which take me to a very familiar and sad place and bring up all the same feelings I have each time I lose someone.

Dan, a forty-three-year-old gay man who lost a lover of twenty years to AIDS three years ago, wrote:

> This past week has been hell for me. I have been very depressed. More so than at any time since before T.'s death, I think. It finally hit home that I was going to leave this job. It will be at the end of January and I haven't the faintest idea what I want to do. The man I have been dating was incommunicado for over forty-eight hours and then when we did see each other Thursday night for a work-related function, he wouldn't spend the night and wouldn't see me over the weekend because I had family visiting. I was so despondent over the perceived emptiness in my life that I began having thoughts that were running to the suicidal. Thinking things like it would not matter whether or not I was around, there was no real reason for me to continue on, because it doesn't make any difference. There is no one who needs me or wants me in the way I want to be needed or wanted. I have cried more in the last two weeks than I have in a long time. . . . I keep hoping with time and patience things will change, but that does not help me very much right now. I am feeling so very lonely.

Several of Dan's journal entries discussed grieving and missing his dead lover, T.

> Thursday—sorting thru boxes—cleaning—loss of lifestyle! gay pride weekend '79 + days following . . . Saturday. Thought how much T. would have loved their house—how lucky they are.

It was not easy for the men to share feeling depressed, lonely, or overwhelmed. Some men were more able to openly discuss these feelings than others, and some were more comfortable writing them down on the cards but not bringing them up in group. Each time this occurred, group facilitators urged and encouraged the member to bring the story up in group. Several men felt they were the only ones having such strong and difficult feelings and that something must be wrong with them. The facilitators attempted to normalize these feelings and place them in the context of living during an epidemic and struggling to have a satisfying life. This externalization of the powerfully uncomfortable feelings and validation of them through recognition from other group members helped alleviate the feelings of "something is wrong with me."

HIV AS A LESSON

As a result of discussions about losses and the death of loved ones, several men broached the topic of finding meaning from the AIDS epidemic. This was discussed with great ambivalence by the group members. In regard to what can be learned from the epidemic, Joe raised the following concerns:

> I'm somewhat resentful of the books discussed in *The New York Times* (books about self-improvement and spiritual growth) that say this is what we get from AIDS—its purpose.

Mark responded by saying he thought there was some truth in these books and similar statements.

Chris, a thirty-six-year-old gay widower told the group about the death of his lover. In quite an eloquent manner, Chris described hating having to go through losing his lover but "how awful but incredibly expanding" the experience was for him. The awful part for Chris was watching the illness ravage his lover's body and the grief of losing his "life partner." He described the "expansion" as no longer fearing death and being impressed with how his lover faced death. Chris recalled a feeling of peace surrounding the actual event of dying and discovering his own sense of spirituality.

Overall, the groups struggled with the meaning of the epidemic to them individually and to the gay community at large. Some found it helpful to find a lesson in the tragedy. Other men became angry at such thinking and felt it was too close to "blaming the victims" and imposed "morality."

Cultural Implications

The discussions about the meanings to be garnered from the AIDS crisis led to talk about the gay community at large and not just individual lessons learned. Many of the group members wondered if being gay meant more than just "having sex." The pressure to look a certain way and act a certain way was discussed. Some agreed the pressure was communal, and others felt it was more individual. Darryl wrote:

> Gay Culture—how do individuals in the group define it? Who makes up the culture? Is it changing? How so? What/how does the gay culture deal with HIV positives and HIV negatives?

These discussions diverged from the basics of sex and safer sex. The men began asking questions about the direction and future of the gay community. The facilitators noted that this was an extremely important issue because men who had earlier stated feeling there was no place for them in the gay community were now claiming a place and subtly discussing the future of the community they had "reclaimed."

As this chapter has illustrated, HIV status affects even the lives of those who remain uninfected. Much of the following may appear to have little to do with HIV, but in fact, HIV was ever-present, at least as a frame within which the discussions occurred. The examples that follow are important because they mark a transition for the group members from hopelessness about their futures to assuming that they will have a future and taking responsibility for the shape of their future. These men struggled with how to thrive during this epidemic. Only part of their struggle was directly related to how to remain uninfected by the virus that was decimating so many other gay men. The middle and ending phases of these groups were largely characterized by these men wrestling with issues that directly affected their quality of life as gay men who were going to most likely survive this epidemic. This marked a transition from defining themselves in relation to HIV to viewing themselves as people with their own particular needs and issues.

RELATIONSHIPS AND SEX REVISITED

During the middle and later phase of the groups, discussions of sex went beyond safer-sex techniques. Many members took risks in discussing how they had sex, how they used sex, and how they feared sex. This led into discussions of the importance of intimacy and closeness and how these needs were oftentimes confused with having sex. Paul wrote:

> I'm still/again/always obsessed/worried re: whether I want to be single or married. I don't really know which I want—and I'm pretty old not to know which I want. I mean, I like freedom to come and go as I please—I have a very full schedule (AA, gym, The Works, friends)—but I also want Mr. Right (or maybe just Mr. Pretty Good) to be with me. Or maybe just Mr. Pretty Hot Sex All The Time! But what do I have to negotiate to get what I want???!!!

Paul was torn between his fear of HIV, his increasing desire to have sex, and the lack of intimacy in his life. He reduced the conflict to whether or not he wanted to be partnered. He did not have a lover or boyfriend at the time so, for him, the idea of a committed relationship seemed to answer his fears about finding a Mr. Right (a.k.a. Mr. Pretty Good or Mr. Pretty Hot Sex All the Time). His single life was not the one he fantasized about, and his self-image was so low that he felt he had few desirable traits which would help attract a potential partner. On another card he wrote:

> How much longer do we have to use condoms. On my mind: I want to look stable—but what does that look like? Is monogamy it?

Paul's comment about wanting "to look stable" provides insight into his struggle. He did not feel control over his life circumstances, including relationships, frequency of sex, or his employment. He also indicated that it was important to *look* stable as opposed to *feeling* stable.

Dan wrote the following about his new relationship:

> Saturday was the third month anniversary of my meeting R. He wasn't even aware of it and didn't want to come and see me so I went out and had sex.

Dan did not describe what type of sex he had and the circumstances leading up to it. He did describe coping with feeling disappointed by his boyfriend and seeking out acceptance and approval through impulsive, anonymous sex. The group helped Dan realize that his self-reported depression and loneliness, coupled with using sex as a way to cope with painful and uncomfortable feelings, could place him at risk for infection in the future. The last thing Dan shared with the group during the final session was, "I still will have unprotected anal sex if I am the top."

Chris, three sessions after telling the group about his lover's death, asked, "Am I sending something out that makes me not able to get dates?" Chris wondered if his unresolved grief about his lover's death was somehow contributing to his difficulty in dating, while also pondering if the death of his lover would make it difficult for him to become close with another man in an intimate and loving way.

Joe, who in the early group sessions described feeling asexual, later disclosed that he had been sexual with a couple who were his neighbors. When asked how this came about and what things he was doing sexually, he responded he did not have anal sex (which he had told the group was a problem for him to have with condoms) because "I thought, what will I tell the guys in the group?" Several other men mentioned using the group in this type of observing ego manner to curtail risky sexual behaviors. The facilitators used these disclosures as an opportunity to point out that something important seemed to have occurred during the course of the group, since several men had begun to give the group as the reason for not engaging in unsafe sexual activity. In addition, this observation was quickly followed up by helping the men realize they were able to control and monitor their own urges. The real observing ego was their own to use from then on.

After several group meetings, Rick, age fifty-one, slowly disclosed his sexual activity. It turned out that his main sexual outlet was in sex clubs and meeting men anonymously. He "had given up on falling in love." His choice of which sex clubs he visited was dictated by them not allowing anal sex. He revealed feeling unable to avoid the temptation of anal sex if it was around, so this was a self-imposed rule. He further stated he would not go home with one guy, "who was his ultimate fantasy," afraid if he did, he would not be able to control himself and would wind up engaging in unsafe sex.

Turner, who had been sexually abstinent for three years, met a boyfriend while he was in the group. His excitement was contagious, and there were lots of questions about how they met and how Turner was feeling. Turner informed the group that he told his new boyfriend about being in the group and thus being HIV negative. His boyfriend did not discuss his own HIV status in relation to Turner's disclosure. Turner felt it probably meant he too was HIV negative. However, upon hearing Turner's interpretation of his boyfriend's nondisclosure of his own HIV status, the group's mood deflated. Most of the men voiced concerns that Turner's boyfriend was HIV positive and that was why he had not discussed his HIV status. This conversation became upsetting to Turner and ultimately brought the pervasiveness of HIV back into the room. In response to the session about Turner and his boyfriend, Ralph wrote, "Trust—relationships—sex, it's all a mystery."

GROUP ENDINGS

Much of the facilitators' work was to help the men talk explicitly about how living as gay men who were uninfected with HIV affected their self-perceptions, feelings, and behaviors. The facilitators also realized that the men in these groups were often not making connections between how they felt and their behaviors and attempted to elicit and explicitly point out possible connections whenever there was an opportunity to do so. In addition, the facilitators tried to help members learn to control both how they reacted to their feelings and their consequent behaviors to gain an added measure of control over their lives. The facilitators were also cognizant of the need to encourage these men to cultivate an awareness of themselves as part of the broader gay community that included both infected and uninfected men. This was an attempt to strengthen identification with a gay community diversified along serostatus. Toward this end, a significant shift happened in the last few sessions of both groups. A sense of connection, support, and community was evident and is described next.

Support and Strength

In the later meetings, several men stated that being able to hear how other men were handling their sex lives and sexual decision making was helpful and meaningful to them. Others commented that the group gave them a place to be with other men who were different than them but who were also struggling with the same issues. One man commented it was nice to be in a nonsexual place, getting to know people, and "having these type of conversations with other gay men."

Some men made obvious connections to others and found support, strength, and courage. For some, the ability to act in self-actualized ways as proud gay men emerged as a result of their being in this group. In a discussion related to homophobia, Mark, a self-described blue-collar worker, told the story of being harassed on the job. Using a strength he found as a result of attending the group, Mark confronted the harassment directly, and as a result, management warned employees about making antigay slurs. Mark's story inspired other members to share their own incidents of demanding respect.

Ralph, a teacher, related a story in which he was being harassed by an employee of the school district. After a very long battle, he was able to resolve the situation in a formal way with which he was comfortable. Rick related the following story about not tolerating antigay bigotry:

> I like to sunbathe at various public pools in the city. I was at this public pool in between two projects and was decked out as usual, ready for the sun—you know, with the eggshell glasses to protect your eyes—when I heard this kissing sound coming from the distance and it kept going. I eventually looked up and the guy making the sounds yelled, "Hey guy, don't you think you're in the wrong neighborhood?" I screamed back I had a right to be anywhere I wanted and this went back and forth. Eventually I went to the security office, which was even more homophobic and refused to help and even refused to call the police. After ordering them to call, they finally called the police. I had to carry the complaint all the way through political representatives, but eventually it was handled.

Attending these groups helped these participants develop an improved sense of self-esteem that they attribute directly to working through their feelings of discomfort and shame about being HIV negative. All three had made formal complaints and demanded formal resolutions to what they perceived as homophobia and infringements on their rights, something each felt he would not have done prior to attending this group. James, crediting strength he found as a result of the group, related the following incident:

> I went into a deli up on the Upper West Side. Not too unusual a place for gay men to shop. Inside the deli, I was waiting to be helped and the guys working behind the counter were talking in Spanish to a few female friends out front, where I was. I kept waiting and heard them call me a faggot in Spanish. Their problem was that I know how to speak Spanish and knew everything they said. At first I was just going to ignore it, but when I got outside, I said, wait a minute, they have no right in this neighborhood to be calling me names and making me uncomfortable. I just kept thinking of Mark's, Rick's, and Joe's stories from last week and I got more angry. I went back in and asked for the manager. I told the employees who were making the offensive comments why I was upset and that I wanted to report it to the manager, who was not there. Normally, I would have let it drop. But I didn't. I went back two days later, saw the manager, and made a complaint, and he was very apologetic and said he would speak to his employees about the situation.

CONCLUSION

In the first group session, most men could not articulate what made them sign up for the groups. The knew they were struggling, unhappy, and HIV negative. Initially, they did not connect their unhappy feelings to being uninfected with HIV. They did know that they were not feeling comfortable with being HIV-negative gay men within the gay community. Many felt hopeless about their futures and the possibility of remaining uninfected. These men experienced some catharsis from just sharing their experiences, learning that they were not alone in their reactions and feelings, and being validated by listening to other men grappling with similar issues.

Some of the men gained personal insight and growth from the group experience. During the course of attending the groups, Tom began to realize the pervasive impact of his lover's illness. James stated that the groups helped him clarify his wants and helped him feel as if he could "stand up for himself" without being embarrassed. Others regained a sense of possibility in their lives and resumed sexual activity and dating.

The groups provided a forum in which all members began examining how they were currently meeting men and having sex.

In addition to the numerous examples of individual gains and growth as a result of attending these groups, certain members began to make community and political interventions as a result of feeling more empowered as HIV-negative gay men. A few members expressed interest in facilitating similar groups as peer group leaders. Shaun began volunteering politically. Other men referred friends to the next series of the group program. As more uninfected men describe and share their experiences, it will become more accepted that HIV-negative gay men have their own set of unique psychosocial issues and dynamics, both interpersonally and intrapsychically, that must be addressed to ensure the long-term survival of a vibrant gay men's community.

Perhaps the most important outcome to emerge from these groups is the need for AIDS-prevention programs to listen to what uninfected men are saying they experience as HIV-negative gay men and what they need to remain HIV negative. It is only through hearing the diversified realities of uninfected gay men and integrating their needs into the design and implementation of prevention programs that these efforts can ever be successful in stemming the tide of new seroconversions. AIDS-related service and prevention organizations must begin outreach to uninfected men and communicate loudly and unambiguously that how the AIDS epidemic is affecting the lives of men who are not infected is one crucial component of the overall health of the gay community. One way this can occur is for the AIDS-prevention programs that host groups for HIV-negative gay men to incorporate into future prevention strategies the experiences of the men who are represented in this chapter. What has been learned from these groups and the literature so far is that HIV holds a unique relationship to the gay community in the United States, and it has become merged in the political and social identities of gay men. This will most likely continue to occur, as the epidemic shows no indication of abating.

In the early years of the epidemic, people living with HIV and AIDS experienced isolation and alienation as a result of their illness and gained support and strength through support groups. Similarly, the experiences of the men in these groups demonstrated that they too greatly benefit from being in support groups focused on their common experience. By connecting, talking, feeling, and challenging one another in a safe group milieu, HIV-negative gay men questioned environmental, social, and individual responses to AIDS. Because HIV has so defined the realities of gay men, issues that do not seem directly related to AIDS became important topics of discussion issues such as monogamy, use of drugs and alcohol, anonymous sex, marriage, conservatism, homophobia, and even the direction of the gay movement.

The difficulties inherent in remaining uninfected as a sexually active gay man deserve a more comprehensive prevention response than condoms alone. Remaining uninfected is not just about avoiding a virus during sex. When given the opportunity to speak for themselves, HIV-negative men are clear that prevention efforts have to become more sophisticated in addressing their complicated lives. For these men, staying uninfected is more about coping with difficult feelings within a culture that does not address or even often recognize these feelings and realities. These groups have demonstrated that to be effective prevention strategies they will need to address gay culture as well as gay sex. HIV has permeated not only how gay men have sex with each other but all aspects of living as a gay man today. Contemporary AIDS-prevention strategies need to take a broad environmental approach if they are to be both comprehensive and effective. Just as individual change can lead to cultural change, cultural change can lead to individual change and growth.

REFERENCES

Ball, S. (1996). HIV-negative gay men: Individual and community social service needs. In M. Shernoff (Ed.), *Human services for gay people: Clinical and community practice* (pp. 25-40). Binghamton, NY: The Haworth Press.

Ball, S. (1999). Support groups for HIV-negative gay men. In M. Shernoff (Ed.), *AIDS and mental health practice: Clinical and policy issues* (pp. 85-94). Binghamton, NY: The Haworth Press.

Johnston, W. (1995). *HIV negative: How the uninfected are affected by AIDS.* New York and London: Insight Books, Plenum Press.

Kayal, P. (1993). *Bearing witness, Gay Men's Health Crisis and the politics of AIDS.* Boulder, CO: Westview Press.

Odets, W. (1995). *In the shadow of the epidemic: Being HIV negative in the age of AIDS.* Durham, NC: Duke University Press.

Rofes, E. (1996). *Reviving the tribe: Regenerating gay men's sexuality and culture in the ongoing epidemic.* Binghamton, NY: Harrington Park Press.

Chapter 10

Spiritual Issues and HIV/AIDS in the Latino Community

Eduardo J. Baez

AIDS has had a marked influence on the lives of many Latinos who struggle to deal with the ignorance and fear that continue to exist within the Latino community fifteen years into the pandemic. The role of spiritual beliefs and practices, specifically in the treatment of Latino clients, is a topic that has received limited attention in the professional literature. Virtually nothing has been published on spiritual issues and HIV/AIDS in the Latino community, even though religious and spiritual institutions have long been recognized as primary sources of natural supports for Latinos. The Catholic church has established itself as a focal point of many Latino communities, and its influence has helped determine and define societal norms. Belief systems such as *Curanderismo* (the syncretism of Roman Catholic and indigenous Mexican beliefs), *Santeria* (the syncretism of Roman Catholic and African/Yoruba beliefs), and *Spiritualism* (a European-based belief system that incorporates the concept of a world inhabited by both good and evil spirits that influence human behavior) also figure prominently in Latino communities, even though they are decried by the mainstream churches (Delgado and Humm-Delgado, 1982; Stevens-Arroyo, 1974). Malinowski (1943) wrote the following regarding the importance of these natural sources of support, which should be considered when working with Latino clients affected and/or infected by HIV/AIDS:

> Both magic and religion arise and function in situations of emotional stress: crises of life, lacunae in important pursuits, death and initiation into tribal mysteries, unhappy love and unsatisfied hate. Both magic and religion open up escapes from such situations and such impasses as offer no empirical way out except by ritual and belief in the domain of the supernatural. (p. 87)

The importance of acknowledging and understanding the role of spiritual beliefs and practices in working with Latino clients is paramount when one considers the strong influence that organized religion has had on their societal, cultural, and familial lives (Stevens-Arroyo, 1974).

Cultural competence has been recognized as an essential element in the treatment of members of diverse communities (Morales, 1989). In working with Latino clients affected and/or infected by HIV/AIDS especially, the role that spiritual beliefs play in their ability to function and cope should be recognized and assessed. This chapter is based on my experiences as a bilingual/bicultural Latino social worker who has worked with clients affected and/or infected by HIV/AIDS in a variety of settings and as a Spiritualist counselor and Santero novitiate.

What are the cultural norms and values with which the client was raised, and how might these help determine the coping mechanisms that the client employs? Was the client raised with the belief that reality contains spirits and ghosts, and if so, how does this determine how she or he views the world? Although it would be a considerable mistake to assume that cultural competence with Latinos can be achieved with one universal approach, there are some norms and values that seem to hold true across the wide spectrum of Latino cultures.

Delgado and Humm-Delgado (1982) recognized the importance of natural support systems as sources of strength in the Latino communities. They identified these as the extended family, folk healers or religious institutions, merchant groups such as *botanicas* (herbal medicine stores) and *bodegas* (Spanish grocery stores), and social clubs. Latinos in general tend to rely heavily on these systems of support and often take a dim view of formal support systems, such as mental health clinics and other human service organizations. According to De la Rosa (1992), "Individuals who receive more support from their natural support systems are less likely to experience serious emotional problems than those who receive little or no support from their informal support systems" (p. 183). Given the high value placed on these natural support systems, it is particularly important to evaluate their availability when working with Latino clients who are seeking social services.

Latino clients affected and/or infected with HIV/AIDS may suffer from a lack of support from the community due to the stigma the disease and its possible causal factors still carry. Of HIV/AIDS within the Puerto Rican community, Bok and Morales (1992) wrote, ". . . the Puerto Rican also tends to be moralistic and traditional in family values and fatalistic toward conditions and events perceived to be beyond the individual's control. Behaviors such as drug abuse, prostitution and homosexuality are generally maligned within the Puerto Rican community" (p. 14). These values hold true throughout Latino cultures and can interfere with the willingness to both provide and seek help when HIV/AIDS is involved (Bok and Morales, 1992). The tendency toward a belief in fatalism within the Latino community is important to note because it directly links to the role of spiritual and religious beliefs in dealing with illness. As a social worker in an outpatient oncology clinic in a Latino community, I was surprised at the number of my patients who believed that their behavior or lifestyle was the primary causal factor in their diagnosis of cancer and how many of them believed that their illness was a punishment from God. The strong moralistic values within the Latino community have left many people infected with HIV/AIDS feeling unsupported as a result of what the community may believe to be a result of abhorrent behavior.

In working with gay Latino clients, I found that a vast majority felt they had little access to natural support systems within their communities. Due to the stigma associated with AIDS, I also found this to be true of many of my Latino clients who were trying to cope with HIV/AIDS, both homosexual and heterosexual. Although the Catholic Church and other established religious institutions are attempting to provide services to people affected and/or infected by HIV/AIDS, I believe that the strong moralistic stance of the community and a history of intolerance on the part of religious institutions has led to many Latinos challenged by the disease to feel unsupported by mainstream churches. The support of merchant groups (with the exception of *botanicas*) and social clubs within the Latino community for people with HIV/AIDS is negligible. Many of my clients have maintained close contact with, and have had the support of, family members, but often this support has been bittersweet due to ignorance about the disease and possible modes of transmission. Despite the apparent lack of support, I found that some of my clients were able to develop coping mechanisms and find support within their communities. Among these were people who practiced alternate belief systems such as Curanderismo, Santeria, and Spiritualism. Given the preference of Latinos for natural systems of support, it would be in the best interest of social service and mental health providers working with Latinos to have an understanding of how alternate belief systems meet the needs of clients and how they can be of assistance in providing necessary social services.

The influence of organized religion, particularly Roman Catholicism, has had a strong influence on the availability of the extended family, merchant groups, and social clubs to provide support for Latinos facing the challenge of AIDS. It does not, however, hamper the ability of traditional folk healers to do the same. Traditional folk healers and belief systems such as Curanderismo, Santeria, and Spiritualism, continue to exist and be practiced throughout Latino communities in the United States and in Latin America, despite the attempts of mainstream churches to eradicate them.

These alternate belief systems have roots in Christianity and allow practitioners to maintain a connection to the organized religions in which they were raised. It is not uncommon for believers in Curanderismo, Santeria, and Spiritualism to also be members of a mainstream church and fully access both of these systems of support. It is important to note that not all Latinos are exposed to these belief systems. Similar ones, however, are present throughout Latin America and represent an amalgam of traditional belief systems and healing methods with the belief systems of colonial settlers.

Latinos who practice these alternate belief systems often find a supportive network of friends and experience familial bonds among fellow believers. The holistic approach found in Curanderismo, Santeria, and Spiritualism allows believers to participate in all aspects of their healing and imparts a sense of control in their lives. Although these belief systems do not offer a cure for HIV/AIDS, they can provide much-needed support for Latinos who may otherwise feel abandoned and hopeless within their communities.

Social work training taught me the concept of being "where the client is at," but there was surprisingly little training in culturally specific work. Both of my field placements involved working with predominantly Latino clients. It was clear in my process recordings that many of my interventions were based on observed behaviors. I found that I needed to relax professional boundaries to create a more friendly environment to engage my clients. I used my observations of their body language and vocal inflections, as well as my clinical knowledge, to formulate questions that would elicit information about their emotions and feelings. When I tried to follow the generic approach I was being taught in school, my clients were less forthright in discussing personal matters and remained focused on concrete issues and concerns. I found that although my field supervisors considered my work slightly unorthodox my clients responded well to my directive, familial style.

My approach was an adaptation of the counseling style I learned from my family members who were Spiritualist. "Clients" were treated in a friendly manner and were put at ease through gestures such as offering something to drink and "small talk" prior to their *consulta* (a Spiritualist counseling session). This served to establish a sense of trust and familiarity and also provided me with information about the client before the actual session.

Curanderismo, Santeria, and Spiritualism have been studied as natural mental health systems in social work and psychology literature because they incorporate a counseling aspect in the treatment process (Delgado, 1977; Gilestra, 1981; Harwood, 1977; Perez y Mena, 1977). In Latino culture, a high value is generally placed on the role of elders and/or respected persons (such as traditional healers) within the community as persons who offer guidance and counseling. When patients visit a traditional healer, they usually present with a specific physical or emotional problem that they want solved. Their expectation of the "treatment process" for emotional issues is short-term, with quick results, and they expect to be guided through the process. Many Latinos bring this same expectation into therapy.

In my work with Latino clients affected and/or infected with HIV/AIDS, I have found that the initial meeting determines whether they will engage or not. For Latinos, interpersonal relationships are formed based on a sense of trust. Creating a warm ambiance is essential; social service providers can accomplish this by simple gestures, such as shaking hands with clients, asking them to be seated, and offering them something to drink. Clients in turn may engage the worker in some preliminary "small talk" and, in later meetings, bring the worker a small token of appreciation such as food or a plant. All of these are formalities which Latinos consider common courtesies and which indicate a respect and understanding of tradition. Understanding and participating in these small gestures can go a long way toward establishing a sense of trust.

Traditional healers use a holistic approach in their counseling and usually address matters of mind, body, and spirit in their sessions. They are directive in their counseling approach and engage clients in question-and-answer sessions that will elicit the presenting problem as well as guide the formation of the treatment plan. Every session with a traditional healer ends with the recommendation of some course of action that is meant to address the problem at hand. Clients are expected to actively participate in their healing and to report progress, which helps determine the course of treatment.

As both a social worker and a Spiritualist, I have learned to appreciate and respect culturally accepted norms and values used by traditional healers in their work and to incorporate them into the provision of social services. Following the model of traditional healers has helped me in my work with Latino clients, whether they use traditional healing methods or not. I have found that my clients respond best to a directive approach in therapy which incorporates traditional norms and values.

In my practice, knowing a person's belief system has been a key to successfully working with them. Even if clients do not adhere to any particular religious or spiritual beliefs, their lives are affected by the beliefs of their families and the community at large.

I have found that by assessing the investment that the client has in her or his beliefs and by working with those beliefs, the quality of the interaction is enhanced. This is substantiated by the work of Ghali (1985), who found that practitioners who used spiritual values in treatment and modified their technique accordingly were the most satisfied with their interactions with Puerto Rican clients.

Understanding the client's belief systems can give the practitioner great insight into internalized conflicts the client may have. In my experience, probing into the belief systems of my clients during the initial phases of therapy is considered less intrusive than asking about their family dynamics. One of the universal tenets of Latino culture is that family business remains in the home and is not to be discussed with strangers. This belief can frustrate attempts to elicit information and requires that a level of trust be established by the therapist. Since religious and spiritual beliefs are closely linked with all of the natural support systems, initiating discussions about belief systems often leads to the client disclosing about issues such as family dynamics, community support, and personal perspectives on life.

Although being bilingual and bicultural might serve to enhance work with a client, it will not do so if the worker is judgmental and insensitive. Social service providers should keep the following in mind when working with Latino clients affected and/or infected by HIV/AIDS:

- In most cases, the natural aversion that Latinos may have for formal systems of support has been greatly reduced since the client is seeking services. You are in the position of providing assistance: avoid making judgements and keep an open mind to cultural differences and norms.
- Remember that the initial meeting is very important in engaging the client and that the best approach is to present the work to be done as a joint effort. Try to go at the client's pace, but if time is limited, use the initial meeting as an introduction and set up an appointment for as soon as conveniently possible.
- When speaking about interventions, try to engage the client in short-term goal-oriented work until some level of trust has been established. This gives the client the opportunity to assess the potential benefits of working with you. This also allows for the formation of a good working relationship.

- When making your psychosocial assessment, encourage the client to talk about personal beliefs. You will more than likely have to initiate this topic, which can most easily be accomplished by asking the client directly what her or his beliefs and practices are. Ask the client to help you understand a belief, norm, or value if you are not clear as to the meaning.
- Give the client the option to work with you or not. This will allow the client to commit to the working relationship. If possible, give the client a stress reduction tool or a measurable task to complete before the next meeting. This is in keeping with the treatment practices of traditional healers and will give the client an incentive to engage the counselor.

For social service professionals working with Latino clients challenged by AIDS, understanding the client's belief system in its cultural context will aid tremendously in determining the course of treatment. The role of religion and spiritual beliefs in determining the client's perspective on life is paramount and determines how clients respond to major events. The stigma associated with AIDS in the Latino community has caused a sense of isolation and abandonment for many who are affected and infected, while increasing the need for support. Some have turned to traditional healers in an attempt to connect with a spiritual element while creating a new family of like-minded believers, thus increasing available natural supports. Therapists working with Latinos coping with HIV/AIDS must recognize the role that spiritual beliefs play in their lives and be respectful of them in the treatment process.

REFERENCES

Bok, M. and Morales, J. (1992). Cultural dissonance and AIDS in the Puerto Rican community. *Journal of Multicultural Social Work, 2*(3), 13-26.

De la Rosa, M. (1992). Natural support systems of Puerto Ricans: A key for well-being. *Health and Social Work, 13*(3), 181-190.

Delgado, M. (1977). Puerto Rican spiritualism and the social work profession. *Social Casework, 58*(8), 451-458.

Delgado, M. and Humm-Delgado, D. (1982). Natural support systems: A source of strength in Hispanic communities. *Social Work, 27*(1), 83-89.

Ghali, S. (1985). The recognition and use of Puerto Rican cultural values in treatment: A look at what is happening in the field and what can be learned from this. New York University. *DSW*, June. Unpublished doctoral dissertation.

Gilestra, D. (1981). Santeria and psychotherapy. *Comprehensive Psychotherapy, 3*, 69-80.

Harwood, A. (1977). Puerto Rican spiritism: Description and analysis of an alternative psychotherapeutic approach. *Culture, Medicine and Psychiatry, 1*(1), 69-95.

Malinowski, B. (1943). *Magic, science and religion.* Garden City, NY: Doubleday.

Morales, E. (1989). Ethnic minority families and minority gays and lesbians. *Marriage and Family Review, 14*(3/4), 217-239.

Perez y Mena, A. (1977). Spiritualism as an adaptive mechanism among Puerto Ricans in the United States. *Cornell Journal of Social Relations, 12*(2), 125-136.

Stevens-Arroyo, A. (1974). Religion and the Puerto Ricans in New York. In E. Mapp (Ed.), *Puerto Rican perspectives* (pp. 119-130). Metuchen, NJ: Scarecrow Press.

Chapter 11

HIV/AIDS Mental Health Services
to Black Men

Darrell P. Wheeler
Dale V. Miller

In this chapter, we will discuss the need for tailored HIV/AIDS health and mental health services for black men that address historical, cultural, sexual, and systemic agendas. We firmly believe that if HIV/AIDS mental health services in the United States are truly going to benefit black men these issues must be addressed within the treatment context. Our discussion is not about gay, straight, bisexual, or questioning men, but rather it is about men who are black, who are in the United States, and who are facing an onslaught of health and human crises, HIV/AIDS included. This chapter, although targeting mental health providers, is also intended for anyone who values the worth, dignity, history, and ultimately, the lives of black men.

Historically, most HIV/AIDS prevention services have been designed for specifically targeted and identifiable groups (e.g., gay men's services, services to women and children, for blacks, and for men who have sex with men). This perspective reduces the multiplicity of black humanity to one or a few readily identifiable and differentiating statuses (e.g., race, gender, and sexual orientation)—an egregious error. HIV/AIDS services formulated on this model do little to promote or support the full expression of human experiences, thus they are limited in their capacity to meet the client where he is at in the context of his ever-changing life.

Although many commonalities exist that affect black men's experiences with HIV/AIDS, great diversity is also present. Mental health professionals seeking to work with black males must recognize the need to see both the unifying and unique aspects of the men whom they are serving. For example, services to black men, as discussed in this chapter, are not solely intended to be applicable for, or to reference, economically and politically disadvantaged black male groups. Economic resources, education, employment, and groups of affiliation can all affect the course and outcome of services. However, in writing this chapter, we believe and affirm that certain core common experiences have had a significant impact on the collective experience of black males in the United States. It is these experiences and their resultant effect on the therapeutic process that are the essence of this chapter.

THE AFRICAN DIASPORA IN AMERICA

When delivering HIV/AIDS mental health services to black men in the United States, providers encounter and must concurrently address multiple psychosocial and spiritual issues that are inextricable from the biomedical and public health needs of this population. Problems, such as poverty and drugs, that providers must consider when addressing the specific needs of such populations have already been noted. We wish to further emphasize a few that are particularly important. The first is the practice of technology transference—transferring successful designs and models from population to population without considering the specificity with which they were or were not designed. Intervention instruments designed by and for gay white men are premised on a very specific social and cultural commonality—whiteness. Implicitly located within many programs and services trans-ferred across populations are the presumptions of race neutrality and that distinctions based in class, gender, and race transfer to populations social-ly marginalized and culturally located as other.

The process of technology transference then finds successful programs and services slightly modified or "blackened" to meet the needs and address the differences presented by black consumers. Most often, this modification involves a focus on racial identity, which lumps all black men together as one group, despite differences both obvious and subtle. Some black men may then feel repelled by, rather than invited to, participate in programs because of cultural insensitivity, a perceived lack of authenticity, or that undefinable quality of "realness" that is so important in contemporary black popular culture. As British cultural critic Stuart Hall (1996) points out, media in the West have a poor record of conceptualizing the diversity of black populations. We observe a similar effect in relation to HIV/AIDS services that position black clients as members of a monolithic black com-munity. For example, the authors have seen prevention and education mate-rials targeted to black men that are produced by community-based organiza-tions in our area which treat the rich diversity of New York's black communities as essentially one community. One large AIDS service orga-nization's representations treat black men as one single group—gay identi-fied, African American, and middle class, while ignoring the very large black immigrant communities in the city. This same organization, through its substantial market presence in other communities, has in the past incorporated technology transfers from group to group without negotiating the cultural specifics necessary for success across ethnic and social groups.

Ostensibly transferring HIV/AIDS services across groups without regard for social and cultural specificity has had and continues to have dire consequences for black populations, locally and nationally. Slower declines in AIDS case diagnoses in black populations, as demonstrated by recent CDC statistics (1995, 1996, 1997, 1998), call into question the efficacy of this practice (see Figure 11.1).

FIGURE 11.1. CDC Cumulative AIDS Case Diagnoses by Race, 1994 to Mid-Year 1997

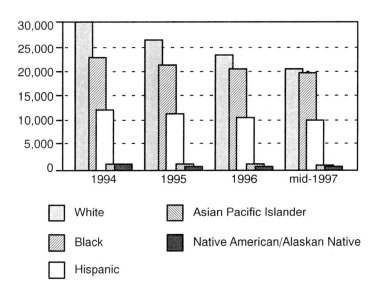

White	29,910	26,508	23,341	20,327
Black	22,838	21,184	20,199	19,611
Hispanic	12,016	11,137	10,337	9,908
Asian Pacific Islander	518	477	480	444
Native American/ Alaskan Native	518	198	166	179

Fairly stable to slight decreases in AIDS case diagnoses for black men in the face of the dramatic decreases for white men are a testament to both the ineffectiveness of the practice of technology transfers and to the need for providers to understand and negotiate the specificities of subgroups within diverse black populations. Technology transfer and the race neutrality premise also ignore the range of experiences and identities of the dominant white population in America, though the influence of race ideology universalizes white identity to such an extent as to minimize the importance of white ethnic diversity in the United States in relation to AIDS services (with the possible exception of white Latino men).

The growing diversity of black populations in America poses significant challenges for providers. The twentieth century has produced large migratory flows of African diaspora peoples throughout the West. In the United States, these flows have a dramatic impact on the delivery and efficacy of HIV mental health services for black men. Within the United States, the historic social and cultural factors that have affected the economic and social mobility of black Americans also produce barriers to access for black immigrants. Identity is also an integral consideration, as it complicates the existing complex of issues providers must navigate for black consumers. Identity then becomes the second problem providers face, both racial and sexual identity. Race and socially constructed racial identity are, according to Omi and Winant (1986), sociocultural factors that have had great impact on American society. In addition to social problems such as discrimination and prejudice, the physical and mental health of black people in the United States is significantly affected by the social practices that definitions of black(ness) and white(ness) produce. A recent study by Fichtenbaum and Gyimah-Brempong (1997) highlights the role of race in the delivery of health services and access to health care for blacks in America. Ideologies of race and racism (Massey et al., 1993; Sanjek, 1994) set the stage for social constructions and cultural meanings of difference and the maintenance of differential health care and life expectancies for black people in America. A definition as black has historically meant a life of unequal access, injustice, and marginalization in America. Are we seeing these sociocultural phenomena again, in the post-civil rights and "postrace" era, in relation to HIV/AIDS?

The sociocultural realities (U.S. Commission on Civil Rights, 1995) of continuing disadvantage and difference in many areas, including housing (Hirsch, 1983), jobs for youth (Sullivan, 1989), planning (Davis, 1990), and conceptualization (Fainstein, 1993), must be brought to bear in program design and service delivery for HIV/AIDS in black communities. When program planners place an understanding of the construction of race and race ideology in the U.S. cultural context in dialogue with racial and cultural bias (Bliebtreu and Meaney, 1973), the intersection of cultural competence and good design produces an effective tool to address contemporary health problems in black communities that are historically rooted.

As cultural critics have outlined the problems with representations of black subjects and the politics of identity (Hall, 1996; West, 1993; Fuss, 1995), we must now reconsider and expand the identities of the black populations served by HIV/AIDS health care systems. In New York City, the diversity of black male populations to be serviced include African Americans and immigrants from the Caribbean, South America, Africa, and Europe. Several black agencies exist that service distinct populations within the black community in the city. Niche marketing is evident in agencies that provide services predominantly to Caribbean-identified black gay men, black-identified gay men, gay-identified black men, etc. Often comprised of members of differing ethnic identifications, they recognize that deploying a "one size fits all"* strategy, using anthropological markers of similarity, ignores the psychological, social, cultural, and political realities of these vastly different men. Heterogeneity is therefore critical for providers to recognize and consider. Distinctive cultural practices, values, and behaviors must be negotiated when developing services for "black men." Recognizing heterogeneity is important not only for immigrants but for African-American men as well, as differences occur across and within class, region, multiethnic, and sexual identifications. Increasingly in the United States, there is a blurring of racial lines and individual identifications across ethnic lines. Golf star Tiger Woods, singer Mariah Carey, and movie star Halle Berry are but a few popular culture icons that attest to multiethnic identification and to the need for providers to deconstruct ideologies and focus on localized cultural specifics when transferring or designing services. Cultural identity is an important aspect of mental health service-delivery paradigms. Writers from both psychology and social work have provided a wealth of information about the role of culture, cultural understanding, and cultural competence in serving black communities (Martin and Martin, 1995).

SEXUAL ORIENTATION AND IDENTIFICATION

Addressing sexual and substance use behaviors (which is less likely to connote social status) rather than a singular focus on identity when working with black men may be more congruent with the individual's world-

---

*Reference to an analysis of focus groups conducted by Darrell Wheeler and Dale Miller, authored by D. Michael Poulson, "One Size Does Not Fit All."

view and life experiences. An understanding of this is essential if AIDS prevention and mental health providers are to be effective in reaching populations of black men in need of these services. In Jeffrey Weeks' (1991) discussion of what he terms a "relationship paradigm," we find a concise conceptualization providers may use as a starting point: stress relationships rather than identities when addressing sexual behaviors. Focusing on sexual identity as the starting point for black men may alienate them because two other important domains, within which they coexist, are ignored—sexual orientation and experiences.

Sexual identity may represent the psychological integration of these domains and exist simultaneously with them, while integrating gender ideology. Sexual experiences may be framed or influenced by social, psychological, and other factors, both intrinsic and extrinsic (situational sex, for example). They may be spontaneous and need not be motivated by deeply felt desire. Sexual orientation toward men, women, or both, on the other hand, is more likely a predetermined status or one that is less amenable to willful change (Bem, 1974; Spence and Helmreich, 1978; Hacker, 1990; Wofford, 1991). Ultimately, a composite definition for gender identification (behavior, orientation, and identity) is suggested as a more appropriate solution to this dilemma.

Application of a more global definition of sexuality allows for incorporation of gender and sexual ideological constrictions that have real life effects. When social and cultural forces are not congruent with these gender and sexual constructions, dissonance between practice and identity may ensue. Contending with the inability to meet sex-linked cultural norms can create stressors in the lives of young black men. Although many of the barriers to meeting these roles result from discriminatory practices, often retaliation or response is not directed at the sources of the barrier but rather is rechanneled inwardly. Responses to these stressors are varied and inconsistent. Researchers have shown that these responses may manifest in self-destructive behaviors (intentionally or unintentionally). Sexual exploitation, of self and others, and the concomitant risk for HIV infection, is one such probable outcome (Karon, 1958; White, 1984; Poussaint, 1990; Thomas, 1991; Brown, 1990).

In environments in which the active acknowledgment of gay, bisexual, and MSM orientations and lifestyles are too threatening or produce community sanctions, getting black men to rally around labels presents a major barrier to HIV/AIDS services. This we found true doing prevention/education work and research in a black community-based agency in New York City; the stigmatization of gay and bisexual identity led to decreased help-seeking and risk-reduction behaviors from gay-identified sources and likely continuation of risk for HIV infection.

Labels such as "gay" or "bisexual" may have utility for trend watchers or providers, but they may have much less use in the lives of the black men whom mental health professionals are trying to reach regarding HIV/AIDS services. At times, the use of "gay" may carry unrecognized stigmatization along racial lines, such as the homophobic identification of "gay" with a specific white gay male identity and set of behaviors as portrayed in the media. These associations may be far removed from the life experiences and realities of black communities. Internalized homophobia is a strong disincentive to HIV/AIDS help-seeking behaviors. Gay is also a troublesome complication to black male gender constructions, calling into question the fragile masculinity ideologies and constructions of all men. Perhaps as a result, very few black male "leaders" and public intellectuals openly discuss the complexities of being black, male, and sexual, beyond reinscribing heteronormativity, patriarchy, misogyny, and nationalist dialogues.

Critical cultural studies debates in black Britain, involving questions of sexuality and gender among other variables, by writers such as Stuart Hall, Kobena Mercer, Paul Gilroy, and others, have prompted greater discourse on subject formation and identity but generally have not penetrated beyond the academy in America. A few black American intellectuals have taken up this work, among them Phillip Brian Harper, Kendall Thomas, Cornell West, and Robert Reid-Pharr. Filmmakers Marlon Riggs and Thomas Allen Harris have examined homophobia, patriarchy, and health concerns related to these constructions and have ignited significant cultural controversies doing so. Black America has yet to grapple with masculinity and gender constructions in a sustained dialogue or to begin to closely examine homophobia, patriarchy, and health concerns related to these constructions. In the larger culture, scholars such as Michael Kimmel, Michael Kaufman, Robert Connell, and others have begun the work of unpacking the histories and tracing ethnographies of masculinity and gender constructions so that we will more fully understand how these factors play social, cultural health roles. Black men's internalization of these ideologies presents barriers to providers that must be overcome in nonthreatening manners. As Levant and Majors (1997) have shown, black men in the United States maintain more traditional masculine ideologies and aspire to more traditional roles than other groups. Although there may be some change in the late 1990s, these ideologies still exert powerful influence in the lives of black men. The use of stigmatized labels destabilizes these ideologies and may push these men away from providers who attempt to apply them.

The distance between practice and identity became apparent during a focus group for young men in Harlem. As the group discussed behaviors that placed them at risk for HIV infection, there were several instances in which participants' boasting about sexual conquests had undercurrents alluding to homosexual practices. Many of the young men participating described incarceration experiences and their lives engaged in hustling since their release. (Unemployment was and remains a large factor in the lives of young, urban black men). Though no one stated explicitly their homosexual experiences, their "double lives" were clearly evident. This closeted sexual behavior, described as "on the down low" in the vernacular, is highly illustrative of the power of ideologies and social sanctions against homosexuality to deny and/or reconstruct risk behaviors despite a knowledge of how HIV is transmitted. Hearing how these men described and referred to sexual behaviors during the focus group became a prime opportunity to use appropriate slang or vernacular for their risk behaviors. We are now able to disseminate this same language to providers as tools to more effectively engage men from this urban community.

Providers must understand that sexual orientation—that predetermined status which is less amenable to willful change—need not align with contemporary politically correct identifications, as may happen in other communities. The disavowal of gay identification by homosexually active black men is frequently regarded as indicative of confusion concerning sexual orientation and sexual identity. In our experience, the confusion lies in the attempt to apply a label that may bear cultural weight that black men are unwilling to assume or may simply be a refusal to label behaviors and to fall into the identity-politics paradigm. Sexual behaviors and experiences are not the defining being for some black men but are instead components of myriad behaviors performed.

RACE, SEXUALITY, AND HIV/AIDS

Based on the preceding discussion, it should be evident to the reader that race and sexual culture are intersecting domains that must be adequately addressed in HIV/AIDS counseling efforts for black men. Before we go on to discuss specific practice issues, a look at the epidemiology of AIDS among males may help to reinforce the need for the practices that will be discussed later.

Data from the Centers for Disease Controls' HIV/AIDS Surveillance reports for the past several years provides a wealth of information about the risk factors associated with the spread of HIV and AIDS. Mental health providers can use this information in the formulation of services to their clients. In reviewing this information, Figures 11.2 through 11.4 show a stark representation of differences in risk categories for men from varying racial backgrounds. These tables present the percentage of AIDS cases reported in CDC's end of year surveillance reports for 1994, 1995, 1996, and the mid-year report for 1997.

Although many risk factors are presented in the surveillance reports, the authors will highlight three categories we believe are particularly important for mental health providers working with black men—heterosexual exposure (Figure 11.2), men who have sex with men (Figure 11.3) and risk not reported or identified (Figure 11.4). In reviewing these figures, three points become extremely clear. First, for black men, heterosexual transmission has increased slightly in the past three years and is consistently higher than that reported for any other racial group. Second, there appears to be a fairly consistent frequency of exposure among black men who have sex with men,

FIGURE 11.2. Percent of Cases—Heterosexual-Identified Risk by Year and Race

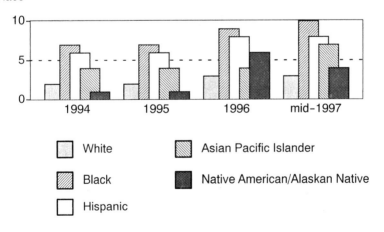

White	2	2	3	3
Black	7	7	9	10
Hispanic	6	6	8	8
Asian Pacific Islanders	4	4	4	7
Native American/Alaskan Native	1	1	6	4

FIGURE 11.3. Percent of Cases—MSM-Identified Risk by Year and Race

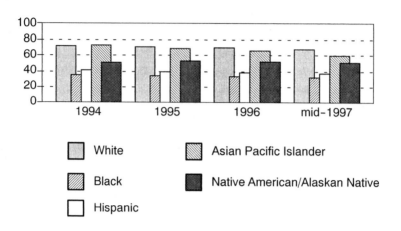

White	72	71	70	68
Black	35	34	33	32
Hispanic	41	39	38	37
Asian Pacific Islander	73	69	66	60
Native American/Alaskan Native	51	53	52	51

and this number is dramatically less than that for white men who have sex with men. Finally, and likely the most alarming observation, is the consistent and growing number of cases with no reported or identified risk factor for black males. In fact, these numbers suggest that for all racial/ethnic groups there is a trend toward increasing numbers of AIDS cases without a reported or identified risk group. This final point is so startling because prevention, intervention, and the theories and perspectives upon which they are built so often assume an identifiable risk pathway around which services can be developed. For example, in the early years of the AIDS epidemic in the United States, the recognition among white gay men that they were at increased risk of infection was a galvanizing tool and may have contributed to the improved status of gay white men in recent reports on AIDS deaths and morbidity. The data here support, as noted earlier in this chapter, the notion that labeling may be an ineffective way of targeting HIV/AIDS mental health, prevention, and intervention services for black men. As is painfully obvious from these numbers, an increasing number of men are

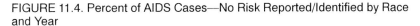

FIGURE 11.4. Percent of AIDS Cases—No Risk Reported/Identified by Race and Year

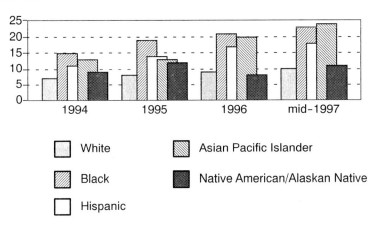

White	7	8	9	10
Black	15	19	21	23
Hispanic	11	14	17	18
Asian Pacific Islander	13	13	20	24
Native American/Alaskan Native	9	12	8	11

either choosing not to reveal or identify, or they do not know their exposure category. Any of these scenarios has dire consequences for the development and implementation of HIV prevention and education services. Although a discussion of substance use in black communities is beyond the scope of the present work, it is well worth stating that the issue of substance use and abuse, particularly injecting drugs, has also been seen as a major contributor to the AIDS epidemic among black men. The factors related to HIV/AIDS exposure and transmission clearly manifest in ways that suggest the need for different responses in different communities. What then are the practice issues for mental health providers working with black men?

PRACTICE IMPLICATIONS

Systemic Issues

Based on empirical evidence and personal experiences, we now move into a discussion of practice issues. We begin with a bold proclamation that the vast majority of contemporary American mental health and health service models are not constructed to be useful to the black male experience. This statement at first sight may appear too global. However, close examination of the most current health care statistics, hospital reviews, and reviews of provider training programs clearly tell us that black males (and women of all races) are not faring well in the current U.S. health care industry. The underpinnings for this current situation have deep historical roots. That contemporary health and mental health care models do not seem amenable to embracing the presenting needs of black men is no accident. Popular media and medical science have portrayed the black man in many unflattering ways, from buffoon to demon. These perspectives have done little to promote understanding and much to damage already tenuous relationships between clients and providers. One result has been the underutilization of health, and particularly mental health, services in proactive and preventive styles. The absence of black men in many health care settings provides the space for others to perpetuate stereotypes about these men that often result in self-fulfilling encounters when services are sought.

The effects of a system that is itself a formidable obstacle to a population are numerous and far reaching. Mental health providers must acknowledge the power and privilege differentials between themselves and clients—regardless of the providers' race. These power and privilege dynamics may not seem to be a major agenda for providers, which is part of the benefit of having power and/or privilege. The effect of unchecked power on clients who present when they are vulnerable can be devastating. The providers' use of words, methods of introducing helping steps, and physical actions can all convey messages about the perceived worth of, and respect for, clients. The perspective that clients hold from the earliest moments of the helping relationship can dramatically shape the outcome of the process.

Gender Issues

Gender differences also affect help-seeking and utilization practices. Although the present work is specific to the issues of black men, some mention of gender differences seen in treatment is warranted. These gender differences may be even more salient among groups in which gender roles are more rigidly reinforced. Studies have shown that women are more likely to seek health care earlier and more consistently and to use these services more regularly. Mental health services designed on the typical one-hour-per-week format, with an exploration of problems and rapid movement to change, may not be the best model for work with men—especially men unfamiliar with or leery of the therapeutic milieu. When therapeutic services are consistent with the sociocultural, political, and spiritual realities of the men being served, the likelihood of productive outcomes is increased. Developing standing relationships with black men over time has a facilitative role in health care. Because black men may not base their decision(s) to use health and mental health services solely on health status, providers' ability to understand and relate to the men is a more powerful predictor of using services in the long run. Increased treatment usage has been observed when the same provider meets consistently with the client, as opposed to a different professional being introduced at each treatment session. Also, congruency between provider and client demographics has been associated with increased treatment usage. This latter point is more difficult to overcome in the current system. Among mental health providers there is a particular dearth of minority men available in these professional roles. Even with this imbalance in numbers of providers available, it is still more likely that a minority provider will serve underserved populations (Xu et al., 1997).

Providers' Cultural Competency

Cultural factors have a powerful role in the development of health care perspectives, beliefs, attitudes, and practices. Maria C. Julia (1996) writes:

> The effectiveness of health care providers in reaching and working with multicultural populations rests heavily upon the sensitivity, respect and understanding paid to ethnic diversity. The barriers to providing appropriate services to ethnic populations are a lack of appropriate informational materials concerning resources, rights, and responsibilities for multiethnic groups, compounded by a shortage of trained bilingual, multiculturally educated personnel among health care provider organizations. The subsequent lack of culturally responsive service affects client behavior, access and outcome. (p. 4)

The transition to culturally responsive service efforts identified here requires an active process on the part of providers and provider systems. The action phase of the multicultural learning experience is nested in multicultural skills development.

Because cultural forces affect so many of our daily routines (e.g., what and when we eat, how we dress) and extraordinary life events (celebrations, holidays, etc.) we sometimes become blind to the effect of our own cultural perspectives on others. The power of culture is a force acted out in almost all human interactions. This powerful force, as with any element in a precise equation, needs to be accounted for if we are to truly understand the workings of the elements in concert. Too often, however, the attention to culture is ignored, glossed over, or relegated to a meaningless status.

For many health and mental health providers, professional development training reinforced ignoring this element or giving it little more than lip service in the pursuit of loftier "professional" goals. The skills associated with developing multicultural competence are no less important than the skills developed in professional pursuits. Developing a conscious awareness of diverse cultural perspectives is only one step in the process. Diversity is knowledge about material differences and their historical, sociological, and anthropological bases. Competency is about the knowledge as well as the skills that are needed to deal successfully with human differences—racial, ethnic, and sociocultural. The ethical, social, political, and professional reasons for implementing multicultural training in health care settings are compelling. Two questions currently face professional practice and training programs: (1) How are we implementing the cultural competence imperative? and (2) How proficient are workers in acquiring multicultural competence? This emphasis on culturally competent practice is critical, given that ethnic and racial minorities are expected to constitute over one-third of the population by the end of the twenty-first century (Bureau of the Census, 1990). Moreover, it is expected that, in cities such as New York and Los Angeles, the ethnic/racial compositions will outnumber European Americans (i.e., the white majority). These demographic changes, coupled with the underutilization or overutilization by various ethnic/racial minorities of social, health, and mental health services, reinforces the need for effective training of culturally competent practitioners (Cheung, 1991; Vega and Rumbaut, 1991). Recognition that all people are ethnocultural beings is a first and major step in the process of developing cultural competencies. It is easy to forget that our cultural experiences, particularly when they are the same or similar to the dominant group's, are not the only valid expressions of culture that exist. This ethnocentrism can be useful as a unifying and integrating social and psychological tool, but it can, and often does, become a stumbling block to intercultural experiences.

In the helping roles, professionals often are trying to convince patients of the need to adopt new or different practices toward healthier outcomes. This process can be likened to cultural assimilation, which requires mutual consent. Problems can and do frequently occur when ethnocentric perspectives prevail, and the result is perceived client resistance, "noncompliance," or a sense of disrespect. The goal of professionals is to provide sound health care, which is itself a cultural artifact. Rooted in an understanding of quality health care, the professional often attempts to bring patient groups into the realm of dominant thinking regarding health care practices. The process of assimilation (change) is most often the expressed desired goal. However, the process of making these changes is never as simple as presenting facts and observing change. Acculturation, on the other hand, implies a process of gradual adaptation. There is much to be said for acculturation, but this too has its limitations. Ultimately, professionals must realize that the process of developing dominant cultural perspectives and practices on health care is just that—a process. Interventions must acknowledge the importance and relevance of the patient's cultural inheritance, drawing from the patient group needed information about these practices and perspectives.

Quite simply, cultural competence skills should be developed in the rapport establishment, assessment, intervention, and evaluation phases of the helping process. More explicitly, these skills can be developed and utilized in at least the following ways:

- Recognizing the relevance of culture in health care beliefs and practices
- Being able to discuss culture—the dominant and the indigenous—including active recognition of the strengths and resilience characteristics the client brings to the therapeutic interaction
- Using an understanding of culture to frame assessments—avoiding pathological perspectives when differences in worldviews are really at work
- Framing interventions that acknowledge cultural perspectives and provide pathways to adopting new perspectives
- Monitoring, assessing, and documenting outcomes to promote replication and avoid negative occurrences

Avoid Stereotyping

In the therapeutic relationship, providers should avoid sweeping generalizations about the client based on observed or perceived statuses (e.g., ethnicity, sexual orientation, and social class). At first glance, this statement may seem to undermine many points stated thus far. However, as we noted earlier, in an effort to be culturally sensitive, providers want to avoid promoting labels and/or stereotypes that are not applicable to the client. Toward this end, active and earnest discussions with the client about issues of culture and cultural categorizations may be beneficial to both the provider and the client. For the provider, this discussion can clear up areas of doubt and/or misinformation. For the client, it may provide a much-needed opportunity to express issues and concerns about the helping process that have not been addressed because they were overshadowed by real and perceived provider barriers.

CONCLUSION

The authors have attempted to clarify the necessity of focused and specific attention to the needs of black men in HIV/AIDS mental health services. Rather than attempting to list all the possible therapeutic tactics for addressing the needs of these men (which would be a near impossible task), we have focused on developing an argument for why these differences exist, how they affect the HIV/AIDS epidemic among black men, and strategies for developing appropriate interventions.

The historical backdrop of black and white, dominance and oppression, power and privilege has been suggested as a major issue affecting the black male psyche. This backdrop applies, in many complex interactions, for all men acculturated in America. These issues, as we have argued, can create major barriers to engaging and working with the target population. In approaching these issues with clients, the mental health provider cannot be an objective and distant participant. Providers, seeking to develop real and meaningful professional relationships with their clients, will have to address their own histories and recognize that the therapeutic interaction has a context which is itself a significant element in the success or failure of the clinical relationship.

In addition to the racial/ethnic aspects of work with black men in HIV/AIDS mental health settings, the issue of learned and practiced sexual orientations, identities, and behaviors is a critical element. Based on empirical and anecdotal supports, black men in general appear to hold more traditional gender role perspectives. Using behaviors to suggest orientations and identities may be an inappropriate approach to working with black men—especially those who do not identify as gay, bisexual, or MSM—an approach has taken on great popular appeal in HIV/AIDS work. These perspectives should not be minimized in the clinical process. Inattentiveness to this caveat can undermine the clinical interactions.

Cultural competence and not just a recognition of cultural difference has been suggested as the desired goal for the mental health professional. This cultural competence develops over time and through a process. The process is not easily fit into neat packages that can be canned and transferred from setting to setting, person to person. Rather, the process of developing cultural competence may be viewed as a lifelong process that at its best provides an opportunity for worker and client to engage in meaningful and helpful discourse about a difficult and pervasive individual and societal issue. Although understanding specific cultural idiosyncracies is important, a singular focus on difference can lead to supporting stereotypic and damaging worldviews.

From the beginning of the epidemic in the United States, the work of health and mental health providers has not been easy. As we move into another decade of HIV/AIDS in the United States, there are profound epidemiologic changes in populations being devastated by this disease. Mental health and health providers will have to develop systems of care and specific interventions to meet the needs of growing populations who have been historically marginalized in their settings. The tasks will not be simple. Yet, for those of us committed to the worth and value of all groups of people, we know that this work must be done. Aché.

REFERENCES

Bem, Sandra L. (1974). The measurement of psychological androgyny. *Journal of Consulting and Clinical Psychology, 42*(2), 155-162.

Bliebtreu, H. K. and Meaney, J. (1973). Race and racism. In T. Weaver (Ed.), *To see ourselves: Anthropology and modern social issues.* Glenview, IL: Scott, Foresman & Co.

Brown, D. R. (1990). Depression among blacks: An epidemiologic perspective. In D. S. Ruiz (Ed.), *Handbook of mental health and mental disorder among black Americans* (pp. 71-93). New York: Greenwood Press.

Bureau of the Census (1990). *Statistical abstract of the United States.* Washington, DC: U.S. Department of Commerce.

Centers for Disease Control (1995). *HIV/AIDS surveillance—1994.* Atlanta, GA: Centers for Disease Control, Division of HIV/AIDS.

Centers for Disease Control (1996). *HIV/AIDS surveillance—1995.* Atlanta, GA: Centers for Disease Control, Division of HIV/AIDS.

Centers for Disease Control (1997). *HIV/AIDS surveillance—1996.* Atlanta, GA: Centers for Disease Control, Division of HIV/AIDS.

Centers for Disease Control (1998). *HIV/AIDS surveillance—Mid-year report for 1997.* Atlanta, GA: Centers for Disease Control, Division of HIV/AIDS.

Cheung, Y. W. (1991). Overview: Sharpening the focus on ethnicity. *International Journal of Addictions, 25*(May), 573-579.

Connell, R. W. (1995). *Masculinities.* Berkeley, CA: University of California Press.

Davis, M. (1990). *City of quartz.* London: Verso.

Encyclopedia of Social Work, Volumes I and II. (1987). Silver Spring, MD: National Association of Social Workers.

Fainstein, N. (1993). Race, class and segregation: Discourses about African Americans. *International Journal of Urban and Regional Resources,* Vol. III, 1993.

Fichtenbaum, R. and Gyimah-Brempong, K. (1997). The effects of race on the use of physicians' services. *International Journal of Health Services,* 1997, *27*(1).

Fuss, D. (1995). *Identification papers.* New York: Routledge Press.

Hacker, S. S. (1990). The transition from the old norm to the new: Sexual values for the 1990s. *Sex Information and Education Council of the U.S. Report, 18*(5), 1-8.

Hall, S. (1996). New ethnicities. In D. Morley and K-K Chen (Eds.), *Stuart Hall critical dialogues in cultural studies.* London: Routledge.

Hirsch, A. R. (1983). *Making the second ghetto: Race and housing in Chicago 1940-1960.* New York: Cambridge University Press.

Julia, M. C. (1996). *Multicultural awareness in the health care professions.* Needham Heights, MA: Allyn and Bacon.

Karon, B. P., (1958). *The Negro personality: A rigorous investigation of the effects of culture.* New York: Springer Publishing Company.

Levant, R. F. and Majors, R. G. (1997). Masculinity ideology among African-American and European American college women and men. *Journal of Gender, Culture, and Health, 2*(1), 1997.

Martin, E. P. and Martin, J. M. (1995). *Social work and the black experience.* Washington, DC: NASW Press.

Massey, D. and Denton, N. (1993). The missing link. In *American Apartheid,* Cambridge, MA: Harvard University Press.

Omi, M. and Winant, H. (1986). *Racial formation in the United States: From the 1960s to the 1980s.* New York: Routledge.

Poussaint, A. F. (1990). An honest look at black gays and lesbians. *Ebony, 104*(September), 126,130.

Sanjek, R. (1994). The enduring inequalities of race. In Steven Gregory and Roger Sanjek (Eds.), *Race.* New Brunswick, NJ: Rutgers University Press.

Spence, J. T. and Helmreich, R. L. (1978). *Masculinity and femininity: Their psychological dimensions, correlates, and antecedents.* Austin, TX: University of Texas Press.

Sullivan, M. L. (1989). *"Getting paid": Youth crime and work in the inner city.* Ithaca, NY: Cornell University Press.

Thomas, V. G. (1991). The impact of gender identity on health among African American males. From a presentation at the Conference on the Health and Social Behavior of African American Males. Howard University, Washington, DC, October 16-18.

United States Commission on Civil Rights. The Problem: Discrimination (1995). In Paula S. Rothenberg (Ed.), *Race, class, and gender in the United States.* New York: St. Martin's Press.

Vega, A. and Rumbaut, R.G. (1991). Ethnic minorities and mental health. *Annual Review of Sociology, 17,* 351-383.

Weeks, J. (1991). Sexual identification is a strange thing. In *Against Nature,* Concord, MA: Paulo Co.

West, C. (1993). The new cultural politics of difference. In Charles Lemert (Ed.), *Social theory: The multicultural and classic readings*. Boulder, CO: Westview Press.

White, J. L. (1984). *The psychology of blacks*. Englewood Cliffs, NJ: Prentice-Hall.

Wofford, W. Jr. (1991). Finding the right woman for you: Is it sex, love, or obsession? *Ebony Man*, 7(2) (December), 12-13.

Xu, G., Fields, S. K., Laine, C., Veloski, J., Barzansky, B., and Martini, C. (1997). The relationship between the race/ethnicity of generalist physicians and their care for underserved populations. *American Journal of Public Health*, 87(5) (May), 817-822.

Chapter 12

In the Eye of the Hurricane: Clinical Issues for HIV-Positive Slow and Nonprogressors from a Self-Psychology Perspective

James Cassese

The divisions and categories that have been developed to manage our understanding of the confusing, multifaceted epidemic of the acquired immune deficiency syndrome (AIDS) have often been problematic and always insufficient. In the early 1980s, the acronym AIDS replaced gay-related immune disease (GRID). Soon after, AIDS was cleaved into two categories with the introduction of AIDS-related complex (ARC) (Centers for Disease Control, 1987). The imprecision of ARC was gradually supplanted by the more descriptive label, asymptomatic HIV positive. At this point, categorical distinctions were established between absence or presence of illness. Opportunistic infections (OIs) became the defining parameter. This narrow focus, by definition, could not accommodate the emotional and interpersonal complexities that bridge the terms. Emblematic of this binary view, medically diagnosed opportunistic infections ultimately became the sole criterion for the access of benefits and government resources for HIV-positive people until 1993, when a CD-4 count below 200/microL qualified as AIDS (Centers for Disease Control, 1992). For the time, a decisive action had been taken to classify the effects of HIV/AIDS—a symbolic divide and conquer.

As HIV-infected people continued to survive through various degrees and permutations of illness and health, new terms were developed. Long-term survivor, for example, has been used to describe someone who has lived three years since being diagnosed with an AIDS-related OI (Cao et al., 1995). In the constant search to understand and disable the virus, even more categories have been created to facilitate study. Asymptomatic HIV-positive people have been further divided into subcategories. HIV-positive long-term nonprogressors (LTNP) are defined as having been HIV positive for more than ten years with no evidence of AIDS and a CD-4 lymphocyte count of 500/microL or higher (O'Brien et al., 1996).

This search for categories, ostensibly to divide the overwhelming pandemic of HIV into manageable blocks and to predict a progression sequence for illness, has produced some ironic results. Due to its mutability, the virus makes categorization difficult and time limited. Further, HIV-positive people, who are already stigmatized and historically often ignored, now face a series of categories delineated by exclusion criteria that move in one direction. Lab results define medical categories, not people. Although the category of nonprogressor is defined from a medical/biological framework, it also provides a distinctive grouping that enables examination of relevant psychosocial issues.

The emotional complexities of these categories often surface in psychotherapy/support groups for HIV-infected persons. The question of whether to group asymptomatic people with currently or formerly symptomatic people has always been difficult. For example, in those groups with an asymptomatic focus, what happens to the individual who becomes symptomatic? In this chapter, I will use case discussions from one of the groups, as well as from some of the individual patients, in my private practice. The issues and dynamics from the HIV-positive gay male artist psychotherapy group demonstrate a number of points regarding the interface among different people in various HIV-positive categories. Membership in this group does not include length of time since diagnosis with HIV infection. Indeed, the range of time since diagnosis is quite broad, spanning from nine months to over twelve years.

The existing group was ambivalent about new members who were about to join this group, at times expressing eagerness but also anticipating possible interruptions in the therapy process. Anger and hostility was expressed indirectly through the humor of the existing group. Nearing the addition of the new members, it rose to the surface. Existing members joked about "hazing" the new members and having exclusionary requirements. In particular, one group member, Ben, adamantly demanded that the new members fit within the fairly homogenous age range of the existing group. Ben was not yet aware that one of the new members, age twenty-six, would be thirteen years his junior and five years younger than the current youngest member.

Action techniques were employed as a way to level the playing field and give the new members a fair chance. The first session with the new members began with simple "warm-up exercises," each member introducing himself with his name and a gesture. The rest of the group repeated the person's name and gesture. They were then asked to arrange themselves in a circle according to their ages. This required the members to reveal their respective ages to one another. Their emerging anxiety became evident during this exercise. Indeed, Ben and Eddie, the two eldest members, jockeyed for positions, as they were born only a few days apart within the same year. Ben beamed as he took his position as the eldest member. Members were asked to observe where they stood in relation to others, with the offer that they could move to a different place within the age range if they wanted. None of them wanted to do that. Each expressed that they "liked" where they were.

This exercise was repeated, using as the criterion the length of time they had known, from a diagnostic test, that they were HIV positive. Ben expressed resistance to this, becoming visibly agitated. He insisted that he had known he was HIV positive for a long time before he tested. Interestingly, one of the new members, thirteen years younger than Ben, had tested HIV positive when he was nineteen, placing him in the apparently coveted position among those who had known for a long time. To his chagrin, Ben found himself among the more recently diagnosed men.

When the members were asked how they felt about their positions, they expressed some revealing information. Those standing in the more recently diagnosed end of the spectrum reported that they wanted to move toward the other end. One explained that he wanted to be on the other side of the circle "because I think I would have gotten through all this pain of adjusting to it, and it would be just a part of me by then." Another offered that he thought his "fear would be less because I would have been positive for years and know what to expect by now." Those at the other end of the circle expressed contentment with the length of time they had known they were positive for similar reasons.

This group example illustrates a common perspective through which nonprogressors are viewed. They are often seen by others as veteran soldiers, possessing some magical power and fearlessness. Because of the length of time they have been diagnosed, other HIV-positive people may imagine the nonprogressor to have less anxiety about, or to be comfortable with, his or her serostatus. Although this may sometimes be the case, it also separates the long-term nonprogressor from his or her potentially broader HIV-positive peer group. Other non-HIV-positive people may attribute similar powerful characteristics to him or her as well. This view locates the long-term nonprogressor in the metaphorical eye of the hurricane and is reinforced by medical categories.

The psychosocial implications of each of these individual categories range in presentation. However, the bridge between them is often characterized by intense anxiety. The peaks of this anxious terror seem to reduce as the person moves toward the terminal category of AIDS but are often restimulated at each juncture, thus maintaining the long-term nonprogressor at the edge of this anxious bridge.

Ironically, the lines of demarcation between the categories are often subtle markers that do not visibly manifest in the person's everyday life (e.g., the CD-4 count of a nonprogressor versus long-term survivor). In other words, everything may "look okay" on the outside, but what about how he or she feels emotionally? As a result, these categories subtly enhance some of the struggles the nonprogressor faces, (e.g., isolation or anxiety). At the same time, certain issues are not bound by the categories. People who are HIV positive, regardless of the diagnostic category into which they fit, will be vulnerable to (among other issues) discrimination, potential rejection from current or future romantic partners, and thoughts or fears about mortality.

Located in the eye of the hurricane, however, nonprogressors will also face issues peculiar to their experience. This chapter will examine the emotional or psychosocial characteristics relevant to the long-term nonprogressor through a self-psychology lens. The issues raised may also be interpreted through different psychological orientations.

Self-psychology offers an analytic framework that understands motivation as the self's efforts to survive, with survival measured in terms of self-cohesion. Symptomatology, in this view, reflects the self's best efforts to restore homeostasis or ward off threats to self-cohesion. Threats to the cohesive self are understood to include narcissistic injuries, stress, and trauma. The presence of HIV can produce any or all of these threats.

In self-psychology, the individual is understood to manage anxiety and maintain self-esteem through the internalization of self-objects. The term self-object is used to "denote one's experience of another as part of the self " (Rowe and MacIsaac, 1991, p. 30). It can range from a symbolic representation to a concrete relationship. Essentially, a self-object can be anything or anyone the individual uses to bolster his or her sense of self as a cohesive unit and is often idiosyncratic to the person.

This approach considers three main spheres of need, conceptualized as self-object needs. The first need is for mirroring self-objects to affirm the individual's ability to create something of value and validate his or her feelings of pride, accomplishment, or grandiosity (Rowe and MacIsaac, 1991). The extent to which the individual's childhood mirroring self-object needs have been met will be reflected in his or her ability to maintain self-esteem. Grandiosity is an essential element in self-esteem and, if not appropriately affirmed, can produce an extreme of either low self-worth or oblivious narcissism.

Ben, for example, was raised in a low-income rural area in the South. His parents dismissed his artistic skill as frivolous. When a grade school teacher phoned Ben's parents to suggest they take his talent seriously and enroll him in an art program, Ben's mother responded, "How nice of you to say that about my son." In this way, she not only did not validate Ben's skill, but she shifted the focus onto herself ("my son"). However, from Ben's perspective, as he was not skilled at sports or academic pursuits, the one thing he *was* good at was seen as inconsequential. His mother's response to the teacher, although cordial, did not recognize his skill; it only acknowledged the teacher being nice enough "to say that about [her] son." This has caused Ben to have poor self-esteem, which he attempts to bolster through his love relationships and his art. However, his excessive need for reassurances creates conflict in both of these areas. This was, for example, played out in his need to be the eldest member and one of the people who had known their HIV status the longest.

In the second sphere, idealizing self-object needs reveals the child's wish to merge with a "strong, omnipotent idealized adult," which "serves to protect the [self] from too much frustration and stimulation and promotes the internalization of anxiety relieving mental structures" (Rowe and MacIsaac, 1991, p. 40). To the extent that the parental figure is able to tolerate the child's natural mood fluctuations, the child is presented with the opportunity to "merge with the strength and soothing calmness of the parents" (Cornett, 1991). This will influence the individual's ability to tolerate anxiety and express his or her feelings. For example, Eddie's parents were cool and aloof through much of his childhood. He was expected to be quiet in the home, polite outside of the home, and not express his feelings. He was admonished at age seven for wanting to kiss his father good night because "men don't kiss men." He was called names—"crybaby"—when he shed a tear and they treated him warmly when he was stoic. As an adult, Eddie has difficulty naming and expressing the emotions he feels. Most often, he expresses anxiety or fear at the emergence of a feeling. Without feelings as guidelines and his internalized harsh critic self-object (from his parents), however, he has difficulty making decisions. He is unsure of what he wants because he rarely knows what he feels. He fears making a choice because the internalized harsh critic will judge any decision as the wrong one.

The third sphere, twinship self-object needs, considers the individual's need to feel a sense of belonging to a group or community. Appropriately met, it helps the child understand and develop a sense of connectedness in social relationships or, if not met, a pervasive feeling of being "different" or socially inept. This is a need that appears to increase with age, as the individual's need for companionship becomes greater (Rowe and MacIsaac, 1991).

For example, Robert grew up being teased and taunted by his peers at school. They derided his academic abilities. His parents divorced when Robert was young, and he was left to take care of his younger sisters. Combined with this was a burgeoning awareness of his homosexuality, and Robert was left feeling different, an outsider in any environment. What he learned to crave, to yearn for, was to be part of a group. He found that by building his body at the gym and through steroids, the attention placed on him was no longer negative, but indeed positive. He found that he belonged to the degree that he was able to physically maintain his appearance. However, the intrapsychic Robert was locked behind the muscular shell of his external appearance, continuing his longing to connect with others and believing himself incapable of belonging.

In terms of mirroring self-object needs, the long-term nonprogressor is in a complicated position. The long-term nonprogressor has survived a significant length of time in the current AIDS context. His or her very survival may imply actions he or she has taken to maintain good health, a particular genetic makeup, or simply luck. As such, the individual becomes a subject of study, an anomaly who may offer answers to the puzzle of HIV. Others may express admiration for the long-term nonprogressor's strength, knowledge, or skill. His or her ability to survive may become a source of encouragement or even envy for others, transforming this characteristic into a potential positive self-object for the individual as well as those around him or her. Indeed, in the group example provided, Ben wanted his place to be among the other nonprogressors, but by virtue of the date of his test, he was excluded.

However, it would be difficult for the long-term nonprogressor to be able to internalize these affirmations if his or her self-cohesion is loose (whether the result of insufficient mirroring in childhood or the strain of life's circumstances). The individual may dismiss these factors as existing outside his or her control. Further, the long-term nonprogressor may experience guilt over friends and family lost to HIV. This guilt compromises the individual's feelings of pride or accomplishment in his or her situation, further frustrating his or her mirroring self-object needs.

Conversely, the needs or concerns of the long-term nonprogressor may not be taken (by himself or herself or others) as seriously as for those who have been, or currently are, in the throes of illness. This is illustrated by the group case example presented earlier. The members seemed to attribute a power and calm to the people who had tested positive long ago. "I would be used to it by now," one member had imagined. This perception provides fertile material to boost the long-term nonprogressor's self-esteem. The long-term nonprogressor is placed within a context of having others admire attributes that he or she appears to possess, but at the same time, the individual may believe that he or she must keep silent about other characteristics (e.g., fear and anxiety) to preserve that image. This was true of the group members in the example provided, who even after ten years were *not* "used to it." Conversely, the long-term nonprogressor may excessively turn to others for reassurance and comfort for his or her anxiety, thereby causing conflict in interpersonal relationships. The individual may recognize this and defend against this need for affirmation, or he or she may move toward increasingly grandiose expressions of, for example, anger.

When the long-term nonprogressor disguises fears behind a facade of anxiety-free adjustment, a false self may be created or an existing one reaffirmed. This prevents the long-term nonprogressor from being able to fully internalize the positive, self-esteem enhancing self-objects that his or her "category" might offer. The anxiety of being in the precarious position of having one's identity category (i.e., long-term nonprogressor) depend on the health variable may restimulate the discrepancy between the person's external presentation and internal self-esteem. Can the long-term nonprogressor trust in his or her ability to remain in that respective category forever?

The infinite uncertainty in that question, our lack of medical knowledge, and the person's internal struggles may exacerbate an existing imposter syndrome. In the imposter syndrome, the individual fears a revelation of the true nature of the inherent incompetence or "badness" he or she believes to be true of himself or herself. This provokes considerable anxiety as well as, at times, frantic efforts to preserve the false self by denying or splitting off real or suggested vulnerabilities. When these split-off elements are revealed by contradictions between the false and true selves, they may be experienced as psychologically shocking and threaten self-cohesion. Idiosyncratic symptomatology would emerge at this point, as the individual makes efforts to restore homeostasis. The appearance of these split-off or denied feelings may then provoke a judgmental reaction or a dissociative response in the individual. He or she may express impatience with, or demand unrealistic or perfectionistic standards for, himself or herself. As counselors, we can provide support in helping the individual to find adaptive ways of coping with these feelings and restoring cohesion.

This would be particularly important for the individual whose denial or splitting off of anxious feelings is echoed by his or her environment, reinforcing a fragile self-cohesion. The long-term nonprogressor's fear or anxiety may seem less worthy of discussion or even inconsequential in the context of life-threatening manifest illness. Indeed, health care professionals may unintentionally trivialize a long-term nonprogressor's anxious concerns in an effort to be optimistic (especially in the era of protease inhibitors) or as an expression of compassion fatigue. Some AIDS service organizations, such as Gay Men's Health Crisis, limited their group service provision in the 1980s to those who have AIDS. This reduces the number of resources available to the asymptomatic person and further implies that their concerns are less urgent compared to those in the throes of physical illness. Further, particularly in group work with HIV-positive persons, there often exists an implicit hierarchy of health status among the members that parallels the CDC categories of progression.

For example, one of the members of the group, Scott, would become incensed when peers minimized his fears in relation to his consistently high CD-4 and minor viral load counts. This repeatedly threatened his self-esteem as well as his sense of belonging. At the same time, Scott questioned his "right" to complain when others were so markedly ill. These comparisons often provide the individual with the psychic space needed to deny or compartmentalize the severity of the situation, while appearing to discuss it, albeit in intellectual terms.

Recently, Scott's CD-4 count dropped, removing him permanently from the category of nonprogressor. In one session, he reported his outrage regarding a friend who was talking about a fear of death. "I can't believe I'm saying this after having it said to me so many times," Scott reported, "but I was furious at him for even talking about it. With a thousand CD-4 cells and no viral load for all these years—what does *he* know?"

The situation with this patient also demonstrates the assaults on mirroring self-object needs by a shift out of the category of nonprogressor. "Before, it was scary, but there was a comfort in being able to say that I had no symptoms. I could say I was *just* HIV positive. Now I wonder if I'm on the path to illness." For this patient, self-admonition and regret increased his anxiety as he lost his nonprogressor status. Scott's prior compulsive sexual behavior abruptly resurfaced, this time accompanied by a strident rationalized defense fueled by a sexual partner who supported this behavior. Scott appeared to use his sexual behavior to numb his emerging anxiety regarding his health and had found a supportive friend to share in his activities. In this way, he was able to find a way to get his mirroring as well as his twinship needs met in one coping strategy.

Counselors need to be aware of the potential to gratify mirroring self-object needs through our genuine empathy for and curiosity in the patient. Our interest in him or her, our empathically accurate interpretations, and our compassionate interventions serve to affirm the patient's sense of being understood and valued. This may pose particular difficulties for counselors, with regard, for example, to the behavior management disorders (e.g., drug/alcohol misuse, unmanageable sexual behavior). We must be aware that our role provides us with the opportunity to enhance self-esteem as well as the potential to narcissistically injure a patient through our interventions. This is particularly urgent for the long-term nonprogressor, as we may be among the few people to whom he or she exposes his or her vulnerabilities and anxieties.

The ability to tolerate anxiety is influenced by parental response to the child's idealizing self-object needs. To the extent the parent/parent figure can empathize with the child's natural mood fluctuations and soothe him or her, the child is given the chance to merge with someone more powerful than himself or herself. The long-term nonprogressor may serve as this powerful figure in others' lives. The "self-object is the function that is usually provided by a person rather than it being the person" (Rowe and MacIsaac, 1991, p. 31). Serving this function for others may meet some of the long-term nonprogressors mirroring self-object needs, enhancing his or her self-esteem. If the individual's own idealizing self-object needs have been appropriately affirmed in childhood and adolescence, his or her own "category" or length of survival may help maintain self-cohesion.

Conversely, the long-term nonprogressor whose idealizing self-object needs had not been met appropriately in childhood may be at a disadvantage in terms of finding idealizing self-objects. For example, Scott's father was largely absent, and his mother pointedly discouraged Scott's expression of feelings. As a result, he had a profound need for idealizing self-objects. He is constantly searching for some omnipotent figure with whom he may merge and by whom he may be soothed. This plays out in Scott's sexual behavior and his need to idealize nearly any sexual partner as "brilliant" or more powerful or smarter than himself. When he discovers this is not the case, he suffers not only from disappointment but from self-reproach and shame for his idealization. He often prolongs his attachment to these men to avoid this ultimate disappointment and punitive regret.

Further, because of the very narrow, limited subset of people who fit the category, the long-term nonprogressor's ability to idealize and merge with a more powerful figure may be restricted. This may further increase anxiety. For example, Eddie has known he is HIV positive for over twelve years, and his CD-4 count has remained consistently high. Recently, however, the cell count has begun to hover around 500, and his health practitioner has been urging him to make a decision regarding antiretrovirals and protease inhibitors. Eddie's anxiety spikes and turns to panic when he tries to consider his options. He wonders about friends of his who have taken medicine, observing that he has outlived them all. He is not sure that he has made better choices than they did. He is uncertain as to why his health (aside from the CD-4 count) is in no way troubling him physically but does not trust that this will always be the case. He has difficulty trusting his feeling that he will survive. He has no one whom he knows that is in a similar position who might offer guidance and soothing, echoing the lack of positive idealizing self-objects in his childhood.

If the long-term nonprogressor idealizes the imagined strength or invulnerability of the HIV-negative person, the permanent distinctions between them (i.e., HIV serostatus) will locate the long-term nonprogressor at a less powerful position and interrupt the process of internalization necessary to shore up idealizing self-object deficits. If he idealizes another long-term nonprogressor, he risks narcissistic injury should the idealized self-object become ill. If the long-term nonprogressor idealizes the strength of the PWA who has dealt or coped with illness, the implications for strength and omnipotence are similarly complicated.

If the individual's historical idealizing self-object needs have not been met appropriately, he or she will often evidence difficulty with the management and expression of feelings, particularly with respect to tolerance of anxiety. Located in the eye of the hurricane, with illness raging around him or her, the circumstantial provocation of anxiety will have a synergistic effect on his or her already compromised ability to tolerate it. Furthermore, discomfort with one's feelings will often evoke an anxious response when feelings eventually emerge. In the case of the trauma survivor, an emergence of feeling may also provoke a dissociative reaction. Anxiety or dissociation can initiate a feedback cycle, whereby, for example, emerging feelings produce anxiety which elicits dissociation which provokes further anxiety which increases the dissociation. The individual may then suffer from panic attacks and/or be virtually numb to emotional sensation, making it even more difficult to identify, experience, or express feelings. The long-term nonprogressor may report feeling "dead inside," respond with paralysis in the face of decision making (as in the case of Eddie), or be unable to grieve losses.

As discussed, the long-term nonprogressor's anxiety and fear may not be appropriately validated by the individual or persons in his or her environment. As counselors, we must be particularly vigilant to the emergence of feeling states to help the patient identify and express them in a supportive atmosphere. In particular, for the long-term nonprogressor, I have observed common feeling states to often include anxiety and fear, anger and depression, and guilt and loneliness, often obscured by flat or labile affect. We need to create a safe space and maintain the empathic, or "experience near," perspective to recognize the presentation of these issues.

When the patient reports undergoing even routine medical or lab exams, for instance, we need to assess the degree to which the person may be experiencing unexpressed anxiety. When working with an individual who indicates a behavior management disorder (e.g., drug/alcohol misuse, unmanageable sexual behavior, self-mutilation), which reduces his or her anxiety, it is useful to, when appropriate, assist the patient in finding alternate routes for anxiety management. Anxiety may present as an impatient mood or disproportionate worry over relatively minor issues. Stress-related somatic complaints may evoke fear, which becomes attached to the presence of HIV. For example, nervous stress may produce diarrhea, which frightens the long-term nonprogressor. The anxiety may then result in a skin rash. These symptoms may suggest to the person that HIV is at work. We need to be able to tolerate the anxiety ourselves and help the patient find soothing, thereby meeting some idealizing self-object needs.

The issues of category, distinction, and division will have a profound effect on the twinship self-object needs of the long-term nonprogressor. For many HIV-positive people, their mode of transmission (homosexuality, drugs) may have historically had implications for their sense of connectedness. For some gay men, the first time they felt that they belonged might have been with other gays or lesbians as adults. Discovering their HIV status may have been a blow to this nascent sense of connectedness. As the gay man adjusts to his HIV status, he may find a relevant peer group among other HIV-positive people. Being placed in the narrow subset of long-term nonprogressor may once again damage his twinship self-object needs by moving him to another identity category.

The long-term nonprogressor is—by fitting that category's criteria—labeled different. An identity distinction is made between him and others. First, the gay man feels different growing up. In adolescence or adulthood, he finds a subset of the population into which he fits. With the advent of an HIV-positive diagnosis, he is then placed in a smaller subset within that subset. With the label of HIV-positive nonprogressor he is again relocated, this time within an even smaller subset within a subset.

Beyond the historical intrapsychic issues, we need to be aware that (in terms of numbers) the narrower subset exists for health (e.g., nonprogressor) and the broader subset exists for illness (e.g., PWA). For some, this may provoke an unconscious movement toward the larger group. In the case of Robert, after testing HIV positive, he reluctantly observed that his new status was an admission ticket to join his friends, most of whom were positive. Although he had a sense of belonging, he also had an over-whelming regret *that* he belonged.

However, this classification into a small subset may offer relief for the long-term nonprogressor who has felt different from his or her HIV-posi-tive peers. He or she may have felt unlike them due to health concerns or attitude. Being "like" other HIV-positive people may have evoked fears regarding his or her own health. Indeed, the term itself, non*progressor*, offers hope. To have a name, and consequently a validation for his or her difference, may be enormously soothing to the long-term nonprogressor. This individual may feel that he or she has finally found a peer group to which he or she can belong.

The problem with this, of course, is the variable of time. Can we say that the long-term nonprogressor will always be a nonprogressor? How many years will the person have to survive with no symptoms before he or she can breathe a sigh of relief and forget about becoming a PWA? HIV/AIDS, although nearly two decades old, is still young and cunning enough to render time-based categories obsolete. In a few years, will the criteria for a nonprogressor need to be further refined to be limited to those who show no signs of disease progression for fifteen years instead of ten? Will the category be as imprecise as ARC is now?

This has been one of the most frustrating elements about HIV/AIDS: there are no absolutes. Our attempts to label or name it have been con-founded by its ability to present in myriad ways and mutate in others. In response, we need to recognize that the categories which exist represent our attempts to define and conquer the syndrome. People's health issues may fit the diagnostic *medical* criteria, but we must never lose sight that these are simplistic, broad criteria. As such, they cannot do justice to the unique individual.

Although I have offered some clinical observations which may apply to the categories, we must always keep in mind that people are fluid; catego-ries are not. In our ongoing struggle to make sense of HIV/AIDS, to medically master it, our focus must include the psychosocial issues that accompany it and, at times, exacerbate its effects. We must avoid a per-spective that considers the individual within a progression sequence which moves people down a line toward illness. Instead, we must recognize people as capable of moving in any direction, in whatever order they can and will. The categories that have been named by the medical community are not based on psychosocial issues. It would be likely that psychosocially some nonprogressors share more in common with some long-term survivors, and some long-term survivors may have more in common with some PWAs. As opposed to organizing our thinking about where they are in the AIDS spectrum, we must be sure our thinking follows and empathizes with the individual first. The category is simply a descriptive term that is relevant to the nonprogressor and by which he or she may be loosely grouped, with certain issues anticipated but not predicted.

REFERENCES

Cao, Y., Qin, L., Zhang, L., Safrit, J., and Ho, D. (1995). "Virologic and immunologic characterization of long term survivors of human immunodeficiency virus type 1 infection." *New England Journal of Medicine, 332*(4): pp. 75-79.

Centers for Disease Control (1987). "Revision of the CDC surveillance case definition for acquired immunodeficiency syndrome." *Morbidity and Mortality Weekly Report, 36* (Supplement 1S):1S-15S.

Centers for Disease Control (1992). "1993 revised classification system for HIV infection and expanded surveillance case definition for acquired immunodeficiency syndrome." *Morbidity and Mortality Weekly Report, 41*(RR-17):5.

Cornett, C. (1991). "Self-object intervention in brief treatment with patients inappropriate for traditional brief psychotherapy models." *Clinical Social Work Journal, 19*(2), Summer: 131-147.

O'Brien, T. R, Blattner, W., and Waters, D. (1996). "Serum HIV-1 RNA levels and time to development of AIDS in multicenter hemophilia cohort study." *Journal of the American Medical Association, 276*:105-110.

Rowe, C. and MacIsaac, D. (1991). *Empathic attunement.* New York: Aronson.

Chapter 13

HIV Care for Male-to-Female Pre-Operative Transsexuals

James Grimaldi

INTRODUCTION

The AIDS epidemic has forced American health care to change and customize its delivery to special populations. Beginning in the 1980s, HIV-positive gay people advocated for their rights in hospitals, health care, and research. AIDS-prevention professionals continue to fight on behalf of injection drug users for needle exchange. Now, in the second decade of this epidemic, another population, male-to-female transsexuals, emerges with its own set of needs. Although they have been affected since the beginning of the epidemic, whether infected through unprotected sex or shared needles, their medical and psychosocial needs were very often ignored. This chapter will attempt to illustrate biopsychosocial issues of mental health practice intrinsic to HIV-positive, pre-operative, male-to-female transsexuals, based on my experience in two medical settings in Manhattan.

I met my first transgendered patient in a large New York City hospital in 1993. She was all alone. She faced discrimination and ridicule on a daily basis from both staff and other patients. The changes in her body terrified her. She was unable to obtain female hormone treatment from her HIV physician and was subsequently in the process of reverting back to her former male physical state. She felt ashamed by the chest hair that began sprouting over her breast implants. Often she was unable to look at me and explained that she had trained herself long ago to avoid direct eye contact with anyone who could hurt her. She cried often over the loss of her feminine beauty and would show me pictures of herself before AIDS.

She was unable to return for follow-up care as an outpatient upon hospital discharge because she felt ashamed of further AIDS-related physical changes. We maintained telephone contact for several months. She wanted me to remember her as she looked in the hospital. She would describe herself as painfully alone. She trusted neither hospitals nor doctors because they could not give her the hormones that she needed to remain feminine as her AIDS illness progressed. Her biological family had abandoned her long ago. She cut off communication with her transgendered friends because she feared that they might gloat over the loss of her beauty. She gradually isolated herself more and more; she died alone in her apartment.

She inspired me to use everything in my reach as a professional social worker to stop this from happening to any other HIV-positive transgendered individuals. Therefore, in September 1994, I left Mount Sinai Hospital and found a job at a more progressive hospital, the center for Special Studies at New York Hospital Cornell Medical Center. Here I was able to begin the process of approaching HIV-positive male-to-female pre-operative trans-sexuals who were socially and emotionally isolated, some of whom were sex workers, in an effort to provide them the same psychosocial supports offered to all other HIV-infected individuals in an outpatient HIV center. These patients had all presented with poor records of medical compliance and stated feelings of isolation and discrimination.

I decided that the best way to gain their trust was to develop a transgender subcommunity within the larger HIV hospital community, that is, a group to address their unique needs. The group provided a safe environment for clients to give one another mutual support (about transgender issues and hormone therapy), develop communication skills (to protect against future isolation), and address concerns of prejudice from transgenderphobic health care providers and patients. (Transgenderphobia is an irrational fear of a transgendered person.) Group members educated one another on safer sex, the challenges of condom use to female self-perception, the risk of violence from sex customers and police, and discrimination from entitlement workers and potential employers. This HIV transgender support group has met more than 120 times over the course of three and a half years and continues to involve a pool of sixteen members for a semiweekly group.

DEFINING TRANSSEXUAL

Health care professionals must understand who a person is before they can meet his or her needs. A transsexual is an individual who suffers gender dysphoria (discomfort and sadness about one's gender) to such an extent that the individual desires and seeks a physical (i.e., secondary sexual characteristics) change to resemble that of the opposite sex. This chapter refers to my work with *only* male-to-female transsexuals. A male-to-female (MTF) transsexual is an individual who feels female but was born with testicles and a penis and desires/seeks to change her appearance to match what she feels on the inside (by growing breasts, removing the penis, etc.). Pre-operative (pre-op) and post-operative (post-op) refer to the stage in an individual's gender transition, that is, whether they have undergone sexual reassignment surgery or not. A pre-op transsexual has not had the surgery, while a post-op transsexual has had the surgery.

Mainstream society often misuses the word "transsexual" to label different types of individuals who break traditional norms of gender and sexuality. Therefore, society often confuses a "pre-operative male-to-female transsexual" with a "transvestite," a "cross-dresser," a "drag queen/king," a "hermaphrodite," and sometimes even a "homosexual." Most MTF transsexuals resent being compared to drag queens. Drag queens are men who wear flamboyantly feminine costumes, makeup, and hairstyles, while signaling an unmistakably male body beneath. MTF transsexuals do not feel the need to overstate their female attire because they invest greater effort into simulating a female body beneath the clothes.

Table 13.1 summarizes the differences between these terms. This table accounts only for those individuals born with male reproductive organs.

Many people over the course of history have desired bodies of the opposite gender, but the means were unavailable to change their gender. Technological advancements in the twentieth century (such as hormone reassignment, sexual reassignment surgery, electrolysis, silicone injections, tracheal shaves, and breast implants) have supplied people with the

TABLE 13.1. Diversity Within the Male-to-Female Transgender Community

INDIVIDUAL	GENDER (feels like a)	SEXUALITY (wants sex with)	REASON (why she desires a female appearance)
transsexual	woman	man	to match her inner feelings
transvestite	man	woman	for an erotic high
drag queen	man	man	for sex only, to attract male sexual partners
female impersonator (gender illusionist)	man and/or woman	man or woman	for artistic purposes (theater, performance)
hermaphrodite male (intersex)	man and/or woman	man or woman	born with both female and male reproductive organs

medical means to alter their physical gender. "HIV" is also a recent phenomenon, emerging only in the last quarter century. Therefore, these two
recent scientific phenomena have existed within our lexicon for a limited
time. People still fear their novelty. An HIV-positive, pre-op, MTF transsexual struggles on a daily basis to articulate her needs, within both scientific and professional heath care communities that have few answers.
Courage, persistence, and creativity are her strengths. The unbiased psychotherapist can help the client access these strengths to help her manage
her responses to HIV illness.

COUNTERTRANSFERENCE

Graduate school and postgraduate training teaches professionals to be
aware of countertransference so that the worker's belief systems do not
interfere with the client's needs. However, discrimination against a transgendered individual is so prevalent in contemporary society that it would be
unrealistic, even presumptuous, to assume that mental health professionals
are immune to these prejudices. Thus, the vast majority of professional
health care workers are transgenderphobic. The first and most important
step in helping a transgendered client is for the worker to assume responsibility for his or her personal feelings toward gender. By identifying and
confronting this prejudice, transgenderphobia becomes clearly identified as
the worker's problem, not the client's. Everything people learn about gender
originates in infancy, based on a dichotomy of opposites—yes versus no;
hot versus cold; wet versus dry. Of these dichotomies, the most significant
is female versus male. Gender usually determines whether a child plays
with a Barbie doll or a football. If a boy plays with a Barbie doll, children
will often tease him, and eventually, embarrassed parents will attempt to
discourage the nonconforming gender play. Biological gender determines
which bathroom individuals should use. Girls use the door with the stick
figure in a dress. Boys use the one without a dress. Thus, children find their
place in either camp. Once in a camp specifically defined by gender, the
vast majority of children feel safer, and most individuals have thus formed
an important building block of their identity.

This categorization between male and female gives people a sense of
control over the chaos in the outside world and control over their emotions
inside. No matter what happens (losing a job, a home, a loved one), people
still have their gender as one constant in their life. It is a constant that
directs many of life's choices and anchors people through the waves and
upheavals that life sends to everyone. However, imagine the emotional
turmoil of the individual who wakes up with thick stubble on his face and

a high-pitched female voice, dark chest hair covering full D-cup breasts, and long luxurious hair surrounding a large shiny bald spot. Most people would find these scenarios intolerable because it robs them of what feels comfortable. When a baby is born, most people take for granted that it will be either a boy or a girl and remain that same gender for the rest of its life.

Gender-dysphoric individuals have the courage to break these rules, overtly blurring the boundaries between male and female categories. Homosexuals disrupt these boundaries, but it is not visual. They transgress gender rules behind closed doors during sex, where most people cannot see. However, a transgendered individual breaks gender rules on the street, in front of everyone, by wearing the opposite gender's clothes. Suddenly, the building blocks of most people's identity come crashing down when confronted with a transgendered person. It is common to feel momentarily lost when encountering a transgendered person and to resent that person for disrupting a sense of security.

Transgenderphobia is not limited to the heterosexual community. Many homosexuals who have experienced tremendous discrimination in their lives develop strong aversions to transgendered individuals because of internalized heterosexism and homophobia. They fear that heterosexual society will confuse them with a drag queen on a float during Gay Pride parades. Some gay men feel that they conform to the gender rules, at least in public, and are very threatened by transgendered people. Some of my gay professional colleagues have even stated, "I don't get a pre-op male-to-female transsexual. They cannot sit on the fence forever. They must choose which camp they want to belong to. They're either gay and male or straight and female. They can't have it both ways. "

Most people do not realize that they may be jealous of a transgendered individual's ability to explore his or her gender identity. Most people never indulge in exploring gender identity and gender-related boundaries. Perhaps this explains why so many people are curious whether a transsexual has had sexual reassignment surgery. "Does she still have a penis, or did she get rid of it?" is the first question most people ask me about a transgendered client. This curiosity is not wrong but perhaps simply represents a momentary desire to live vicariously through that transgendered person's courage and ability to manipulate his or her body and identity.

One final note, those of you (who are not transgendered) who will advocate for your transgendered clients' rights to have equal quality HIV health care may encounter prejudice from colleagues. Colleagues may marginalize you and fantasize that you cross-dress on weekends. You can use your feelings and reactions to your colleagues presumptions to empathize with your clients' isolation. Moreover, you will realize the importance of connecting with other professionals who have similar ideals and the importance of connecting your isolated transgendered clients with their peers, while providing them access to quality, individualized, and sensitive professional services.

BATTLING SOCIAL ISOLATION:
THE SUPPORT GROUP PROCESS

Group became a necessary tool to help HIV-positive, MTF, pre-op transsexuals in my hospital clinic. Prior to joining the HIV group, these patients presented individually as isolated and mistrustful. They did not seek out our services voluntarily. Most had been in denial of their HIV diagnosis and had avoided any reminders of their health condition, such as doctors and medicines. Others had been unaware that they were infected. However, a serious opportunistic infection and hospitalization forced them all to face their illness and interface with a hostile medical setting. They were all discharged from the hospital with follow-up appointments in our outpatient HIV clinic.

Many had missed their first medical appointment and had rescheduled several times because they feared that staff would ridicule them. Patients especially dreaded a physical examination, the moment at which a doctor would see both their female breasts and penis. Many had experienced negative and painful scenarios in doctors' offices prior to their HIV diagnosis. Those who made it to their appointments were noncompliant regarding their medications. Some would agree to take the prescriptions and then discard the pills at home. Others would disregard the medication regime, missing doses for long stretches of time, which placed them at risk of becoming resistant to protease inhibitors and other antiretrovirals.

During individual sessions, all the patients felt safe enough to reveal to me their doubts about medication and their leeriness about doctors. Individual counseling allowed them to express their feelings, but it did not alter their behaviors. Clients repeatedly told me that no one could understand their feelings, except other transsexuals. It became increasingly clear that only peers could help these clients change their behaviors. Thus, the idea for this group was born.

Many of these clients had survived terrible hardships and continued to thrive. I realized that by using a traditional social work approach of identifying clients' strengths, I could use these strengths that they had developed as transgendered people, as sex workers and teenage runaways, for them to help one another. I therefore created a group to address the issues that only other MTF pre-op transsexuals could tackle: building a transgendered community within a medical setting; advocating for transgender rights within hospital and entitlement systems; coping with discrimination; increasing trust for clinic staff; increasing compliance with medication and appointments; coping with physical violence from sex work customers and police; increasing condom use; decreasing needle sharing among injection hormone users; coping with changes in self-esteem as HIV erodes female physical beauty; safeguarding female physical appearance throughout illness; protecting gender selection in hospitals, nursing homes, home care, and funerals.

Most of what I will describe is based on empirical data, that is, observations of, and interactions with, my clients over the last four years. (My observations cannot apply to all HIV-positive transgendered people. Their purpose is to simply assist social workers in meeting their clients' needs.) The transsexual individuals whom I met all struggled to trust anyone because they had experienced discrimination in most of their personal and professional relationships. The lucky ones had role models to teach them how to develop trust, intimacy, and communication skills. Most of these clients did not have any role models or relationships with other people whom they trusted.

Contemporary American society teaches people to devalue gender nonconformity and thus to devalue transgendered people. Society has taught transgendered people the same lesson. Therefore, it is inevitable that many transsexuals have internalized transgenderphobia. They express transgenderphobia by devaluing one another, especially those who exhibit both masculine and feminine physical characteristics. This was my first obstacle in forming a support group. For instance, Sonia refused to join the group because she developed an aversion to another member's deep masculine voice. Sonia felt that she would be unable to sit in group without hurting that member's feelings. She stated, "I just wanna go up to her and tell her that it's a lost cause. You'll never pass for a woman. Get out of the club. You make us look bad." Gender transition is based on changing one's physical appearance to match the inner female feelings. It is therefore inevitable that members judged themselves and one another upon appearance. When they looked at one another, it was as if they were staring into a mirror. They turned away from those whose appearance displeased them; they respected and revered those who looked beautiful.

Initially, my main task as a group leader became protecting all members from hurting one another. To accomplish this, I redirected expressions of their anger away from one another and toward me. For instance, many groups began with a friendly tournament of flinging insults at one another, comments such as, "You forgot to wear mascara," or "Your falsies are showing." But these lighthearted barbs soon mushroomed into hurtful put-downs. Before it reached this point, I would ask members to redirect their anger and insults toward me "because I don't want you to hurt one another." Sometimes they would take my suggestion, and other times they would not. No matter whether they complied with my request or not, they soon realized that I would continue to be their social worker, even if they were trying to push me away with insults or, as they term it, "shade." Sometimes they would create distance between themselves and me by ignoring my presence in the room, cutting me off during conversations, and not allowing me to speak. To myself, I interpreted these behaviors as messages that clearly told me they were in control of the group, just as they were in control of their bodies. I let them know that these behaviors would not deter me from continuing our professional relationship.

In addition, I fostered a family atmosphere in the group to replace the families that had abandoned them long ago. I did this by serving meals at every session to simulate a family dinner, including special events for Thanksgiving and Christmas. I celebrated each member's birthday with a cake and candles. Members reacted strongly to the birthday cake. Mona broke into tears and said, "No one ever gave me birthday cake." Leslie confessed, "I always boast about my busy social life to you all. But the truth is that I have no friends." Gradually, members lowered their defenses and risked exposing their vulnerabilities and other feelings.

A more complex illustration of the group process occurred when, Diana, a glamorous sex worker, developed a friendship with another member, Gabriella, an impoverished and socially isolated individual. The two women hit it off so well that they began phoning each other between sessions, exchanging stories, laughing, and crying, until one day Diana stated, "I like you Gabriella." This may seem a benign statement to some, but to Gabriella (who had never had a friend in her life), the statement was devastating. Gabriella misinterpreted the statement as a declaration of erotic love and not of platonic friendship, and she confronted Diana: "Diana, I'm your equal, a female in search of a dominant heterosexual man. Instead you treat me like one of your boyfriends just because I can't afford your expensive clothes, makeup, and hormones."

Diana felt rejected by the group, hurt, targeted for her sexuality, unable to escape the world of her sex work, and she refused to return to group. I encouraged both members to express their anger toward me. Gabriella was able to tell me, "You let me down. You promised that they would treat me like the woman I am." Similarly, Diana confronted me, "You lied to me. You promised that I wouldn't get hurt."

Months later, Diana was hospitalized. I encouraged the group to visit her in the hospital. Diana was extremely happy to see us. Gabriella and Diana hugged, and Diana exclaimed, "That's the first hug of the day." We soon realized that Diana's family had abandoned her, at which point I encouraged the group to become Diana's surrogate family and emotionally support her through the hospitalization.

The group process began with transgendered individuals being scared to join because they did not know how to trust. They feared being hurt, and they feared hurting other transsexuals. Once they joined, dynamically, they set themselves up to be rejected, which reinforced their experience of the world abandoning them and themselves rejecting any efforts at closeness and intimacy. One task of the group leader was to become extremely active in motivating "other group members" to show the "rejected group member" that she was indeed "lovable." If the worker can gain a member's trust after she has experienced rejection in the group, then the worker succeeds in beginning to change her lifelong perception of herself.

I also organized several recreational outings. I approached theater and music organizations for ticket donations. These organizations often wanted to help HIV people and were transgender-friendly. The group was therefore able to move outside the hospital environment and into the world. The group attended classical music concerts and shows in traditionally conservative venues, such as Carnegie Hall, Lincoln Center, and Broadway. They initially felt self-conscious when other spectators stared and whispered but soon realized that they could count on one another and me for emotional support. They developed strength in numbers. This even helped heal some of their past painful experiences as individuals in public settings.

SAFEGUARDING GENDER IDENTITY THROUGH THE AIDS ILLNESS PROGRESSION

Since gender transition revolves around changing one's physical appearance to match the person's inner feelings, and HIV illness progression erodes physical appearance through wasting syndrome, Kaposi's sarcoma lesions, and a variety of other opportunistic infections, HIV disease progression works at cross-purposes with the gender transition process. A primary focus of the HIV mental health professional with transgendered clients is to help safeguard gender identity through the course of AIDS illness. As HIV robs clients of their physical ability to independently maintain their female physical appearance, the worker must help transgendered clients locate transgender-friendly nurses, home attendants, and family who are willing to maintain the clients' female appearance. This often proves to be difficult. Before I began the group, I would often go myself and help clients maintain their feminine beauty, by assisting them with shaving, makeup, and hair. Once the group was formed, I would travel with the group members to patients' hospital rooms and encourage members to help with these grooming tasks.

An illustration of this issue occurred when Diana (mentioned earlier) was hospitalized. She would often say, "Female beauty is like a badge of honor and prestige. When you don't have the education, skills, and status that money can buy, I find that being a female beauty can give them to me." Diana's physical beauty was arresting. Being transgendered, she had avoided depending on anyone for help. However, when AIDS robbed her of her physical independence, she was no longer able to bathe herself. The first home health attendant was a man, who flew into a rage when Diana answered the door. "Why didn't you tell the agency that you dressed in women's clothing. You some kind of freak transvestite!" he yelled.

The agency then sent a female home health attendant. As Diana disrobed to enter the shower, she was depending on the physical support of the attendant for safety. Instead, the attendant recoiled with disgust at the sight of Diana's female breasts and male penis. Diana fell helplessly, as the attendant berated her, "Why didn't you tell me you were a man?" I advocated for Diana's right for a transgender-friendly attendant at each hospital discharge. Eventually, Diana was unable to live independently. Since her biological family had abandoned her and she had no partner, she needed placement in an AIDS nursing home. I advocated on a daily basis with the nursing home to place her with a female roommate, but the nursing home did the opposite. Diana was devastated because nursing home staff treated her as a man. Her heterosexual male roommate would insult her during the day and masturbate facing her at night. Throughout this period, the group and I visited her regularly. Members would sometimes take over for the nurses and wash the diarrhea from between her legs. Diana appreciated this gesture immensely.

Before she died, Diana requested a special favor from the group. She asked the group to go to her funeral and make sure that her family buried her as a woman. The other members and I traveled to the funeral home armed with a dress, women's shoes, and makeup. When the minister referred to Diana by her former masculine name, members advocated on the patient's behalf. As we traveled back from the funeral, members discussed fearing that their turn to die was next. However, this experience had reassured them that the group would protect their female gender, even into the grave.

HORMONE TREATMENT

A transgendered individual may develop an identity crisis and major depression if her physicians are transgenderphobic and subsequently refuse to prescribe hormones. As mentioned earlier, my first patient would cry for hours as she helplessly watched the chest hair sprout over her breast implants. It was her worst nightmare come true. Social workers need to advocate for their transgendered clients' right to receive hormone treatment. Often this is a challenging process. Most medical schools do not offer courses on hormone replacement. When doctors graduate, they have not learned which hormone to prescribe, the dosage, the side effects, and how to appropriately monitor liver function tests. Although learning resources are scarce, they do exist. A social worker or a transgendered patient can direct the physician to read resources regarding medical and hormonal treatment for MTF transsexuals (see list at end of this chapter). Social workers can also refer doctors to other physicians in the community who already prescribe hormones to transsexuals (for instance at the local gay and lesbian community center of a large city).

HIV physicians routinely prescribe testosterone and Oxandrin to HIV-positive men with wasting syndrome. There seems to be much less reluctance to prescribe hormones to traditionally genderized HIV-positive patients. This seems to reflect a strong cultural bias that is based on both transgenderphobia and heterosexism and needs to be questioned whenever encountered. Social workers and transgendered patients need to take every opportunity to broach the issue of countertransference with all professionals on the health care teams. Protease inhibitors herald a new age in HIV care. As with many other HIV-positive people, transsexuals are living longer and healthier lives between hospitalizations. State-of-the-art HIV medical treatment mandates that pre-op transsexuals centralize their medical care, that is, integrate hormone therapy into their overall HIV medical treatment. This creates a complicated scenario, one best illustrated by the following case.

Alex was born a male but felt female since childhood. Her mother neglected Alex's nine younger siblings and forced Alex to care for them. At the age of eleven, Alex was already wearing a maternal uniform (frock and aprons) as she cleaned, cooked, and changed diapers. She ran away from home in her mid-teens after being sexually abused by her stepfather. Alex was forced to wear a male uniform to maintain her job as a janitor and financially support herself. She could only wear female clothes and makeup during weekends. She lived an isolated existence from the age of twenty to forty, unable to trust outsiders with her lifestyle, unable to find and connect with other transsexuals. Alcohol became her coping mechanism.

After neighborhood teenagers took a dislike to her female attire and assaulted her with a baseball bat, she became disabled and, during this hospitalization, was diagnosed as HIV positive. At the age of forty, Alex suddenly had full-blown AIDS and realized her life span was limited. She chose to make a gender transition before she died. She decided this upon entering an outpatient HIV clinic. Her doctor refused to prescribe female hormones, claiming that he had no idea what drugs to prescribe or the correct dosages. He referred Alex to a psychiatrist for evaluation. Alex felt that the clinic was assessing whether she was a "true transsexual" or a personality pathology who was about to make irreversible changes to her body that she would later regret. She felt as though she had lost control over her body. It no longer belonged to her; it belonged to psychiatry. Psychiatry had a different agenda from Alex's. Since the 1970s, most psychiatrists have been taught to help transsexuals accept their body image instead of helping them achieve gender transition. This is the approach Alex's psychiatrist took with her. Therefore, Alex felt misunderstood by her psychiatrist since his goal was not to help her pursue gender transition.

Alex joined the support group the year she found out she was HIV positive. There she met other transsexuals for the first time in her life. Alex's peers normalized her feelings and assisted her through the steps of gender transition. The group helped her choose a female name, Gabriella. They also told her about venues outside the HIV clinic where she could get hormones. Therefore, Gabriella turned to the black market to obtain her hormones since Medicaid refused to pay for them without the approval of her HIV physician. Gabriella was forced to return to work to afford these drugs, which were essential to her overall sense of well-being. Employers refused to hire Gabriella in her female identity. The only profession that was not off-limits to her was sex work. Sex work placed Gabriella at high risk for violence from both sex customers and police. She also placed herself at risk of being reinfected with HIV by her customers if a condom broke—if she used condoms. Her customers were also at risk of being infected with HIV.

Without a physician's guidance, Gabriella doubled and even tripled her hormone dosage in an attempt to accelerate breast growth. No one was monitoring her liver function tests to make sure that she was not harming herself. Gabriella then turned to injection hormones because she felt they would work faster. She placed herself at risk of sharing needles and becoming reinfected with more strains of the virus. I never stopped advocating for Gabriella's right to centralize her medical care in her HIV clinic. After four years, she received her first hormone prescription from her HIV physician, who is finally able to track her dosage and monitor her liver function tests.

At the dawn of the twenty-first century, the transgender community is empowering itself by advocating for client-centered health care that meets its unique needs. A desperate need exists for scientific research on the effects of hormone therapy on HIV-positive transgendered people so that physicians can become knowledgeable about, and feel comfortable in, prescribing hormones to this population. So far, there is no evidence that hormones actually worsen a transsexual's HIV/AIDS disease progression at the medical center where I work. Five of my patients who began hormone therapy after they were diagnosed HIV positive did not develop opportunistic infections regardless of whether they were on antiretroviral combinations and prophylaxis. Another one of my patients with AIDS stopped her hormones for a year after developing pneumonia and being intubated for a month. When she restarted female hormones in conjunction with triple combination therapy, her CD-4 count subsequently jumped from 62 to 592 over a six-month period.

FINANCES

Gender transition is extremely expensive. The entire process can cost between $100,000 to $150,000 (to pay for sexual reassignment surgery, breast implants, electrolysis, long-term hormone treatment, tracheal shave, silicone injections, and legal fees to change a name). A transsexual person must make a large salary to afford these procedures. Since most employers are transgenderphobic, few options are open, outside of sex work, for earning the kind of money needed to finance the sex change. When AIDS disables the transsexual client, she is no longer able to cope with the stresses of a sex clientele and thus loses her income.

AIDS physically disabled many of my group members and prevented them from working. They were no longer able to afford the expensive procedures delineated earlier that would enhance their female appearance. Suddenly, they were forced to survive on a fixed budget that barely paid for food. They mourned the loss of their financial independence and the ability to make choices with their money. Many clients felt controlled and resented feeling this way. They were angry at having a disease that robbed them of their health and their ability to change their gender. Being trapped within a budget paralleled being trapped in an anatomical male body and was often a topic of discussion in the group.

Most of the group members feared applying for disability benefits because many entitlement workers are transgenderphobic. They often ridicule transsexuals. Some members missed their face-to-face interviews with disability and welfare workers to avoid humiliating treatment and discrimination. This meant that they lacked the ability to pay for food, shelter, and medical insurance. Again, social workers and other mental health professionals need to repeatedly advocate on behalf of HIV-positive transsexuals to entitlement agencies.

SEX WORK

Therapists and case workers need to address their countertransference and their colleagues' countertransference toward sex work. Many people oppose sex work (or, as it is otherwise termed, "prostitution") for religious, political, and philosophical reasons. When any client who is a sex worker senses a health care provider's judgment about how she earns her money, she will not reveal her profession. This drives the HIV epidemic further underground in this population. The patient is in danger of being reinfected, and she may transmit the virus to her customers. The following example illustrates how a clinic can easily lose a transgendered client who is a sex worker. Georgina was a fifty-five-year-old MTF pre-op transsexual sex worker. She attended our outpatient clinic for two months and suddenly dropped out. I later ran into her on the street. She explained what had caused her to stop attending the clinic:

> I didn't feel safe telling my doctor anything, especially how I make a living, night after night behind Grand Central Station, giving blow jobs in alleys and carrying a knife in my purse for protection. He never asked me how I caught pneumonia. So I never told him about giving blow jobs outside in the middle of winter at three in the morning. He never told me to wear a condom on my penis. I think he wanted to believe that I didn't have one. He didn't even examine me fully naked. He seemed afraid of me. My body freaked him out, even if he never saw it. He requested that I keep my clothes on. I got the message. I missed one appointment because the police picked me up during a raid. But I couldn't tell him or the receptionist that I missed because I was in jail. I was afraid they'd ask me why. I'm sure he's relieved that I never came back. It's easier just to forget it. I sniff my coke: that got me through Christmas.

Safer Sex

An important role of mental health professionals in HIV is safer sex education. Some MTF transsexuals use condoms; others do not, just as in both the heterosexual and homosexual worlds. However, transgender culture poses its own set of unique obstacles to condom use, including female self-perception, violence from customers, financial incentives, and affirmation from sex customers. Case examples best illustrate the complexity of these issues.

Female Self-Perception

When I have sex with my boyfriend, I hike up my skirt, sit over him, bob up and down as he enters my asshole. For those few moments, it's like a fantasy come true. I am the woman I've always wanted to be. The hell I'm going to stop to stick a condom on his penis. That would mean turning on the lights, fumbling around, both of us paying closer attention to each other's anatomy—me noticing the penis taped over my abdomen and the testicles tucked between my legs.

Violence from Customers

I dated a man who tried to stab me after he climaxed during sex. I couldn't report him because I feared the police would accuse me of provoking him. I have spent too many nights on the pavement picking up the contents of my purse after the cops dumped them out on the sidewalk. Once a guy pushed me into a washroom stall and tried to strangle me at my friend's wedding. I guess these men tried to kill me because they hated themselves. All I know is that I can't tell them what to do, and that includes putting on a condom. I'd be too scared. I'd have to keep an eye on his hands, knowing that if he reaches down he could pull out a knife. You're trying to convince me to use a condom so that I can live more years. But if he slashes my throat I won't make it through the night.

Money

He'll pay me triple if he can do it without a condom. And do you know how cold it is during winter, circling that meat-packing district at four in the morning? Sixty dollars means I can go home and get me my hormones. And he probably already has HIV if he wants to do it without a condom. And anyway I already have the package.

Affirmation from Customers

I started out in prostitution to pay the rent and food. But I stayed in it because I found people who accepted and appreciated my body. Don't underestimate how much that means to me. While everyone else slammed doors in my face, my johns make me feel attractive and desirable. I'd be too afraid of losing him if I asked him to wear a condom. I know he can find another girl like that who will do it without a condom. And I'll be alone again.

Traditional safer-sex arguments (that work with less oppressed groups) lose their effectiveness on an MTF pre-op transsexual client. These arguments discount the harshness of her reality and rob her of her feelings. The danger of reinfection is not a persuasive reason to engage safer-sex techniques for most MTF clients with whom I have worked. Planning for a longer and healthier future becomes irrelevant when she is barely able to survive the moment. Moreover, why would she trust that a health care professional was invested in the health of her body, if most of society fears it? In addition, if the only person who finds her body desirable refuses to wear a condom, it is completely understandable that she will be quite reluctant to give him up.

Once clinicians grasp the scope of this particular dilemma, they realize that possible solutions are complex. They cannot hope to convince a client to give up the four incentives (listed previously) unless they can replace them with something else. One option that has helped some clients begin to employ safer-sex techniques was attending an ongoing structured support group. This transgender-friendly community, with social structures that praise the client's body and identity, helped some transgendered clients grapple with options concerning safer sex.

Mental health professionals can help HIV-positive MTF pre-op transsexuals begin to engage in conversations about safer sex, keeping the following four points in mind:

1. Workers can advocate for a transsexual client's legal right to press police charges against violent customers. I have accompanied a client to the police station because she would not go on her own. I also referred her to the local antiviolence project. She was subsequently able to broach the subject of condoms with her customers because she could count on me and the police to defend her rights.
2. Workers can build a resource of transgender-friendly employers so that the client has job options in addition to sex work.
3. Professionals can create transgendered support groups so that caring HIV-positive transgendered peers replace the affirmation of exploitative sex customers. Some of my clients have listened to safer-sex education when it came from their peers rather than me.
4. Workers can instruct MTF transsexuals on safer-sex options. Since male condoms challenge female self-perception, MTF transsexual

clients were less apprehensive about female contraceptives, such as inserting female condoms in their rectum and using vaginal spermacidal foams that contain nonoxynol 9. Moreover, the process of purchasing these female contraceptives in a store enhanced their female self-perception in public.

LIFE REVIEW: A GROUP PROCESS

As with all terminally ill people, reviewing one's life goals and dreams is an important clinical task for AIDS workers to engage in with their clients. Pre-operative MTF transsexual clients living with AIDS may also use clinical mental health sessions to take inventory of their lives once they realize that their time is limited. The way my support group most often discussed loss was in relation to how HIV robbed these individuals of the opportunity for sexual reassignment surgery and to die as anatomical women. All the clients struggled with intense grief when they discovered that American surgeons will not perform sexual reassignment surgery on HIV-positive people. Members expressed their anger at the medical system. They felt doubly stigmatized, being HIV positive and transgendered. Some were prepared to fight the medical establishment to obtain the surgery before they died. Others felt helpless and unable to engage in this struggle against the medical establishment and paralleled this feeling with their powerlessness against the HIV virus raging through their bodies.

The thought of dying with a penis and testicles horrified my group members. Most had dreamed of dying with breasts and a vagina. Some had even visualized themselves in a coffin, wearing a specific outfit and jewelry. This image comforted many members, especially when they had initially struggled with their HIV diagnosis. One member stated, "After the doctor gave me the news that I was positive, the only thing that got me through it was the dream of getting the surgery and becoming a complete woman. I entered life as a boy. But I was going to exit as a woman."

Discussing their HIV or AIDS diagnosis hurled group members back into the past, to a time when they were HIV negative. Many members regretted not pursuing the surgery before they were infected. Some members emotionally attacked themselves for having become infected, replaying over and over the moment at which (they believe) they became infected, trying to change the ending of the memory (by using a condom, bleaching a hormone needle, stopping an unprotected sexual encounter). During her final hospitalization, shortly before dying, one member explained to the group how she had become obsessed with an old friend who had succeeded in obtaining the surgery:

She keeps popping into my mind. She was positive too and knew that
the surgeons wouldn't touch her. So she convinced an HIV-negative
friend to impersonate her and take the HIV test in her place. I admire
her for not letting anything stand in her way. She got to die as a woman.
I remember I was seeing a psychiatrist at the time who convinced me
that I'd regret the surgery. But my friend would say to me, "Diana, you
are so foolish!" Now I'm dying of AIDS and it's too late.

These painful realizations and discussions brought members closer together. Emotional defenses seemed irrelevant, as members witnessed their
peers dying with such sadness, anger, and frustration. They rallied around
one another to guarantee that they would all die as women. They made a
pact to go to one another's funerals and ensure that biological families and
church congregations would not dress their corpses in masculine clothes.
As members made these promises to one another, their relationships became more intimate. Instead of mistaking intimacy for erotic love (as in
the first year of the group), members translated intimacy into more comforting terms, into female-enhancing terms. Members viewed the "maternal relationship" as the ultimate female relationship. Consequently, they
felt comfortable becoming surrogate mothers to one another. More experienced members adopted younger members as their daughters. The mother-
daughter relationship safeguarded members from any erotic feelings and
underlined every member's female identity. Recently, one member looked
around the group and stated, " I have two mothers in this room. Gabriella
is my hormone mother. Gina is my other mother. And Gabriella has two
daughters, Crystal and me. It's like we've become a family."

This form of nurturing demonstrates how these HIV-positive, pre-
operative transsexuals cope with devastating losses from HIV. They express intense anger for justifiable reasons. Instead of feeling defeated, they
develop adaptive mothering skills. These strengths belie society's stereotypical view of them as "freaks." Their ability to nurture one another is a
means to embrace all they want in life in the face of AIDS and, ultimately,
to die with as much dignity as possible.

CONCLUSION

I hope that this chapter has humanized pre-operative HIV-positive transsexuals for the reader. A transgendered person deserves good HIV care just
as much as any other person. Society's prejudices should not stand in the
way of her receiving the most sensitive and sophisticated medical and
psychosocial care possible.

The professional HIV community needs to respond to the needs of the transgender client in several ways to help create transgender, client-centered HIV care that will integrate hormone treatment into HIV medical care. Educating health care staff on transgender issues is one crucial first step toward this end. Research needs to be conducted into the interaction between hormone treatment and the HIV-infected transgendered client. In addition, there should be a concerted effort at outreach to HIV-positive MTF transsexuals to help them access state-of-the-art medical care. Mental health professionals and clients need to seek out opportunities to work together in pioneering outreach and customized care for this client population. In addition, workers can help their transgendered clients by developing therapeutic relationships with them and creating transgender support groups to battle isolation. Advocating on these clients' behalf with medical, legal, and governmental institutions is also essential. By seeking out transgender-friendly employment resources, therapists can help these clients find ways of supporting themselves outside of sex work.

One of my goals is to offer transgendered clients dignity and individualized HIV treatment. All clients deserve this, especially those who struggle with life-threatening illness. I challenge all health care providers to move beyond their discomfort with gender ambiguity. How is a transgendered person's loss of beauty any different from an HIV-positive man's loss of muscle mass? How is the rage of a pre-operative transsexual who cannot obtain sexual reassignment surgery less valid than any other person's rage at being denied the opportunity to accomplish his or her major life goals because of AIDS? The members of this particular HIV group demonstrate a capacity to mother one another that equals any other individual's parenting potential. My clients' stories prove that transgendered people are *not* to be feared. They are strong and courageous. They battle incredible discrimination. They are survivors. They adapt and find ways to meet their own unique life goals, and by doing so, they have the capacity to teach and inspire us to do the same with our lives.

BIBLIOGRAPHY

Futterweit, W. (1980). Endocrine management of transsexuals. *New York State Journal of Medicine,* July, *80*(8), pp. 1260-1264.

Meeks, G. (1994). Progesterone and progestins. *Endocrine, 2*(6), pp. 31-43.

Rivlin, M. E. (1994). Estrogens. *Endocrine, 2*(6), pp. 15-30.

Valenta L. J., Elias, A. N., and Domurat, E. S. Hormone pattern in pharmacologically feminized male transsexuals in the California state prison system, *Journal of the National Medical Association, 84*(3), pp. 241-250.

Chapter 14

Internalized Homophobia in the Psychotherapy of Gay Men with HIV/AIDS

Maria R. Derevenco
Ronald J. Frederick

INTRODUCTION

Although much has been written about psychotherapeutic work with HIV-infected gay men, less attention has been paid to internalized homophobia and its implications for this work. This paucity of theoretical and technical discussion is the likely result of pressures on clinicians to attend to the crisis aspects of HIV/AIDS, which leads to oversight of broader intrapsychic issues. Such a phenomenon is illustrated in the following case example, as David, a fifty-year-old gay man, and his therapist are confronted with the possibility that the patient may be HIV-infected:

> Throughout the first two years of treatment, David was unable to talk about his risk of HIV infection and presented himself as unconcerned, though a highly active sexual past made infection a likely possibility. He rationalized that his asymptomatic condition was reassuring. At the beginning of the third year of treatment, David reluctantly acknowledged growing concern, as he had started having night sweats and shortness of breath. As he and his therapist began to look at the possibility of David's being HIV positive, both developed a sense of dread that something terrible was about to happen. At the time, the therapist suspected that this was related solely to HIV fears, and most interpretations were in line with this hypothesis. As treatment progressed, it became clearer that the dread was due in large part to David's pending acknowledgment of abhorred aspects of

himself—his homosexuality, which he equated with femininity. In addition, the therapist had his own anxiety and HIV-related fears, his concern for the patient, and his own unconscious enmeshment in projective identification through which he contained the patient's warded-off anxiety, which all contributed to the narrow focus of inquiry. Once the therapist began to make sense of his own anxious feelings, he was able to broaden his focus from HIV issues to an exploration of David's sense of self and of his internal object representations. Intense self-loathing and shame about David's sexual orientation, disavowed feminine identifications, and identification with the aggressor emerged prominently.

The term homophobia, first used by Weinberg (1972), refers not only to the fear of homosexuals and homosexuality but also to all negative attitudes and prejudices against gay people. Internalized homophobia is the gay person's repudiation of thoughts, feelings, desires, and sexual behaviors involving same-sex partners. It regularly results in shame, guilt, anger, and tendencies toward self-punishment (Friedman, 1991; Malyon, 1982).

Shidlo (1994), in a review of the literature, distinguishes between conscious and unconscious internalized homophobia and suggests that, based on existing prevalence data, 25 to 33 percent of gay men have experienced conscious negative thoughts or feelings about their sexual orientation. Since these data are derived from self-report measures, they reflect only the conscious aspects of internalized homophobia. For the most part, the gay studies literature defines internalized homophobia as a product of gay persons' growing up in an antihomosexual society, governed by the stigmatization and denigration of homosexual identity, desire, and relationships. Herek (1990) termed this ideology "heterosexism" and cited survey results showing that about two-thirds of Americans exhibit homophobic attitudes. The focus in the gay studies literature seems to be on the role of social norms in generating homophobia, external and especially internalized homophobia. Although intuitively appealing, this does not fully account for either the existence of societal homophobia or for the complex psychological processes whereby societal opprobrium shapes the development of gay youth and is transmuted into psychic reality.

MANIFESTATIONS OF UNCONSCIOUS
INTERNALIZED HOMOPHOBIA

Numerous writers have described the effects of antihomosexual social norms as expressed through parental/community disapproval. Gay youth's sense of identity and of psychological integrity, self-esteem, cognitive, defensive, and relational patterns, as well as superego development, are thought to be affected (Cabaj, 1988; Driggs and Finn, 1990; Herek, 1990; Isay, 1989; Malyon, 1982; Nicholson and Long, 1990; Shidlo, 1994; Weinberg, 1972). Obviously, unconscious internalized homophobia can only be inferred and can only be observed as it is expressed symptomatically, as with any other unconscious mental content. In the following case examples, we attempt to illustrate the often elusive effects of the unconscious component of homophobia in gay men who are overtly comfortable with their homosexuality.

> Ted, a gay man who had been HIV positive for many years, often stated that "there was nothing wrong with being gay" and that he felt proud as a gay man. Yet he maintained that most gay men were "too in-your-face" about being gay.

> Fred, a man in his sixties who had been in a monogamous relationship for twenty-five years, revealed to his therapist that he had never had anal intercourse "since only women are penetrated, and both my partner and I feel like men."

These statements express unconscious internalized homophobia and contain, in various forms, concomitant devaluation and idealization of these men's sexual identities and the defensive denial and projection of intolerable aspects of the self.

> Albert, a health professional who continued to work with AIDS patients even after his own HIV infection because of his desire to alleviate suffering and to contribute to the gay community, became quite depressed after a period of therapeutic gains. While trying to identify the sources of his depression, it was revealed that he was engaging in promiscuous, unprotected anal sex during weekends at a gay resort. During those episodes, he felt "empty, not himself, driven," and afterward was filled with shame and remorse for possibly infecting others.

In Albert's case, unconscious homophobia manifested as periods of ego fragmentation, experienced subjectively as emptiness. He was attempting to "fill himself," literally and symbolically, through frenetic sexual activity that was morally unacceptable to him and only increased his sense of shame.

> David, the patient discussed previously, was made very uncomfortable by any discussion of his health. He felt that he would begin to

"shut down," not wanting to "be like other gay people who seem to complain a lot about their health." Illness, or thoughts about it, were an indication of weakness, equated with his depressed, hypochondriacal mother. His resistance to HIV testing seemed to be fueled, in part, by his aversion to experiencing himself as anything like his mother—weak, fragile, helpless, or in other words, feminine. He would rather be like his father and disregard or neglect bodily needs.

Howard, a forty-five-year-old, HIV-positive, gay male patient recalled that his introduction to other gay people took place in his early teens at a drag club close to home. This experience evoked conflicting feelings. On one hand, he enjoyed and felt comfortable being with the club patrons, as he felt accepted and could be himself. On the other hand, he thought the more effeminate men and the drag performers to be weak and strange. It bothered him to feel that he was in any way like them. From this time onward, he presented himself to the world as being excessively proud of being gay. He engaged in street fights with people who ridiculed him and often became physically threatening as he demonstrated the extent of his masculinity.

These two patients constructed a counterphobic identity by warding off aspects of themselves that they perceived to be weak or feminine.

INTERNALIZED HOMOPHOBIA AND HIV/AIDS

HIV/AIDS often becomes a container for deep-seated internalized homophobic material, which vastly complicates the clinical work in the treatment of gay men with HIV/AIDS. As Odets (1995) stated, "AIDS has given many gay men the opportunity to shift familiar and traditional guilt about thinking, feeling, or living homosexually, to guilt about having HIV, not having HIV, or not doing enough to help others survive" (p. 104). Abramowitz and Cohen (1994) suggest that HIV/AIDS can feel like a "present day retribution or confirmation that the self is bad, defective, unworthy, and unlovable" (p. 215). Since in the initial phase of the epidemic AIDS was largely confined to the gay community, it was identified as a "gay disease." Though this is no longer the case factually, the equation of homosexuality with AIDS persists symbolically, for gay men and for society as a whole.

In a strange parallel to what Odets (1995) refers to as the "homosexualization of AIDS," there seems to have occurred a symbolic "infection" of the gay identity by AIDS so that there is a bidirectional equation of homosexuality and AIDS. For example, we have encountered in our clinical work several gay men who, even though they have never had unprotected sex, nevertheless believe that they have AIDS simply because they are gay.

Other patients court disaster, convinced that AIDS is their fated destiny as gay men:

> Jay, a man in his mid-thirties, who was an openly gay community leader, felt throughout his childhood that he was "different." After an adolescence spent in a religious all-boys school where he had numerous same-sex experiences, Jay fell in love and married a woman who shared his interests. A few years into the marriage, he met an openly gay man, fell in love, divorced his wife, and entered a monogamous relationship that was to last till his partner's death. Gianni was diagnosed HIV positive about six years after he and Jay committed to each other, and he died within two years, leaving Jay heartbroken and beset with guilt about surviving his beloved Gianni. As he emerged from a severe clinical depression, and seemingly having worked through his survivor's guilt, Jay started engaging in unprotected sex with a boy of his acquaintance who was a teenage prostitute. This exposed him to severe legal and financial risks, not to mention HIV exposure. As this behavior was being explored in treatment, issues about warded-off femininity, heterosexual longings, and self-hatred began to emerge, and Jay terminated therapy abruptly and unadvisedly. In his last session, he expressed his strong belief that nothing was going to prevent his dying of AIDS.

The incorporation of AIDS into male homosexual identity has obvious implications for psychotherapy. In particular, we are concerned with the potential for ignoring unconscious internalized homophobia in these patients, as a diagnosis of HIV infection is devastating to any individual. Ample evidence now exists of the negative psychological impact of such a diagnosis, including anxiety, depression, suicidal ideation, social isolation, etc., regardless of the individual's risk factors. Gay men, although contending with some of the same psychosocial issues experienced by others infected with and affected by HIV, have been additionally stressed as they have seen their social networks disappear and their sexuality further stigmatized. A unique stressor identified for gay men is the emergence or reemergence of internalized homophobia (Linde, 1994; Nicholson and Long, 1990).

In individuals who present as comfortable with their gay identity, unconscious homophobia may not be readily apparent, especially in the early phases of psychotherapy, as witnessed by the case of David, presented at the beginning of this chapter. This phenomenon may present a challenge for both the clinician and patient, particularly when HIV takes center stage. AIDS and its specter of death can easily preempt the exploration of other, seemingly less compelling issues in psychotherapy. AIDS-related fears and anxieties, in patient and clinician alike, may distract both from focusing on underlying issues such as unconscious homophobia.

CLINICAL IMPLICATIONS

Questions frequently asked in supervision and in case conferences refer to the conflation of gay identity and AIDS and to the difficulty of untangling such issues with patients and determining the "right" focus of therapeutic inquiry. It has been the experience of the senior author, from direct clinical experience as well as from supervision, that a potentially lethal illness, be it AIDS, cancer, cardiac or terminal kidney disease, tends to draw the clinician into a "crisis intervention" mode of thinking, aimed at alleviating psychic discomfort in the immediate term. Although this focus may be appropriate in the very beginning phases of therapy, once it is determined that the patient's demise is not imminent, and some measure of stability has been resumed, the clinician is well advised to begin focusing on the meaning of the illness for this particular patient, at this particular time.

We contend that the therapist/analyst needs to inquire in detail into the patient's experience of HIV/AIDS, identifying, examining, and making sense out of the related affects and associations, attending to HIV-related issues as he or she would any other clinical material. A clinical examination of the consciously and unconsciously assigned meanings of HIV/AIDS will most likely uncover unconscious internalized homophobic material, with all that this construct entails. The cases of David and Howard highlight several important issues. Both cases illustrate the salience of shame, which is invoked by self-representations unacceptable to the homophobic part of the self. Though both men were consciously comfortable with their gay identity, further exploration revealed intense unconscious homophobia and conflicted, contradictory self-representations. The negative self-representations were associated with maternal identifications perceived as passive and weak. The trainee-therapists working with these patients experienced intense anxiety and heightened, unfocused terror of HIV infection. This is common, in the senior author's experience, for male and female trainees regardless of sexual orientation.

The therapist's own internalized homophobia and discomfort with femininity and passivity can lead to countertransference problems (Isay, 1989; Frommer, 1994). Whether the therapist is male or female, gay or straight, countertransference is likely to manifest as counterresistance to the exploration of patient's experience of gender and of homosexual identity:

> Julie, a psychology trainee in the process of coming out as a lesbian, was assigned the case of Hun, a young Philippino man newly diagnosed with AIDS. Although they established rapport and began therapeutic work, Julie was uneasy with exploring her patient's sexual experiences and sexuality. In supervision, she became aware of a possible mutual sexual attraction, which had led her to retreat emotionally from her patient. This also precluded any exploration of patient's and therapist's conscious and unconscious homophobia. As this was being worked on in supervision, the trainee-therapist became more aware of her patient's resistance and was able to perceive her own contribution to his discomfort about discussing homosexuality.

We agree with Frommer (1994) that the proper focus of treatment is not to locate the "etiology" of the patient's homosexuality in early experience. However, if internalized homophobia is to be resolved, the patient needs to gain an understanding of the role of early identifications and their defenses against them and of the fact that these occurred in the context of a homophobic relational environment. The clinician, whether gay or straight, must strive to keep in mind the multifaceted nature of unconscious internalized homophobia in both therapist and patient, since culturally transmitted taboos are always enacted through interpersonal relationships, in which individuals incorporate and disavow them at the same time. Treatment of gay men infected with and affected by AIDS should not be confined to dealing only with issues related to HIV. Internalized homophobia, and particularly its unconscious manifestations, require therapeutic vigilance in regard to transference and countertransference phenomena. Such vigilance will enable the patient to work through the conflicts that thwart his ability to live a more satisfying life.

REFERENCES

Abramowitz, S. and Cohen, J. (1994). The psychodynamics of AIDS: A view from self-psychology. In S. A., Cadwell, R. A., Burnharn, and M., Forstein (Eds.), *Therapists on the front-line: Psychotherapy with gay men in the age of AIDS* (pp. 205-221).Washington, DC: American Psychiatric Press.

Cabaj, R. P. (1988). Gay and lesbian couples: Lessons on human intimacy. *Psychiatric Annals, 18*(1), 21-25.

Corbett, K. (1993). The mystery of homosexuality. *Psychoanalytic Psychology, 10*(3), 345-357.

Driggs, J. H. and Finn, S. E. (1990). *Intimacy between men.* New York: Penguin.

Friedman, R. C. (1991). Couple therapy with gay couples. *Psychiatric Annals, 21*(8), 485-490.

Frommer, M. S. (1994). Homosexuality and psychoanalysis: Technical considerations revisited. *Psychoanalytic Dialogues, 2*, 215-233.

Herek, G. (1990). The context of anti-gay violence: Notes on cultural and psychological heterosexism. *Journal of Interpersonal Violence, 5*(3), 316-333.

Isay, R. (1989). *Being homosexual: Gay men and their development.* New York: Avon Books.

Linde, R. (1994). Impact of AIDS on adult gay male development: Implications for psychotherapy. In S. A. Cadwell, R. A. Burnham, and M. Forstein (Eds.), *Therapists on the front-line: Psychotherapy with gay men in the age of AIDS* (pp. 25-51).Washington, DC: American Psychiatric Press.

Malyon, A. K. (1982). Psychotherapeutic implications of internalized homophobia in gay men. In J. Gonsiorek (Ed.), *Homosexuality and psychotherapy* (pp. 59-69). Binghamton, NY: The Haworth Press.

Nicholson, W. D. and Long, B. C. (1990). Self-esteem, social support, internalized homophobia and coping strategies of HIV+ gay men. *Journal of Consulting and Clinical Psychology, 6*, 873-876.

Odets, W. (1995). *In the shadow of the epidemic: Being HIV-negative in the age of AIDS.* Durham, NC: Duke University Press.

Shidlo, A. (1994). Internalized homophobia: Conceptual and empirical issues in measurement. In B. Greene and C. Herek (Eds.), *Lesbian and gay psychology: Theory, research and clinical applications.* Thousand Oaks, CA: Sage.

Weinberg, C. (1972). *Society and the healthy homosexual.* New York: St. Martin's Press.

Chapter 15

Dying Well:
Counseling End-Stage Clients
with AIDS

Michael Shernoff

There is no debating that death touches every individual and family and that contemporary American society is unmistakenly a death-denying culture. For confirmation of this fact, consider the terms used as euphemisms for dying: "gone to meet his or her maker"; "gone on to a better place"; "made his or her transition"; "passed on"; and numerous other expressions that avoid the word "died." Unfortunately, social workers and other mental health professionals are often no better prepared to deal with the death of a client, a loved one, or their own imminent dying than any other individual. Yet, it is precisely during the period immediately after the diagnosis of a life-threatening illness such as AIDS until shortly before death that individuals and families can greatly benefit from skilled mental health interventions. This work helps all concerned express the feelings and fears they are experiencing, balance hope with the realities of having a life-threatening illness, prepare for the end of life, ensure that the dying person will be in as much control of his or her life as possible during the final part of life, and say good-bye to those people who are closest.

Until clinicians have faced and worked through issues concerning their own mortality, it will be extremely difficult to work effectively with individuals and families who are struggling with end-of-life issues. For the purpose of this chapter, the term family is not limited to biological family or a legal marriage but also includes same-sex partners, unmarried opposite-sex partners, and friendship groups that function as primary support systems for the person with AIDS (PWA) who is at the end of his or her life.

If the mental health professional has not examined personal beliefs and feelings surrounding death, he or she will not be able to initiate discussions about this with patients. A professional's inability to discuss directly a client's impending death and the dying process can only create a sense of secrecy or shame in the patient, who may not have anyone else with whom to discuss these feelings and all of the corresponding issues. My experience indicates that although initially uncomfortable for clients, discussing questions about death, dying, and end-of-life practicalities provides relief for clients who are very ill. One useful way to introduce the topic is to ask the client what he or she believes happens after death, and if those beliefs are comforting.

When an individual has a life-threatening illness such as cancer or AIDS, it is often difficult for all concerned to determine when the person has made a transition from living with this illness to starting to die of it. It is often even more difficult to tell when the people around the individual should acknowledge that dying has entered the relationship (Marks, 1995). A skilled social worker can be an invaluable asset to an individual and his or her family in this phase of the life cycle. At a certain point, different for each individual, we must all let go of living well and begin to consider the concept of "dying well." As Marks (1995) notes:

> this can be a very attractive concept for both client and counselor: many associate the dying process with all the worst things, from pain to mental deterioration. But what does it mean to die well, and how can counseling near the end of life promote this outcome? In addition how can people who are living truly understand what it means to the body and mind to let go of life? (p. 2)

This chapter will address concrete ways that social workers can be of valuable assistance in ensuring that clients at the end of their lives have the opportunity to "die well."

Psychotherapy with people with AIDS who are at the end stage of their illness generally occurs in one of two clinical situations. The first applies to an individual who has been in some form of ongoing counseling prior to entering the final phase of life. In the other case, a client seeks out a mental health professional as a direct result of being diagnosed as HIV positive or as a result of having deteriorated physically due to wasting or an opportunistic infection. AIDS has challenged social workers in private practice as well as those who are employed in hospitals, nursing homes, hospices, visiting nurse services, community-based AIDS organizations, and other home health care agencies to become prepared for working with people who are dying and their loved ones.

Few social workers or other mental health professionals receive specific training in counseling people who are at the end of their lives. The art of assisting people who are dying and their significant others is founded upon the professional's ability to be comfortable with helping people directly confront some of life's most painful issues and decisions. Asking a client questions concerning the choice to begin or discontinue a particular treatment and what the ramifications of that choice are helps the client examine what he or she values about his or her life. Working with PWAs who are dying and their loved ones requires the ability to engage in conversations about quality of life, spirituality, dying, and death. This ability is needed in all AIDS work and is a valuable clinical skill to possess in all aspects of practice with any client population. Although dying patients who are in ongoing psychotherapy will usually still want to do some intrapsychic exploration, the author's experience is that the content of sessions usually focuses increasingly on practical issues related to death, unfinished business with important loved ones, and feelings accompanying the knowledge that their lives are ending.

The clinician's experiences with death and dying and his or her related personal belief system have the potential to shape clinical work with patients who are at the end of their lives. For instance, does the clinician believe that death is final, or does he or she envision some kind of life after death? When working with a client who is dying, the professional needs to inquire about the patient's spiritual beliefs and the comfort he or she may derive from traditional religious beliefs and institutions. If the clinician does not subscribe to a traditional belief system, it may be difficult for the therapist to understand and empathize with just how comforting and important religion may be to a client. Conversely, some mental health professionals may have difficulty in understanding some clients' complete indifference to any potential comfort found in spiritual or religious tenets.

Health care professionals must do everything in their power to ensure that the needs of dying clients are met. For example, aggressive control of pain and anxiety. As Follansbee (1996) states, "the dignity of a peaceful death, without pain, fear or futile therapy can be realized only if time is spent in its preparation" (p. 6). Most people fear dying alone. Thus, all therapists can be of enormous assistance by ensuring that clients are not alone at the time of their deaths. The remainder of this chapter will elaborate on the mental health professional's role as assistant to clients during this time of enormous vulnerability and transition.

Rose (1996) notes that it is not always clear when someone is dying. Sometimes, when a person has been in a serious and steady decline with wasting, disorientation, and other symptoms and infections, it can be difficult for the closest caregivers to see, or admit, what is going on. Rose further states, "If this is the case, it can make a tremendous difference for physicians, friends or mental health professionals to speak the truth, acknowledging the approach of death gently but clearly" (p. 1).

CATEGORIES OF DYING

Follansbee (1996) describes four categories of dying, two of which are primarily psychological and two of which are primarily physical. For social workers to intervene effectively with people living with or dying from HIV or AIDS, an understanding of these categories is very helpful, especially when helping a client conceptualize where he or she is on the continuum of the process of dying. Follansbee states that in response to any initial diagnosis of a potentially terminal illness an individual may begin the *psychic* category, the process of accepting death. *Sociologic* dying, the second category, involves the withdrawal from people and activities. *Biological* dying is the loss of those characteristics that constitute being "human," for example, personality. Finally, *physiologic* dying represents the failure of the body's organs, the state that most of us recognize as death. Follansbee explains, "the terminal phase of dying involves all four of these processes, although the psychological aspects may begin months or years before the physical processes noticeably progress" (p. 5).

Follansbee also notes that "everyone experiences all these categories, although people differ in their attention to any one of them" (1996, p. 5). Many people will not focus on psychic or sociologic aspects until they face the biologic and physiologic stages of dying; others will never be able to distinguish the psychic from the physical aspects. He cautions that "confusion may arise when patients and providers use the term dying to describe different categories: the patient focuses on the psychic or social aspects of the process while the provider may focus on the biological or physiological aspects" (p. 5). For people with any life-threatening illness, dying often begins when he or she is diagnosed. Yet physicians and other health care providers may not recognize the dying process for several years. "This discrepancy may lead to misunderstanding or conflict. By introducing the above-mentioned categories of dying, social workers can help patients recognize the difference between living with a terminal disease and dying from it" (p. 5).

PREPARING FOR SERIOUS ILLNESS

As people develop symptoms of advanced AIDS, they increasingly lose control over their bodies and lives. One task of counseling is to help people living with HIV and AIDS recognize what they can control. An individual's physical and mental deterioration has an effect on him or her as well as the people with whom he or she lives. Family therapy can be a valuable tool to help family members adjust to the changes that the progression of a loved one's illness has on the family structure and dynamics. Clients living with a progressive disease such as HIV/AIDS require help in planning for hospitalizations and debilitating illnesses. It is best for the clinician to raise the difficult and painful issues discussed next long before any associated problems arise. This ensures that the client is still well and is therefore more likely to have the necessary physical and psychic energy to plan for the ensuing difficult realities. Social workers need to question and often challenge clients' unwillingness to discuss concrete plans or desires for a living will or treatment options. It is helpful to stress to the clients that by addressing these issues now they can ensure that they will have a measure of control over what happens to them later. Obviously, this has the potential to confront a client's denial; thus, the clinician must be prepared to be the target of the client's anger in response to initiating such necessary queries.

Professionals must overcome their own discomfort about discussing preparations for the end of life to help clients, their families, and loved ones accept this eventuality. Issues to address now, with all clients, but especially with those who have a life-threatening illness such as AIDS, include will preparation, medical proxy, and living will. Even if clients are only in the beginning stages of disease progression, therapists should emphasize the importance of addressing these difficult issues immediately. This is certainly true if the client is a single parent and has not made provisions for child care, if the client becomes too ill to actively parent, or for child custody following death.

Crucial Points to Specifically Discuss with Clients

1. Which hospital is to be used in the event of an emergency? Who in their support system is aware of this?
2. If clients live alone or with small children, who is the contact person, even in the middle of the night, to provide transportation to the hospital and/or to care for children or pets during a crisis?
3. Clients need to maintain a current and complete list of all prescribed medications and dosages that should be brought to the hospital during an emergency admission.
4. Clients need to discuss advance medical directives that include whether they wish to be kept alive if there is no reasonable hope for recovery or for a good quality of life.

5. A living will should be prepared. These directives need to be written down and given to the physician and brought to the hospital to be placed in the chart at the start of each hospitalization.

6. Clients need to designate a health care proxy (a family member or close friend) and ask this person if he or she will be able to ensure that the client's wishes will be followed even if those wishes are contrary to what the proxy believes is best.

7. Clients need to be asked, "What do you want done in the eventuality that your heart stops beating?" If a client does not wish to be resuscitated then a "do not resuscitate" (DNR) order needs to be written and placed in his or her chart. Clients need to be reminded that they can always revise these instructions if any of their feelings change over the course of their illness.

End-of-Life Issues

"Few people who are not profoundly depressed speak about being ready to die or welcoming it, except if they are in the advanced stage of a terminal illness. People with AIDS who have become debilitated after going through extensive treatments often speak of being ready to die since they no longer have a meaningful quality of life" (Rabkin, Remien, and Wilson, 1994, p. 147). It is imperative for the therapist not to judge these feelings and to elicit how the client feels about approaching the end of his or her life.

Funerals and Memorial Services

Dying clients can be greatly empowered by urging them to discuss what they wish done with their bodies after they have died. Do they want to be cremated or buried? Have they written this down? It can be comforting for some people to plan their funeral or memorial service, to specify who they wish to speak, what music or prayers should be recited, and where the service should take place. Similarly, confronting these details may be too stressful for those individuals who cannot face what making those plans means in terms of accepting their health status. If the client has been able to address these issues during a professional session, the next step is to urge him or her to discuss these details with family and loved ones and to prepare a written document that includes these wishes. If the family or loved ones refuse to discuss these issues with the client then the worker should urge the significant others to come in for counseling sessions to help them work through their feelings of denial, sadness, and discomfort.

These family sessions can help members see that understanding the wishes of their loved one will make it easier for them to carry out these wishes after the loved one has died. A useful intervention is to restructure the reality from one of morbid preoccupation with the unpleasant inevitability to one that allows the dying person some control over his or her life. It is also useful to explain to the loved ones that because the ill person loves them, he or she does not want them to have to guess about procedures during the extremely stressful period following death.

Medical Proxy

It is especially important to have several sessions with the terminally ill individual and the person he or she has designated to act as medical proxy. Assigning a medical proxy allows the dying person to take care of loved ones while ensuring that wishes will be carried out if he or she becomes unconscious or unable to speak or make decisions on his or her behalf. There is enormous stress inherent in having the responsibility of making life and death decisions for another individual. Not everyone who is very close to a dying person will feel able to act as the medical proxy; it is therefore urgent that the specifics of the dying individual's wishes in terms of life support and end-of-life care issues be explicitly discussed with the designated medical proxy. The worker needs to ask the medical proxy whether he or she feels able to carry out orders to discontinue treatments or life support, even if this decision is contrary to the individual's personal wishes and beliefs. The proxy needs to be encouraged to voice all doubts, fears, and concerns, especially those involving authorizing the medical team to "pull the plug." If the proxy is unsure of his or her ability to have treatments or life support terminated, and this is the expressed wish of the ill person, then the proxy should be encouraged to withdraw from this important position. The proxy who is honest about being unable to comply with the ill person's wishes should be supported for helping ensure that the sick person can then proceed to locate an individual who will be willing and confident in the ability to shoulder these responsibilities. Once a proxy has expressed willingness to function in this role, then a few more joint sessions are helpful. The patient can express explicit wishes to the proxy and the proxy then repeats the decisions, and the instructions are written down so there is no ambiguity about these crucial matters. It is also useful for these two people to share their feelings about the need for a medical proxy and to express the aspects of their relationship that allow it to include this level of intimacy and trust.

PAIN MANAGEMENT

As Rabkin, Remien, and Wilson (1994) state, "Most people fear that they will be in excruciating pain as they near death from a terminal illness. Clients need to be assured that they will not suffer. Most major hospitals have physicians who are pain management specialists who can consult with the patient about helping him or her remain comfortable at this phase of the illness. Some people prefer to be unconscious, others wish to be alert, but sedated and pain free" (p. 73). People need to be taught to explicitly describe how much pain they are experiencing and to clearly communicate this to the physician. Pain can be effectively controlled even if the client decides to die at home. In addition, therapists can help clients who experience pain by teaching them the techniques of self-hypnosis and visualization.

Weiss (1991) states that:

> actively chemically dependent patients with AIDS usually require generous amounts of medication while in the hospital. Medical and nursing staff often withhold the very medication these patients need, making them even more irritable and difficult to manage. Making patients comfortable with adequate opiates or sedatives helps them feel they are being heard, enhances their trust, and improves the working relationship between the chemically dependent patient and staff members. (p. 46)

All therapists need to be alert to this situation and be prepared to advocate for chemically dependent patients who are not being adequately medicated. Conversely, some patients who are in recovery have unrealistic expectations regarding using any painkiller that they once may have taken illicitly when they have a legitimate medical need for analgesic medication. Social workers and nurses need to remind people that they did not get sober to suffer and that taking prescribed medication to alleviate pain is not the same as abusing drugs.

CHOICES IN DYING

One major issue for dying people is their diminished ability to control their fate. Clients who are near death can be greatly empowered by discussing with social workers where they want to die. Many clients may not realize that whether to die at home, in the hospital, or in a hospice is a decision that they and their loved ones can, and should, consciously make together in consultation with the physician. It can be enormously helpful if the therapist raises the issue and explains the concept of hospice care. One useful intervention is to suggest that an intake worker from hospice visit the client and his or her family to describe the program in detail. These discussions should involve at least two different sessions. The first session should be with the client alone to explore all of his or her feelings about this emotionally laden issue. The second session should include the people who are part of the client's support team, if there are any, to explore all the emotional as well as logistical and practical considerations.

It can often be difficult for all concerned to acknowledge that "enough is enough." It is an essential and completely appropriate role of the counselor to encourage the client to explore his or her feelings about whether to cease treatments or to continue fighting for extra time. It is not the worker's role to give permission for one choice or another. Dying can be a quality time for the terminally ill person as well as for the loved ones. The worker should ask the client questions that will offer him or her options and some control over the process. Rabkin, Remien, and Wilson (1994) correctly note that it is far easier to believe in the right to choose the timing of one's death when the person is actively dying and when the remaining time is likely to be hours or days. The strength of this conviction is tested when the person is not acutely and severely ill, but untreatable, and may have weeks or months before an inevitable death. Such a person may be able to survive physically but with such chronic discomfort and restricted horizons that he or she sees no reason to remain alive. Is this person entitled to say "enough is enough"? Many health care providers who work with terminally ill people believe so. IV morphine is often started once the client has decided to discontinue medical procedures or drugs, with the double purpose of alleviating pain and possibly accelerating the impending death.

People with AIDS and their providers have been on the vanguard of the assisted suicide debate. Many people with AIDS discuss wanting to have the means to end their lives or to discontinue treatments if they feel that their lives have become intolerable. Psychotherapy's role is to encourage patients to discuss these feelings and to help the patient evaluate whether he or she is depressed. Conversations with terminally ill people that focus on when they might wish to either stop treatment or actively end their own lives are never one-time discussions; they need to occur throughout the progression of the disease. When patients receive treatment for depression, most regain the psychic energy required to continue fighting for their lives. Most patients view going blind, becoming incontinent, becoming demented, or being in unbearable pain as defining an intolerable quality of life. Not all terminally ill individuals who wish to die are depressed. When symptoms of illness and pain are treated and controlled, hope is restored and life once again becomes valued.

As peoples' illness progresses, it is striking to note that many terminally ill individuals are currently living lives that others, and they themselves, once considered intolerable. The question for therapists working with dying clients who discuss wanting help ending their lives is not whether we think suicide is OK but rather have we done everything in our power to assure each of our clients that his or her life is precious and that considering assisted suicide is an understandable option. (Michael Holtby's two chapters in this book provide in-depth discussions of the issues inherent in "self-deliverance" and how to differentiate this from suicidality.)

Crucial Questions for Counselors to Ask a Dying Client:

1. Do you feel that you are going to die soon? If so, how do you feel about this?
2. How will you know you no longer wish to continue medicines, treatments, or supplemental feedings? (It is important to reflect to the client that what he or she feels is intolerable may in fact change. Most surveyed people with AIDS felt that blindness, dementia, and incontinence were hallmarks toward discontinuing life.)
3. Do you prefer to die at home, in a hospice, or in a hospital?
4. Whom do you wish to be with you?
5. Would you like to have a clergyperson make a final visit?
6. Is there anything you have not said to your loved ones?
7. Is there anything else you need to do or complete?
8. Have you thought about letting go, since it seems that you are suffering a great deal?

Once IV morphine has been started, a person may become unable to communicate. Therefore, prior to the beginning of a morphine drip, the professional should look for opportunities to facilitate conversations between the dying person and his or her loved ones and family members. It can be both enormously helpful and comforting to the significant others of a dying person to have a professional make the following suggestions:

1. Is there something you have not said to your loved one?
2. Are there specific things you need to say to him or her?
3. Have you told the person that it is okay for him or her to go now?
4. Tell your loved one what specific things or events will always make you think of him or her.

5. Remind him or her of a special moment you two shared that will be with you forever.
6. Say "I love you," and thank the loved one for the relationship you had.
7. Say "good-bye" and express how much you will miss him or her.
8. Give assurance that although you will miss him or her greatly, that you will eventually be all right.

Although working with individuals who are dying can at times be exhausting or stressful, it also has the potential to be invigorating and can bring countless personal as well as professional rewards, not the least of which is demystifying death and dying. As Gaies and Knox (1991) point out, "By confronting with dying clients the fragility of life and the value of each day, health care professionals begin to confront the vulnerability of their own lives and to acquire a deeper appreciation of living" (p. 1).

REFERENCES

Follansbee, S. (1996). The dying process. *FOCUS: A Guide to AIDS Research and Counseling, 11*(2), pp. 5-6.

Gaies, J. and Knox, M. (1991). The therapist and the dying client. *FOCUS: A Guide to AIDS Research and Counseling, 6*(6), pp. 1-2.

Marks, R. (1995). Editorial: Dying well. *FOCUS: A Guide to AIDS Research and Counseling, 10*(8), p. 2.

Rabkin, J., Remien, R., and Wilson, C. (Eds.), (1994). *Good doctors, good patients: Partners in HIV treatment.* New York: NCN Publishers.

Rose, A. (1996). HIV and dying: The challenges of caring. *FOCUS: A Guide to AIDS Research and Counseling, 11*(2), pp. 2-4.

Weiss, C. (1991). Working with chemically dependent HIV-infected patients on an inpatient medical unit. In M. Shernoff (Ed.), *Counseling chemically dependent people with HIV illness.* Binghamton, NY: The Haworth Press, pp. 45-53.

Chapter 16

Psychotherapy, Counseling, and Self-Deliverance

Michael E. Holtby

Don was a company CEO when he went on disability. His intention was to preserve and strengthen the level of his health by an early "retirement." He had not experienced an opportunistic infection but was having difficulty taking AZT, which caused anemia and nausea. We spent months preparing for the day he would tell the board of directors and his staff of thirty employees that he had AIDS and had to retire. He had grown up on a ranch in Montana, and he faced coming out as gay and HIV positive to his rural family. To his surprise, all of these events went very well, with much support from those around him. However, two months after leaving his job, he became suicidal. Don had few interests beyond his work, and without it he felt lost, with no reason to live. Needless to say, I was very concerned and feared I would have to hospitalize him. I went so far as to draw up seventy-two-hour hold-and-treat papers and discussed his case with the inpatient intake team. Fortunately, Don did not need hospitalization; he pulled out of his depression and lived a productive life for another four years before dying of multiple infections and weight loss.

Don's case illustrates our traditional role as mental health professionals that has involved an ethical obligation to intervene when a client is "a danger to self or others." In a recent study of the suicide risk among people living with AIDS, researchers (Mancoske et al., 1995) found—from Louisiana's vital statistics (1987-1991)—PLWAs were 134.6 times more likely to kill themselves than were members of the general population. This conclusion focused upon the lack of services for PLWAs, noting that rural areas had twice the suicide rate of New Orleans: How many of these suicides were preventable with basic mental health and social services (Mancoske et al., 1995)?

This analysis lacked differential diagnosis. Much difference exists between Don and someone who clearly has only weeks left to live in making a decision to determine the circumstances of death. This chapter is *not* about clients like Don, whose primary problem is clinical depression that can be treated through antidepressant medication and counseling. What I want to explore here is our obligation to support our clients for whom suicide is "rational" and may be more appropriately called "self-deliverance."

Mancoske, in response to my article in *Social Work* (Holtby, 1996b), referred to me as "one obviously seasoned in the trenches" (Mancoske, 1996, p. 325) but dismissed my views to "lingering despair within the helping professions" (p. 325) and "being overwhelmed by the pandemic" (p. 325). The first part is true; the statements about my motivation are not. I do not despair because I do not believe death is a failure. I am not overwhelmed because this is a time of hope (with the antiviral cocktails now available) but also because I believe healing does not necessarily involve life at all costs and circumstances. Mancoske cited Hitler's Germany, when helping professionals facilitated euthanasia for the handicapped as part of the "final solution," saying, "Only if families found hope and advocated for these doomed children did the children survive the extermination camps" (Mancoske, 1996, p. 325). I am appalled that such a comparison is made to considerations about self-deliverance. I believe I *am* an advocate for my clients who want the option of suicide as insurance against unbearable pain and suffering. Regarding hope, I have seen the destructiveness of refusal to accept the inevitable and medical reality, particularly in the face of desperate insistences to "hang on" or judgments about "giving up."

I also believe I do not have a right to impose my values upon my clients. In Mancoske's first article, he and his co-authors stated, "Although autonomy is encouraged, it is limited when an individual's good is threatened, as with suicide" (p. 784). This is true for suicide, as I would define it (see Table 16.1), but not in instances of self-deliverance, in which the question is not whether to die but how and when. In these instances, who are we to presume what is in the individual's best interest? As mental health professionals, we have a higher standard to live up to—*the client's right to self-determination.*

The following statement was issued by the American Psychological Association in 1997:

> The American Psychological Association does not advocate for or against assisted suicide. What psychologists do support is high quality end-of-life care and informed end-of-life decisions based on the correct assessment of the patient's mental capacity, social support systems and degree of self-determination. . . .
>
> The role of the psychologist working with a terminally ill patient who wishes to end his or her life is not to control the patient's

decision, but to attempt to ensure that his or her decision-making process is rational, well reasoned and free of coercion. (1997, p. 3)

The statement from the APA also delineated the following issues as part of the psychologist's role in helping terminally ill patients make end-of-life decisions:

- Protect the clients rights.
- Support the family and significant others.
- Do not allow physicians to affix a mental illness diagnosis if inappropriate.
- Help evaluate if the patient has the capacity to make a rational decision.

The 1993 National Association of Social Workers (NASW) Delegate Assembly reinforced social workers' commitment to client self-determination as the "key value," specifically as it relates to end-of-life decisions:

Social workers should be free to participate or not participate in assisted-suicide matters or other discussions concerning end-of-life decisions depending on their beliefs, attitudes, and value systems. If a social worker is unable to help with decisions about assisted suicide or other end-of-life choices, he or she has a professional obligation to refer patients and their families to competent professionals who are available to address end-of-life issues. (NASW, 1994, p. 59)

A colleague wrote to me about his belief that it is the client's right to take his or her own life under such circumstances but described a "don't ask/don't tell" policy. He clearly states to his client that if the client wants to end his or her life, then the client must stop talking with him about doing it. He explains that if the client is not discussing it with him, then he cannot intervene. I believe this is abandoning our clients at a crucial time. Not only should we help clients explore all the feelings and ramifications of their behavior, we should make sure they are well informed and prepared to kill themselves without violence or crippling attempts and, further, to do it in a way that minimizes endangering their loved ones legally and emotionally. Finally, I believe our equal consideration of *all* end-of-life options can actually *increase* the chances of a natural death.

I recently had breakfast with a colleague who is considering helping her best friend die. She is relieved to have me to talk to, knowing I will make sure she is well informed and emotionally supported rather than judged or prevented. That, I believe, is our role.

I also believe supporting self-deliverance does not mean personally assisting. I concur with the NASW policy statement in this regard:

> It is inappropriate for social workers to deliver, supply, or personally participate in the commission of an act of assisted suicide when acting in their professional role. Doing so may subject the social worker to criminal charges. If legally permissible, it is not inappropriate for a social worker to be present during an assisted suicide if the client requests the social worker's presence. (NASW, 1994, p. 60)

My views about abandoning our clients when they need us most have been greatly shaped by one of my own cases, in which my client, Bill, helped his partner (Greg) die. It was only after that event that he came to see me—for PTSD. Greg had wasting syndrome; he had lost eighty pounds, had severe diarrhea and incontinence, and was so weak he could not hold a book to read. He had been told he could live another two months or more in this condition. He repeatedly pleaded with Bill to help him die, as well as everyone else who came to visit him. He pressured Bill with anger and withdrawal. Finally, when Bill relented and agreed, Greg became a changed person—elated, "like he'd just won the lottery."

This couple did not have a mental health professional's support at this point. They did have a hospice nurse but felt the hospice philosophy and policies prevented seeking support from this source. A friend who was an RN did help by providing pills for an overdose. As an afterthought, she had suggested, "Just to make sure, you can put a plastic bag over the person's head." Greg had said, "That's fine; whatever it takes. I just don't want to be here anymore." She gave no explanation of how long the drugs would take or the proper use of the plastic bag.

It is the middle of the night, and Greg has taken all the pills—but he seems only to be sleeping peacefully. Bill is worried that Greg's daughter will wake up in the morning and come downstairs. He believes they are running out of time. I will let Bill tell the rest of the story in his own words:

> I think when it got to about 3:00 or 3:30 in the morning I started freaking out thinking he was still alive. He was very much alive and breathing just fine, and so I tried to wake him up, and I guess I started panicking, and I guess I said to him, "Do you still want to do this?" And I swear in my mind he said, "Yes"—mumbled the word yes.
>
> So I waited about another hour, and then I thought, I have to do something soon, because once it becomes morning, and then his daughter comes down, and he's not gone, and it could be—well, who knows what would happen? I was afraid that the amount of medica-

tion, if it didn't kill him, would put him in a coma or would make him a vegetable, and then he would die naturally anyway, after how many days, but I didn't want them to know. I didn't want anyone to know. Because I really thought I was getting away with murder, and I was terrified. I remember at the beginning the blinds weren't closed, out to the backyard, and there really isn't any way anybody could see in because we had a big tree, and the garage was back there. Then I remember when I finally did decide to use the plastic bag—that was probably about 4:00, 4:30 in the morning—then I closed the blinds completely, but I kept looking around the whole time, because. . . .

The first time I did the plastic bag, I put it on top of his head, and I made sure there were no airholes, and I laid on top of him over a pillow. I don't know how long—it seemed like it was forever—and I swear, I put my ear to his chest and I felt his nose and stuff and there was no movement. So I took the plastic bag and I hid it—I don't even know where. Not that that would've done anything. And I went back in, and all of a sudden he goes [gasp], and it's like he was just holding it in and stuff. I thought he was gone, but he wasn't, and so he was taking this big deep breath. So at that point, I really freaked out, and I got two plastic bags, and I really made sure that they were tight, and I got a pillow, and I just lay on top of him.

It was really strange, but there was no going back at that point. So it probably took more than five minutes. I really wanted to make sure the second time, because I wasn't going to do it again.

I'm sure he was drugged enough to where there probably wasn't any pain or consciousness on his part. He was making a move; at the very end he made a movement and a sound of gasping for breath, because the whole plastic bag was really molded to his face because there was no air. His legs might have tensed up a little bit, moved up a little bit; his arms might have moved just a little bit, but no . . . no struggling. Definitely no.

And then I couldn't tell because my heart was beating so fast, and I kept hearing something, and I thought: Is that his heart or is that my heart? I had to call a friend with a stethoscope, and he confirmed Greg was gone because I couldn't tell.

I picture that person laying on top of Greg with two plastic bags and a pillow, and it just doesn't seem like it was me.

I believe this whole scenario was too ill-informed, too ill-prepared, too violent, too traumatic, and too unsupported and isolated for both Greg and Bill. It did not have to be this way.

On the other hand, I do not believe the answer was to hospitalize Greg because he was a "danger to himself or others." In fact, a hospital would have been the *worst* place for him to end up. A recent study published in *JAMA* (Seneff et al., 1995) monitored 9,000 critically ill patients at five major medical centers. The findings suggest that many patients painfully linger for days or weeks in intensive care units—despite living wills and medical directives. *Newsweek* quoted Dr. William Knaus of the University of Virginia Health Sciences Center, one of the study's authors, as concluding, "the system doesn't know when to stop" (Cowley and Hager, p. 74).

Hospice care would have been a good alternative, allowing for pain management without preventing the natural dying process. Greg did have a hospice nurse, who did not realize at the time the sense of panic he was experiencing over his lingering life. This nurse later told me if he had known he would have advised Greg to just stop eating and drinking. He predicted Greg would have died within days in his weakened condition. This, in fact, was what happened to Bill when his time came.

Yet hospice is not always an acceptable answer. Intolerable pain and suffering is a subjective concept and not just a matter of physical pain. In fact, I believe suffering is derived primarily from emotional rather than physical distress. In Greg's case, it was a fear of lingering for an interminable period with diapers, diarrhea, and deadening weakness and fatigue. Here again, there is a role for us as mental health professionals: if we can ameliorate emotional distress, we can minimize the suffering.

This was the case when Bill's life was at its end. He was filled with anxiety, which caused insomnia and agitation. When he checked out of the hospice, I received a panicky call from his partner (whom he had met after Greg's death and had now been with three years):

"Bill's going to kill himself, and he wants me to help. I said I would."

"When?"

"Tomorrow."

"Wait a minute, slow down here," I said. "How are you going to do it?"

John replied, "Bill wants me to put a plastic bag over his head, cover his face with a pillow, and then sit on him until he stops struggling."

"Bad idea!" I said, "It is likely you will be charged with manslaughter; let alone what it would do to you emotionally. I'd be treating you for post-traumatic stress disorder! It's too violent and may not actually work."

"What can I do?" John asked. "He is totally obsessed with finding a way to die before he gets too sick and weak. He is still 160 pounds, and he thinks if he dies naturally, it will take months."

I was able to intervene with Bill by getting him to accept a plan that involved waiting until the Canadian Right to Die Society could send him an "exit bag" (a cellophane bag which is to be placed over the person's head and secured around the neck to ensure suffocation). In this way, he did not need to involve John, and we had time to talk about what pills to take and how to avoid throwing them up in the process of taking them. I had purposely built into the plan a delaying tactic to test his resolve. Bill used the option of self-deliverance as a security blanket. With the knowledge that he did not have to fear the lingering death he saw Greg go through, he turned his attention to living his last days rather than being preoccupied with how he would die. John took him in a wheelchair to the botanic gardens, and the two of them had several nice talks about their time together. Bill subsequently was readmitted to hospice and died there peacefully and naturally. Near the end, he experienced alternating periods of delirium and lucidity. He sat up in bed at one point and anxiously asked John, "Did it come?"

"What? What?" John asked.

"The bag," Bill replied.

By then of course, it was too late to use the bag, but it was—to the end—a comforting thought. A week after Bill died, his "exit bag" arrived in the mail.

As I hope you can see from the foregoing examples, there is a difference between self-deliverance and suicide. Part of our role as clinicians is to be sensitive to these differences and adjust our interventions accordingly (see Table 16.1). Of course, it is never as clear-cut as the table suggests. This is where our ability to assess the issues and level of functioning of our clients comes into play.

Two final considerations must be emphasized. The first has to do with pain management. The medical profession has tended to underdose and not be sufficiently responsive to their patients' complaints about pain. On the other hand, hospice personnel have generally become experts at dealing with pain. Richard Baer, RN, from Hospice of Metro Denver has frequently asserted, "It's not always blissful and peaceful, but always workable." Thus, if your client's desire for self-deliverance is based primarily on unrelenting, unbearable pain, the symptoms need to be addressed. It is quite likely that with palliative care there will be no further motivation to use this option. This was underscored by the U.S. Supreme Court Decision in 1997 that ruled physician-assisted suicide was not a constitutional right. However, there was the inference, particularly in Justice Sandra Day O'Connor's opinion, that adequate pain management was.

The second consideration is fear. In the example of Bill, his self-deliverance desires had to do with his fear that he would linger for weeks or

TABLE 16.1. Differentiating and Assessing Suicide and Self-Deliverance

Suicide	Self-Deliverance
1. Generally associated with clinical depression.	1. Client not depressed, although he or she may be physically exhausted from prolonged illness.
2. Generally associated with getting a positive HIV-test result, the first OI diagnosis, or facing disability; yet still relatively healthy.	2. Clearly at the end point of the disease, with multiple OIs, extensive weight loss, etc. (It is no longer a question if the person is dying, more a matter of when and how).
3. Generally an impulsive act, not involving an educated well-thought-out plan.	3. Often involves preparatory reading, e.g., *Final Exit,* and extensive letters and instructions and will left behind.
4. Often is an *attempt,* due to ineffective methods and ambivalence about actual desire to die.	4. Usually lacking ambivalence and clearly meant to end in death by methods used.
5. Obsessive about their focus on suicide, with no willingness to accept an alternative.	5. Will consider hospice care and other options. Often utilize self-deliverance as a security blanket, "If things get bad enough," which is usually *not* used.
6. Has underlying dynamics of shame, or "everyone would be better off without me here." Cannot accept caretaking.	6. Is concerned with the stress on caregivers but has come to terms with being dependent upon them.
7. Is living with a lot of unfinished emotional business.	7. Is resolved with loved ones.
8. Has a desire to be remembered as healthy, in control, and independent. As illness proceeds, this person will withdraw from family and friends.	8. Often very connected to friends and family, who under the right circumstances will support the decision to take one's own life. A plan may involve elaborate "good-byes" with loved ones.
9. A sense of nothing to live for, despair, hopelessness.	9. Not particularly despairing, often exploring spirituality and afterlife issues with professionals and close friends.
10. Dementia or signs of mental incompetence.	10. Mentally competent.

months as Greg had done. This was aggravated by his first roommate at hospice who seemed to be dying in a very similar way. Even more than pain, fear is the vehicle of uncomfortable deaths. Fear is also a factor for many considering controlling how they die. One member of my HIV group was close to dying naturally, was bedridden, and at that point was only able to take small sips of water. The group met around his bed, and he suggested we overdose him with his morphine. His wanting to die in this way was due to his fear that if he died "naturally" it would be with a sensation of choking until he was unconscious or dead. Most of the group had been with partners and friends when they died and were able to allay fears that his passing would be violent. He never brought it up again.

I would like to end with a description of a scenario in which appropriate intervention helped, as did the support of friends, family, and a physician. But its outcome was a "positive" self-deliverance. When Dan died, it was only after a long period during which he prepared—months—for death. His will and medical directives were meticulously completed, as were all other personal arrangements, including detailed instructions for his cremation and memorial service. He left behind letters to all those people close to him, as well as instructions to emergency medical personnel in the event they attempted to intervene. He did not exercise the option of self-deliverance until the level of his health reached the bedridden stage, and he was exhausted from protracted, multiple infections. At that point, he gathered around him his friends and family; candles lit his room, and special music played. He said individual good-byes to all those in attendance. When the time finally came, he injected himself through his catheter with an overdose of morphine. He lay beside his partner of many years and peacefully left everyone behind, resolved and ready for his departure. Who are we to "intervene" and deny him such a death?

BIBLIOGRAPHY

American Psychological Association. (1997). *Terminal illness and hastened death requests: The important role of the mental health professional.* Washington, DC: American Psychological Association, Office of Public Communications.

Cowley, G. C., Hager, M. (1995). Terminal care: Too painful, too prolonged. *Newsweek,* December 4, p. 74.

Holtby, Michael E. (1995). Assisted suicide: Sometimes goes wrong. *Resolute!* April, *4*(3), 10-11.

Holtby, Michael E. (1995a). Fear of dying. *Resolute!* June, *4*(5), 11-12.

Holtby, Michael E. (1995b). Self-deliverance as a security blanket. *Resolute!*, November, *4*(9), 10-11.

Holtby, Michael E. (1996a). Dignity dead in committee. *Resolute!*, March, *5*(2), 13.

Holtby, Michael E. (1996b). HIV/AIDS and suicide: Be open. *Social Work, 41*(3), 324.

Mancoske, R. J. (1996). HIV/AIDS and suicide: Further precautions. *Social Work, 41*(3), 325.

Mancoske, R. J., Wadsworth, C. M., Dugas, D. S., and Hasney, J. A. (1995). Suicide risk among people living with AIDS. *Social Work, 40*(6), 783-787.

National Association of Social Workers (1994). Client self-determination in end-of-life decisions. *Social Work Speaks* (Third Edition). Washington, DC: NASW Press, pp. 58-61.

Seneff, M. G., Wagner, D. P., Wagner, R. P., Zimmerman, J., and Knaus, W. (1995). Hospital and one-year survival of patients admitted to intensive care units with acute exacerbation of chronic obstructive pulmonary disease. *Journal of the American Medical Association, 274*(23), 1852-1857.

SUGGESTED READINGS AND RESOURCES

Available Through Your Local Book Store

Humphry, Derek (1991). *Final Exit: The Practicalities of Self-Deliverance and Assisted Suicide for the Dying.* New York: Dell. A book considered a standard by many about the details and complications of taking one's own life.

Shavelson, Lonny (1995). *A Chosen Death: The Dying Confront Assisted Suicide.* New York: Simon and Schuster. I highly recommend this book, written by a physician and journalist. He interviews in detail a number of people considering self-deliverance—some of whom follow through; others who, in the end, do not. The book includes a good discussion of all the issues involved but is personalized through case studies.

Available Through The Right to Die Society of Canada

Smith, Cheryl and Chris Docker (1995). *Beyond Final Exit.* Victoria, BC: RDSC. Instructions on how to order and use an "exit bag," as well as other ways to die, including fasting.

Smith, Cheryl and Chris Docker (1993). *Departing Drugs.* Victoria, BC: RDSC. In-depth discussion of drugs, dosages, pitfalls, and complications.

Organizations

Compassion in Dying
Ralph Mero, Executive Director
PO Box 75295, Seattle, WA 98125-0295
(206) 624-2775
Fax: (206) 624-2673

ERGO! Euthanasia Research & Guidance Organization
Derek Humphry, President
24829 Norris Lane, Junction City, OR 97448
(541) 998-1873
Fax: (same)
Web site: http://www.efn.org/~ergo

The Hemlock Society USA
Faye Girsh, PhD, Executive Director
PO Box 101810, Denver, CO 80250
(800) 247-7421
Web site: http://www.hemlock.org/hemlock
E-mail: hemlock@privatei.com

The Right to Die Society of Canada
John Hofsess, Executive Director
PO Box 39018, Victoria, BC, Canada V8V 4X8
(604) 386-4583
Fax: (604) 386-3800
Web site: http://www.org/~deathnet/open.html
E-mail: jh@islandnet.com

Chapter 17

"Storytelling" in a Bereavement Support Group for Pediatric HIV/AIDS Case Managers of the Brooklyn Pediatric AIDS Network

David Strug
Craig Podell
Martine Cesaire
Roy Ferdinand
Hillary Kallor
Dorothy Moore
Josephine Walker

INTRODUCTION

This chapter is about the pediatric HIV/AIDS case managers of the Brooklyn Pediatric AIDS Network (Network),[1,2] and the stories they tell about working with sick and dying children and grieving family members. These stories are told in the Network's unique bereavement support group, a safe and empathic milieu for case managers to relate what it means "to live" with HIV/AIDS, not their own illness, but that of the children and the families with whom they work.

Storytelling in this group facilitates the expression of deeply experienced feelings, including loss, rage, hopelessness, love, and joy, as well as

The authors wish to acknowledge the dedicated efforts of all the Network case managers who comprise the total membership of the support group this chapter describes. Network staff, especially Network Director Dr. Hermann Mendez and Project Director Sheri Saltzberg, read this chapter and made very useful comments. Dr. Ruth Ottman provided invaluable editorial assistance.

moral indignation over limited institutional and societal responses to the AIDS epidemic. It plays a key role in helping case managers carry out emotionally traumatic work over time.

Telling one's story to an audience of peers who share similar experiences is extremely healing and powerful. This power derives, in part, from the story's highly metaphorical, image-rich narrative. It also comes from the makeup of the bereavement support group, which is comprised of peers with similar experiences who "mirror" or reflect the feelings of the storyteller. Narrative offers a way to contemplate the ineffable and the abstract by way of the concrete (Mattingly and Garro, 1995), making the technique very relevant to telling stories about death and dying.

Narrative production in this bereavement support group facilitates the expression of oftentimes frightening emotional experience (feelings of rage, loss, helplessness, uselessness) through the use of metaphor that is embedded in social and cultural context. This narrative production allows case managers to access feelings that might otherwise remain inaccessible to consciousness. Storytelling in the group can help the case manager who may be overwhelmed with deep feelings of pain and despair create a plan of action to help children and families cope with the effect of HIV/AIDS.

Storytelling not only reflects the subjective, emotional experience of the case manager, but also reflects the extrasubjective "institutional landscape" (Saris, 1995) in which these case managers work and live. Narrative production, we note, can reflect workers' indignation over inadequate institutional and societal responses to the impact of HIV/AIDS on families, especially poor families. Through their narrative production, group members can express the wide-ranging feelings (anger, pain, sadness) of the individuals with whom they work who themselves are often without a forum for the direct expression of these feelings because of their poverty, alienation, and marginal status in society.

THE BEREAVEMENT GROUP

The Network bereavement support group has been in existence for over five years. It is attended by a total of eleven case managers who work at six different hospital-based pediatric HIV/AIDS programs, at one community-based organization, and at one foster care agency specializing in the placement and care of HIV-infected children. These nine sites are affiliated with the Brooklyn Pediatric AIDS Network of the SUNY Health Science Center, Brooklyn. This group meets at the same SUNY location on a monthly basis. The group facilitator, a consultant, is not a regular Network staff member. Case managers also meet each week at this same location with the Network's case management coordinator, who also attends the bereavement support group. The purpose of this weekly meeting is multiple. It is a source of information that has elements of support, but it is not devoted to bereavement issues per se.

Methods

The coordinator and group facilitator met on three occasions with five of the eleven members of the bereavement group. They asked group members a series of open-ended questions about their work with infected children and their families such as: "How has your participating in the group made a difference in the ways you work with HIV-infected children and their families?" "What is most difficult for you about working with an infected child who is sick and dying?" and "What effect did coming to the group have on you at that difficult time?"

In addition, the coordinator met separately with two of these case managers to talk in depth with them about their work with particular families described in this chapter. All responses were tape-recorded and transcribed. The data presented here come from case narrative responses to interview questions that were subsequently transcribed and analyzed for the purpose of writing this chapter.

Results

Burnout and the Group

Losing children to AIDS, seeing children deteriorate physically, and working closely with grieving, traumatized families all contribute to feelings of burnout or emotional exhaustion, depersonalization, and personal inefficacy (Maslach and Jackson, 1982) among case managers.

The following graphically depicts one worker's feeling of being "burnt-out" resulting from the loss of many children in her caseload over the years due to AIDS:

> I guess everyone has a different level of tolerance about death, depending on how much you've seen. I have seen twenty-seven kids. I have seen more death. I know what I can tolerate. At one point I felt worn down by the multiple deaths, when there were six or seven kids who died in one month. I felt like a compact machine, almost like an accordion; it's a shock; you feel extremely drained by it, then another child [dies]; it's a horrible feeling, and that is when you have to step

back and reevaluate your feelings, and think about how you feel. It's not easy.

The effect of observing asymptomatic children physically deteriorate can also lead to emotional exhaustion:

I felt, "here we go again." I felt angry at everybody. I know this little girl is so special, I felt why her, why *now?* I know they are all going to die; I am clear about that—but why *now?*

Feelings of anger, depression, and helplessness appear in case managers' stories about sick children:

[The child was] crying and shivering and stuff. It made me feel helpless, really helpless; her medication wasn't working, residents were really not empathic. They would say, "She still has the fever," and would walk out. Just another case to them. But to me, this was Y (my patient). [I felt] Helpless and useless. 'Cause there was nothing I could do—talk to her, pray and stuff, and other than that, nothing.

The following illustrates how case managers can identify with the infected child:

I know if I was like that I wouldn't want to live to that point. It's terrible, and you are losing all of the functions of your organs. It's horrible. That's when you see how horrible and disastrous AIDS is, especially for children. Especially for teenagers. It scares them; they are afraid of themselves. It's a horrible sight.

Secondary Traumatization

Workers tell what it is like to work with the suffering family member thereby coping with "secondary traumatic stress" or the stress workers experience when they want to help the traumatized or suffering family member (Figley, 1995):

It is tough, having to come to grips, seeing someone you worked with who was healthy at one point, and has gotten to the point where they are ready to pass on and have to deal with that. With the family members, discussing the funeral arrangements, and having to be there with that family member and seeing them cry, what they have to go through to make those arrangements—it is tough. It is not easy.

Increasingly, case managers must cope with helping orphaned children deal with the loss of biological parents, especially mothers who have died from AIDS. One case manager describes her initial uncomfortable feelings about attending a funeral for the mother of a child on her caseload:

> The mother of my eleven-year-old patient just died. I was a little concerned how my presence at the funeral would be perceived . . . When I approached her, she threw her arms around my waist, and as I leaned over, hugging her back, we were both crying.

Lack of Institutional Supports

Many case managers work at sites lacking adequate emotional support mechanisms for workers; there is little opportunity to talk openly about illness and death with supervisory staff, as the following narrative indicates:

> Where I work they do not know how to talk about a child's death, which is very interesting. Once I cried in front of my supervisor and he just stood there not knowing what to do. He said, "I wish I knew more about death and dying and about kids so I could really help you." I think some of these supervisors are scared themselves to talk about kids and death.

The Importance of the Bereavement Support Group

The bereavement group was established by the Network to help workers talk about the kinds of stressful emotional reactions they experience working with children and families that we have described here. Case managers indicate the group helps them in this regard:

> I think you would get burnt-out quicker without the group. The group is an outlet.

> There would be much more stress without the group, if you did not have somebody to vent to about what is going on, so I can feel free, and get some support and answers. I think the group is helpful, or else I just would have been burnt-out.

INSTITUTIONAL AND SOCIAL CRITIQUE

Storytelling also allows case managers to critique and discuss objectively their perceptions of institutional and societal shortcomings with regard to the AIDS epidemic. For example, the following story, told by one of the case managers, is about alleged medical mismanagement of a dying child by medical staff at her hospital. She began her narrative with a description of her emotional state when she was telling her story in the bereavement support group:

> I just broke apart and tissues were coming from everywhere. Hugs were coming . . . a pat on the back . . . it was like being found. I felt so lost and was drowning, and now I was found. . . . It felt like my heart was made out of stone; that's how strong my feelings were for this kid [her patient], and I felt like I let him down, 'cause he died, and he died in a wrong fashion, and he died begging for water, and afterward I found that he could have gotten the water [from staff]. And they [the nurses] were saying no, no, no [he can't have it].

She then described feelings of support given by the group:

> [I felt] saved [by the group]. It was a nice, nice feeling; it was the same day the child died, and I went to the Network meeting. I felt like I was crawling through mud or something. And to sit there and share, everybody was just wonderful . . . I felt like I was barely making it physically, and I didn't want to go home that way.

Finally, she noted how a plan of action resulted from telling her story in the group:

> The group showed me this place [the hospital] was wrong what they did to him. So I wrote my letter and advocated for him even though he was dead. It was a form of therapy for me, like I asked myself: What are you going to do about it? What happens now? At that time, I had twenty-six cases. It didn't have to happen that way. Was I going to go through the same thing with them? It scared me. What if they all die in the same way? What if they treat all the kids on my caseload the same way?

A BABY NEEDS BURYING

The following summarizes an experience of one of the case managers. It also illustrates how storytelling can transform feelings of pain into a plan for resolving problems that arise in the group, allowing the group to express moral indignation in reaction to society's inadequate responses to the AIDS epidemic.

Z came to the group quite upset and with a dilemma. A very sick, eighteen-month-old baby on her caseload had just died in the hospital. The baby's mother, a woman addicted to drugs, had disappeared and was unreachable. No other family members were available. Z, a new mother, was clearly distraught when she told her story to the group. Z had spoken about the situation with her supervisor at the hospital where she works but felt that her supervisor did not have specific information about how to proceed in such a situation. Z was now bringing the issue to the support group.

"There's no way this baby is going to be buried in a potter's field in an unmarked grave. What's going to happen when the mother comes back? She'll never know where her baby is buried," Z stated to the group.

The group empathically listened to Z's story and identified with her feelings, as case managers who, similar to Z, felt they could not possibly allow the baby to be buried in a common grave.

Members suggested Z make calls to several individuals with experience in handling situations such as this one. Z received the emotional support and information from the other group members that allowed her to leave that day feeling emotionally in control, more optimistic than she began, and more certain of how to proceed.

She followed the group's suggestion during the next week. One person she contacted suggested Z obtain legal authority to bury the baby. Z never did so because the baby's biological mother reappeared and stated she had already made arrangements for the burial of her baby in a private cemetery. But the day of the funeral, the mother did not show up. Z and the funeral director called the state Department of Social Services which determined the mother had given sufficient legal consent for the burial to take place. The mother's presence was not required for the burial to proceed. Z left the funeral parlor certain the burial was to take place later that day.

A week passed, and Z returned to the group to continue telling her story of what had happened. Z began in a calm voice; members listened carefully. Z told of being left alone with the funeral director at the funeral parlor a few hours before the actual burial of the baby was to occur. Two case managers from a city agency abandoned Z there because they did not think the child should be buried without the mother present. Z spoke of how she and the funeral director sat in front of an open coffin that contained the small and disfigured body of the baby.

As Z told her story, and as she heard the emotional response of the other members, she became overwhelmed with emotion. Telling her story before an empathic audience of peers gave Z the opportunity to both experience and express her emotional upset and then to receive emotional support from the group.

DISCUSSION

Looking death in the eye, experiencing shock, feeling emotionally drained, like "an empty accordion," asking, "Why death, again, now?"; experiencing helplessness, uselessness, feeling as if you are "crawling through mud," feeling "lost and drowned," stressed; seeing family members cry—these are some of the ways Network case managers expressed their subjective responses to working with infected children and grieving families in the bereavement support group.

Yet when such powerful and highly metaphorical, image-rich narrative is produced by the storyteller and told to group members who feel the same emotions and share similar experiences, healing and restoration can occur. Burnout may be lessened. By telling a story, the narrator can feel "found, saved."

Narrative, however, not only reflects subjective emotional experience but, as noted before, can also mirror the extrasubjective reactions of workers to the institutional and social context in which they work and live. We saw, for example, how story narrative reflected case managers' reactions to what seemed to be the unempathic response of some doctors to working with infected children, the alleged medical mismanagement of a dying, infected child, the reluctance of many health care workers to talk openly about death- and dying-related issues, and the lack of adequate emotional support for case managers where they work.

Storytelling, as we noted, also allows the narrator and the group to express moral indignation over institutional and societal shortcomings with regard to the needs of children and families affected by the AIDS epidemic. Z's story resonated with the group's deeply felt sympathy for the rights of children, for poor people in general, and for HIV-infected individuals.

Her story tapped the group's angry frustration against the idea of a baby being tossed, like garbage, into a hole in the ground in a city dump. The story and the group's response were strong statements for the right of a mother to know where her baby is buried regardless of whether the mother is drug addicted and whether she has "abandoned" her baby as a result of psychological distress. Z's narrative mobilized the group to support her extraordinary, even heroic, actions.

CONCLUSION

The danger to case managers of not openly addressing their strong emotional reactions to work with sick and dying children and with suffering, traumatized family members (vicarious traumatization) is that it may affect their ability to manage those powerful sentiments, to maintain a positive sense of themselves, and to stay connected to others (Figley, 1995).

Groups such as this are recommended as a particularly powerful way for workers to deal with their feelings. Storytelling is restorative not only because it allows the narrator to experience catharsis but because it allows the storyteller to do so among peers who share similar experiences and feelings. The moral indignation of the narrator ignites that of the entire group.

There are, of course, additional ways for case managers and other health care workers to manage stress, including peer supervision, informal alliances with others at the work site, and taking time off from work, among others. However, a bereavement support group such as the one described here can play a special role for workers coping with stress precisely because it affords an audience for the storyteller to describe powerful feelings, through the use of image-rich metaphor, to individuals who share similar concerns and experiences.

NOTES

1. *The Brooklyn Pediatric AIDS Network,* located at the *SUNY Health Science Center* in Brooklyn, is a federally-funded *Ryan White Title IV CARE Act* project which has been in existence since 1989.
2. The work on which this paper is based was supported with funding by the RYAN WHITE CARE Act, Title IV, MCH-P02047.

REFERENCES

Figley, C. R. (Ed.) (1995). *Compassion fatigue: Coping with secondary traumatic stress disorder in those who treat the traumatized.* New York: Brunner/Mazel Publishers.

Maslach, C. (1982). *Burnout: The cost of caring.* New York: Prentice Hall.

Mattingly, C. and Garro, L. (1995). "Introduction." *Social Science and Medicine, 38*(6), pp. 771-774.

Saris, J. (1995). "Telling stories: Life histories, illness narratives, and institutional landscapes." *Culture, Medicine, and Psychiatry, 19*(1), pp. 39-72.

Chapter 18

Social Work with Hospitalized AIDS Patients: Observations from the Front Lines of an Inner-City Hospital

Barbara Halin-Willinger
Martha Powers
Chris Carlson
Lorna Lee
Mary Beaudet
Miriam Bernson
John Kleinschmidt

In the time since the AIDS pandemic burst upon us, there have been many changes in the treatment of this illness that affect the length of a patient's hospitalization. However, what remains constant is the spectrum of issues facing our patients, including receiving the diagnosis, entitlement referrals, coping and living with HIV/AIDS, and eventually decline and death. Additionally, our patients' lives are often further complicated by substance abuse, character pathology, poverty, racism, and tenuous family supports. Much of the work, therefore, on our inpatient unit can become crisis driven or focused on short-term, goal-oriented interventions. Although this type of work, in and of itself, is effective, the model used by this group of writers, as well as others, encompasses a broader perspective known as "continuity of care." This model allows staff the potential for involvement in the patient's life and the development of a therapeutic relationship over time, as well as for the exigencies of transference and countertransference reactions.

As patients struggle with the devastating effects of HIV/AIDS, so too, although differently, do staff. It is well documented that those who work with PWAs must be vigilant against emotional fatigue and demoralization

(Rando, 1984; Robbins, 1983; Winiarski, 1991). This chapter is the culmination of discussions by a team of social workers and their supervisor about the common and disparate ways each needed and/or sought support. Additionally, their personal accounts are placed in the context of an already existing schematic progression of adaptation to working with the terminally ill from the perspective of the professional caregiver. Our experiences also support the work of Ross (1993), Anderson and Wilke (1991), McCann and Pearlman (1990), and Winiarski (1991), who all discuss the necessity of good clinical supervision to ensure longevity and avoid painful burnout and isolation. Clinical supervision is defined as a place and a person with whom the work can be processed.

HARPER MODEL: RESPONSES AND VIGNETTES

Kübler-Ross (1969) developed a series of stages defining patients' processes regarding their cancer diagnosis that helped clinicians to understand and frame their clinical work. Harper (1977) developed a schematic growth and development scale that described the normative sequence of emotional and psychological progress which health care professionals traversed to reach a comfort level which allowed them to work with patients facing death. Similar to the stages created by Kübler-Ross, in which patients can either fluidly shift from one stage to the other or remain stalled in one place, so too the Harper model needs to be viewed as a process in which professional caregivers will proceed and regress. The model is presented by using illustrations of the authors' personal experiences juxtaposed with case vignettes.

The first stage described by Harper is the use of intellectualization. During this stage, the professional focuses on professional knowledge as a means to decrease latent anxieties of working with the dying patient and facing the resultant death. Within the parameters of the acute care hospital unit and one's adaptation to the setting, we have found that this process takes at least six months.

Chris, on the unit eight months at the time of this writing, is the father of two children who came to social work as a second career. His position on the AIDS unit was his first inpatient experience, and similar to most new workers, he found himself "treading into a new sea of systems, acronyms, and abbreviations." During the entry into AIDS work, paperwork can often symbolize realizable and tangible tasks on the patients' behalf that are more quantifiable than the counseling process often is.

Chris brought to social work his sense of community service and history of activism and of wanting to improve individual and community systems. Although intellectually aware that his "patients' set of circumstances are not mine to fix" he carefully worked on where to enter into each patient's struggle "against the undertow of helplessness" often associated with terminal illness. At the same time, Chris kept his own perspective about such helplessness. Processing these contrapuntal but always colliding forces became the initial goals of supervision and in staff support group.

Chris recalls experiencing much frustration in his first months, as he spent more time learning systems than working with patients. Along with the immersion in paperwork, Chris experienced the overwhelming emotional barrage of the cycle of illness and death. "I still couldn't, professionally speaking, keep track of my practice work, my use of self, and the patients' needs as I wanted to. But I knew I was progressing, both learning more and discovering my realistic limitations. I was establishing a foundation of understanding that we are hand in hand with the larger forces of disease, death, and biology." The mastery of the initial stage facilitates the professional's concentration on the patient in a new way by allowing intense clinical relationships to be formed.

Harper's second stage entails the professional experiencing death on an emotional level while feeling traumatized as they confront the deaths of their patients and the reality of their own eventual mortality. John was hired as an inpatient AIDS social worker after completion of his graduate training, which had included a field placement on an AIDS unit. He had come to social work only after becoming aware of his own HIV seropositivity. John's ultimate disclosure of his HIV-positive status to his colleagues and supervisor was to have ramifications in his professional relationships as well as for his own personal growth.

John began work with Robert when the patient was admitted to the hospital with severe shortness of breath. He was soon diagnosed with Kaposi's sarcoma of the lungs. Robert, a twenty-three-year-old African-American college student, had only recently learned of his HIV-positive status. Robert formed an almost instantaneous alliance with John. Most likely this grew out of Robert's intense anxiety and helplessness as well as his need for mirroring and validation. The close relationship between worker and client was also aided by John's identification, sensitivity, and empathy for Robert. Their work together focused on minimizing Robert's feelings of shame and guilt, his fear of losses, and his need to confront reality and to develop coping strategies. After two and a half weeks of hospitalization, Robert was discharged home. He returned to his family who had not yet settled into an acceptance of Robert's health status or the fact that he was gay. Robert was given John's office telephone number for emergency contact, and within twenty-four hours, he called, complaining of shortness of breath and friction with his family. He was instructed to call the EMS. John returned to the hospital after the weekend to find Robert intubated, with medical personnel frantically trying to help him before he was to be transferred to the intensive care unit (ICU). Within a few minutes, John was made aware that the prognosis was poor.

John's journey and struggle with the impact of his own HIV status was reopened by Robert's situation. In the ensuing hours, John sought support from his supervisor and co-workers at their weekly unit meeting and later at their staff support group. Because John had previously revealed his status to his supervisor, their individual supervisory time was utilized in helping John differentiate his own fears and anxieties from those of Robert. In this way, John could face his anticipated grief and mourning for Robert. This catharsis and processing allowed John to be with Robert and Robert's family in a professionally caring way that did not merge or confuse John's issues and boundaries with the patient's.

Robert's situation provided John with his own watershed experience:

> . . . catalyzing my accumulated losses—friends, patients, self—and it all poured out. Without the support of my peers and the disclosure of my health status to my supervisor, I couldn't have processed this case. Robert's illness allowed me to find a working distance in which to continue without overwhelming emotional vulnerability. The work has since normalized.

In the absence of being able to confront one's own vulnerability, Harper postulates the third stage as "grow or go," in which mastery of self is a challenge. Such mastery involves an increasing acceptance of the realities of death and dying as well as the notion that we cannot make our patients well. Professional caregivers during this stage often vacillate between accepting death and denying its inevitability.

Martha had done a fieldwork placement in a counseling agency where she had worked with PWAs. She spent six months doing inpatient AIDS work with this team, then she was transferred to the program's outpatient clinic, where she spent a year before meeting Cynthia.

Cynthia was well known to the clinic but had avoided medical appointments for several years and was noncompliant with any treatment plans. Martha's first contact with Cynthia occurred as a result of Cynthia's need for insurance clarification. After initial reluctance, Cynthia agreed to meet with Martha. In their ongoing sessions, Cynthia raged about the unfairness of having AIDS and her fears regarding disclosure to her family and friends. She maintained distance by wearing dark sunglasses and leaving sessions when she became too tearful. When hospitalized within a few months of their first contact, Cynthia was seen by another social worker. Upon Cynthia's return to the clinic as an outpatient, she vociferously expressed her anger and disappointment at Martha's not making arrangements to cover her while hospitalized. It became clear to Martha that a strong alliance and transference had developed that could, and needed to, include any social work coverage Cynthia required. From that time on, their meetings were sustained through painful affect, but Cynthia no longer wore her dark glasses.

During a subsequent admission, Cynthia lapsed into a coma. It was during this time that Martha learned about Cynthia from her family. Her source of infection had come from a man whom she no longer planned to marry, but with whom she still lived. She had been raised by her grandmother. Her biological mother, although involved in Cynthia's upbringing, was someone for whom Cynthia held contempt. Both women had recently been told by Cynthia of her illness. In the same meeting with Martha and Cynthia's family, it was agreed that Cynthia's twenty-one-year-old daughter must also be told about her mother's illness. Martha was cognizant of her own profound sadness, not for someone she had known for years, but for someone with whom she had only recently developed an intimate attachment. While experiencing this anticipatory grief, Martha began to realize that professional relationships often engender deeper feelings of connectedness that are not always obvious until the patients are near death.

Quite unexpectedly, however, Cynthia came out of her coma and talked of wanting to return home. As Martha slowly proceeded with the arrangements, she also listened to Cynthia review her losses and failures in her life. Cynthia asked Martha to help her plan her funeral, eulogy, and cremation. Cynthia's health continued to decline during this time, and Martha waited for Cynthia's death.

Through supervision, Martha was able to unblock her feelings and identify her fear and pain as it related to the ebb and flow of Cynthia's deterioration toward death. When Cynthia died, Martha attended the funeral, feeling out of place since the only professional connection to Cynthia's family had been their meetings at the hospital. Martha mourned and reviewed her work with Cynthia in supervision and support group. In both settings, Martha began to let go of Cynthia and to find a place for her feelings, with the realization that she had assisted Cynthia in making peace with parts of her life.

Cynthia's case reflected the omnipresent struggle of professional versus personal self with which Martha had been grappling. Martha believed that "a professional stance always required distance." However, Cynthia's directness, despite her delirium and dementia, called for "my complete involvement. I battled with myself, saying, "Don't put lotion on her leg; don't wipe her brow; don't kiss her on the forehead." But Cynthia brought me right in. There was no way around my full use of self. While Cynthia demanded the human, she needed the professional, and if I had been there halfway, she would have kicked me out of the room." Some staff are not able to traverse this stage and either remain within it, grappling with the issues of professional connectedness to patients, or decide to leave the setting.

The next stage that Harper describes is one of emotional arrival, involving moderation, mitigation, and accommodation. It is during this stage that the worker leaves behind debilitating effects of the previous stages. This is also the stage at which professionals more readily accept death and dying and are not incapacitated by the depression they may feel concerning their own good health.

Miriam had several years of social work experience prior to graduate training. Although not a novice to AIDS work, St. Luke's was her first full-time hospital AIDS employment. An energetic and physically active woman, Miriam likens her work with patients to running a marathon. She often describes the work as requiring her "to pay close attention to the job of putting one foot in front of the other." She seeks to assist each patient in gaining a sense of control over the disease process, as incorporated into the patient-worker contract. This can vary from mourning his/her loss of attractiveness and/or position within his/her social system to planning for the future of survivors or facing the arduous and crisis-filled disease process.

Miriam began her work with Elbia soon after the patient was diagnosed with AIDS. Elbia had grown up in an impoverished region of Honduras. She married early and immigrated to New York City, where she raised her four children while suffering from periodic physical assault by her husband. When her husband was hospitalized with, and later died of, AIDS, Elbia knew she too had become infected. Rather than finding her life made easier by the death of her abusive husband, she found herself a virtual hostage in the family apartment, which her children had transformed into a crack house. In her passivity and shame, Elbia had created a self-imposed prison. She confided to Miriam that being hospitalized allowed her to feel "safe" for the first time in her life.

Over the two months that Elbia remained on the unit, she opened up her life through laughter and tears. She shared a side of herself that she had always kept hidden. She experienced a strong sense of control and destiny regarding death, which had eluded her in her lifetime, from her belief in Santeria. Miriam knew that Elbia related to her and the staff as the transferential "good mother." This was confirmed in Elbia's poignant plea not to be transferred to a nursing home: "This is the only place where anyone has ever cared about me . . . this is where I want to die." Although Elbia initially described her life as devoid of security, self-confidence, and environmental support—aspects of life highly valued by Miriam—by her life's end, Elbia had been able to attain these through the power of the relationship with Miriam and the other staff. As it turned out, Elbia did not have to endure another perceived abuse/abandonment; she died in the hospital. Watching Elbia die was painful for Miriam but is a frequent reality of working with AIDS patients.

Miriam was able to forge a deep relationship with Elbia that helped sustain her through the patient's long and erratic deterioration. The lengthy hospitalization "gave me the time to process things along the way, then to assist Elbia in working through her feelings of deprivation, and to die in peace. I was able to respect Elbia's strengths and remain her ally and partner in the process rather than her caretaker."

In the fifth and final stage of development, Harper refers to deep compassion involving self-realization, self-awareness and self-actualization. A "concern for the dying patient is translated into constructive and appropriate activities based on a humane and professional assessment of the dying patient and the family. They understand and accept that in some instances, living can be more painful than dying" (1977, p. 435).

Barbara, the supervising social worker for this team, met Darren, a thirty-five-year-old African-American gay man, when he was initially diagnosed with Kaposi's sarcoma of the lungs. A call from the physician requested social work intervention due to Darren's "upset reaction" to the news. During the initial consultation, Darren, a handsome young man, lay in bed, covers pulled up to his chin. It was quickly apparent that he was not going to engage in spontaneous conversation but rather needed and responded to gently asked questions, explanations about his medical condition, and statements regarding entitlements.

By the end of the of the first meeting, Darren had revealed that it was his characterological pattern to keep things to himself, "close to my chest." His friend later affirmed that Darren had shared a surprisingly significant amount of information with Barbara. Darren was discharged two days later and contact was sustained by telephone, as Darren struggled with the effects of chemotherapy and the ramifications of Kaposi's sarcoma. In the succeeding two months, Darren was admitted three times for about three days per admission. Although weaker, Darren refused home care. When questioned about this, he indicated that his family, with whom he lived, were available to take care of him. One day, Darren called

Barbara, sounding breathless and as if he were choking. He asked for nothing, was seemingly home alone, and consented to Barbara's calling 911. Barbara later discovered, when she called Darren back, that two family members were in fact at home but unaware of his current state. This was consistent with Darren's keeping his family "out of my business." Darren was admitted to the hospital. The family was grateful for Barbara's intervention, and Darren agreed to home care following this discharge from the hospital.

But time had run out for Darren, and within a week, he was readmitted for the last time. The purpose of Barbara's intervention was to clarify with the physician the need for palliative care, as well as being the compassionate visitor that Darren needed at this time, just two days prior to his death. It was only after Darren's burial that the family verbalized the importance that Darren had placed on his contact with Barbara. This resolved questions Barbara had had during her work with Darren, a reluctant and seemingly disconnected participant in his own treatment.

Barbara struggled with the treatment plan for Darren in his final months. She made decisions with and for him, based on her experience rather than on the explicit information communicated by him. The work with Darren represented for Barbara "much of the skill and expertise I have acquired and internalized over the years. The use of self as well as the continuing process of self-reflection often mesh into an ultimately gratifying experience that provides sustenance for this work."

A MODEL OF HOSPITAL AIDS WORK

How do those of us working with AIDS patients navigate the waters of grief and associated emotional turmoil? What is needed to assist and sustain us as we embark on and continue the journey of working with AIDS patients? Even the most accomplished professional cannot withstand the intensity and constancy of the onslaught of powerful feelings that erupt at varying times during the work, if there are insufficient supports. Even though our relationship with patients is usually peripheral rather than central, as are family and significant others, we too can experience "bereavement overload" (Rando, 1984, p. 430), unless the losses are processed. We can perhaps draw a parallel between PWAs who cope more effectively with their condition through the availability of support and professional caregivers whose potential for burnout is minimized by similar assistance (Rando, 1984; Ross, 1993; Winiarski, 1991).

Webster's New World Dictionary defines support as "help . . . to advocate . . . to maintain with assistance . . . to endure" (p. 593). We postulate that there are different venues of support potentially available for those working with PWAs: departmental, supervisory, collegial, team other than social work, support group, personal therapy, and life-affirming activities. We have found that the combination of any, if not all of these, provides the possibility of maximizing staff's capacity and long-term commitment to the work.

Departmental support: Such support emanates from social work administrators in the form of acknowledgment of, respect for, and validation of the differences and difficulty of AIDS work. In contrast, countertransferential reactions toward PWAs, either on the part of social work or hospital administrators who consider AIDS patients a low priority, can potentially diminish or contaminate a necessary avenue for support.

Supervisory support: Although this will be elaborated upon later in this chapter, other authors, such as Anderson and Wilke (1991) Rando (1984), Robbins (1983), and Ross (1993), emphasize the necessity for adequate support and supervision. Adequate supportive supervision is defined as providing the opportunity for assessment and evaluation of the individual's work performance as well as emotional responses to the work. Working with dying patients evokes varying degrees of emotional reactions and investments. It follows that a grief response and/or decathexis is not only essential but must be legitimized and accepted within the supervisory process to ameliorate or prevent some of the potentially damaging effects of the work.

Collegial Support: Although it is not necessary that staff be homogeneous in terms of race, class, gender, sexual orientation, HIV status, or professional style and capabilities, it is necessary that they respect one another's differences and care about one another. In this way, they not only individually or collectively share in one another's grieving and growth but are available for professional coverage and assistance as well.

Multidisciplinary team support: A variety of perspectives applied to a patient's case can serve all involved, reducing the isolation felt by a worker and providing the patient with a better-balanced care plan. Also, loss and subsequent grieving are more likely to be experienced as a group, potentially allowing for both the acceptance of, and follow-through with, this process.

Support group: The existence of a hospital-based group depends on numerous factors, ranging from the availability of departmental funds to hire an outside facilitator to the willingness of line staff to share their intimate reactions with peers. However, the literature gives credence to the importance of such a group in alleviating the stress of working with PWAs, thus enhancing the capacity of these individuals to continue their work. (Anderson and Wilke, 1991; Grossman and Silverstein, 1993)

Each staff member had different examples about the value of such a support group in doing AIDS work. Whether it was a personal crisis, disclosure, threats of layoffs, discussions of professional difficulties with patients, or the grief of constant loss through death, the group helped pull the team together in a way different from that provided by individual supervision. The group has provided a place for mutual safety where transferences to supervisor could also be clarified.

Personal therapy: Given that AIDS work frequently touches on one's own archaic feelings, the experience of current or previous individual and/or group therapy can facilitate the processing and understanding of those often-felt turbulent reactions.

Life-affirming activities: These can range from spiritual to physical to intellectual to creative to family-oriented pursuits, so long as they expand and enhance the individual's life. For example, Miriam avidly engages in running and rock climbing as a means of regaining her serenity and control. Lorna attends church regularly and is involved in community affairs.

Supervision

The model of social work AIDS case management we are presenting relies significantly on strong supervision that is flexibly concrete, supportive, challenging, therapeutic (intrapsychic), and educational. Kadushin (1985) enumerates three major components of supervision: administrative, educational, and supportive. He further elaborates that:

> one of the major functions of the supervisor is to provide certain emotional supports for the worker. She must encourage, strengthen, stimulate and ever comfort—pacify. The supervisor seeks to allay anxiety, reduce guilt, increase certainty and conviction, relieve dissatisfaction, fortify flagging faith, affirm and reinforce the worker's assets, replenish depleted self esteem, nourish and enhance ego capacity for adaptation, alleviate psychological pain, restore emotional equilibrium, comfort, bolster and refresh. (p. 229)

In a positive worker-supervisor relationship, the supervisor is never far from participating in these functions on a daily basis. At the same time, the authors contend that it is the depth of the supervisor's clinical expertise that will raise the work with PWAs above the level of complex discharge planning to an understanding of the intricacies of the patient-worker relationship. This knowledge can come through understanding the unconscious mirroring occurring within the supervisory process—patient-worker, worker-supervisor—as well as the nature of the transference.

Successful supervision will encompass any or all of the indications described earlier, while acting as a holding environment or container of the worker's myriad affective reactions. It was on the strength of Lorna's trusting relationship with her supervisor that her issues with the patient in the following case discussion could be crystallized, understood, and worked through. This was Lorna's second social work position. After one and a half years on a medical/surgical unit of another hospital, where she had begun to see AIDS patients as part of her work, she sought to engage in this practice full-time.

Lacquana, a thirty-two-year-old African-American woman with full-blown AIDS, was an active crack abuser with a history of noncompliance. She frequently signed out against medical advice (AMA), and sabotaged medical care or discharge plans to which she had agreed. During admissions, she usually related to staff on the unit in a demanding, infantile, and impulsive manner. For some time, she induced in Lorna a sense of anger and helplessness, due to her expressed neediness for interventions and then, ultimately, her rejection of them.

In supervision, Lorna reviewed these interactions while gathering further information about Laquana's life, which had been and currently was saturated with physical abuse and/or abandonment. AIDS was just another cruel blow for this already emotionally deprived and regressed woman. In understanding Lacquana's repetition of the need for, and particularly the fear of, intimacy as it emerged in the therapeutic interactions, Lorna was ultimately able to provide Laquana with a different maternal experience than she had ever known before. The trust in and knowledge from the supervisory relationship was reflected positively in Lorna's work with Lacquana.

Although Lacquana never made any concrete lifestyle changes in the course of her illness, which lasted one year, she was able to internalize Lorna's sense of constancy and dependability. This allowed her to utilize Lorna as her auxiliary ego to discuss her dying process, as her respiratory functioning deteriorated. Lacquana initiated the discussion that resulted in her decision not to be intubated and to die with appropriate comfort care. Perhaps for the first time in her life, Lacquana engaged in adult decision making.

Supervision played yet another role as it assisted Mary, after great personal loss, to clarify her relationship to the field of social work. Mary's decision to become a social worker stemmed from the experience of her mother's death. Her family did not verbalize their loss and bereavement, and Mary believed that social work, unlike advertising, her previous employment, would offer her such an opportunity.

Mary had done a field placement in a hospital neonatal intensive care unit; she then came to AIDS work wanting to expand her skills and intensify her work with terminally ill patients. Within the first months, she experienced several patient deaths and felt sadness for only one, whom she had been able to reach as had no other professional provider. Mary not only felt quite confident about her skills in case managing but also in her ability to go through the losses of cognition and physical deterioration experienced by her patients, which she viewed as "part of the package" of working with AIDS patients. This homeostasis was soon interrupted when her father became ill and was admitted to an ICU and intubated. Mary continued to work, informing her supervisor of her personal crisis. Not unexpectedly, Mary defended against the emotionality of her AIDS work to remain connected to the myriad feelings of her father's crisis and subsequent death. During that time, her excellence at case management reflected the displacement of her need to remain effective.

When Mary returned to work after her father's burial, she resumed her work by arranging timely discharges and efficiently completing documents and forms. Initially, she addressed the loss of her father in supervision, but eventually, this ended. Gradually, Barbara, the supervisor, became aware of a paucity of emotional connectedness in Mary's work with her patients. Due to the sense of a parallel process between the detachment from her patients and Mary's need to protect herself from her own personal loss, Barbara chose not to offer her perception of this impasse. Rather than make a potentially premature and possibly intrusive intervention, Barbara chose to step back and allow Mary to remain in what seemed a protected position, allowing for grieving and healing to occur in Mary's own style. It was a patient situation, however, that jettisoned Mary toward the emotional reevaluation of self that she had begun months earlier.

The patient, Alonzo, received his AIDS diagnosis simultaneously with the results of his HIV test. Alonzo had denied all risk factors despite a diagnosis of *Pneumocystis carinii* pneumonia (PCP). Mary listened to his fears and provided information aimed at comforting him. Since PCP is now usually resolvable, no one—least of all Mary—expected his quick decline. Alonzo was soon transferred to ICU and intubated. He remained on the respirator for two weeks, with chart notations showing his prognosis as declining from poor to dismal. Mary visited him several times despite his inability to communicate with or recognize anyone. After his death, Barbara and Mary reviewed the process of the work and Mary's reaction, helping Mary to clarify what had occurred. The phrase "life imitates art" had transposed itself into "work imitates life." During her father's death, Mary needed to be the "professional" for herself and her family; with Alonzo, she could be the "person," as she relived her father's death and felt the emotional impact of the loss.

After this, Mary "felt ready" to tackle her continuing involvement and struggles with her patients. With several of them, her work reflected an emotional connection to their myriad needs. However, in general, she experienced a sense of frustration, initially attributed to the substance-abusing population with whom she was primarily dealing. Exploration of countertransferential reactions, education, clinical techniques, and support were offered over the next several months. Ultimately, Mary was confronted with the need to clarify for herself whether her continuing ambivalence was stemming from her work with a substance-abusing population, the AIDS population, or a yet to be identified source. Next, she had to evaluate whether to remain in direct patient care. Mary remained working in direct patient care until the summer of 1998.

CONCLUSION

Hospital social work/case management with AIDS patients presents a hybrid of psychosocial needs for which staff must be attuned, skilled, and ever ready to respond. These needs can range from the mixture of a person's receiving an HIV and AIDS diagnosis to a patient's rapid deterioration and death. At the same time, hospital social work demands that staff have the capacity and enjoy being able to react quickly to crisis, "shifting gears" as needed. There is no day in a hospital that is predictable.

It is the authors' combined experience that all this, even multiple deaths, can be managed so long as there is the availability of, and time for, clinical supervision, as well as the presence of the supervisor for, brief consultation as needed to meet the ongoing exigencies of our patients. Despite the supervisor's provision of an atmosphere that meets "the basic psychological needs of safety, trust, power, esteem, and intimacy" (McCann and Pearlman, 1990, p. 137), there is an additional need for the other supports that have been elaborated upon in this chapter. Without these, AIDS social workers may be prone to becoming overwhelmed by the vulnerability and isolation often cited and felt by our patients.

REFERENCES

Anderson, C. and Wilke, P. (1991). *Reflective helping in HIV and AIDS.* Washington, DC: Open University Press.

Grossman, A. and Silverstein, C. (1993). Facilitating support groups for professionals working with people with AIDS. *Social Work, 38*(2), 144-151.

Harper, B. C. (1977). *Death: The coping mechanism of the health professional.* Greenville, SC: Southeastern University Press.

Kadushin, A. (1985). *Supervision in social work,* Second Edition. New York: Columbia University Press.

Kübler-Ross, E. (1969). *On death and dying.* New York: Macmillan.

McCann, L. and Pearlman, L. (1990). Vicarious traumatization: A framework for understanding the psychological effects of working with victims. *Journal of Traumatic Stress, 3*(1), 131-148.

Rando, T. (1984). *Grief, dying and death: Clinical interventions for care givers.* Champaign, IL: Research Press.

Robbins, J. (1983). *Caring for the dying patient and family.* New York: Harper & Row.

Ross, E. (1993). Preventing burnout among social workers employed in the field of AIDS/HIV. *Social Work in Healthcare, 18*(2), 91-108.

Webster's new world dictionary. (1990). V. Neufeldt (Ed.). New York: Warner Books.

Winiarski, M. (1991). *AIDS-related psychotherapy.* Needham Heights, MA: Longwood Professional Books.

Chapter 19

African-American Women Still Remain Invisible: Are Mental Health Professionals Doing Enough? Clinical Cultural Competence Issues

Ednita Wright
Evelyn Blackburn
Susan Taylor-Brown

INTRODUCTION

More and more African Americans are being taken from their communities trapped in the clutches of the HIV disease. We are losing our sisters, brothers, sons, daughters, and partners at an alarming rate (McKenzie, 1991, p. 125). Current statistics indicate that the number of HIV/AIDS cases continues to rise steadily, with no plateau in sight, and women are increasingly being diagnosed with the disease. In 1994, 14,081 of the reported AIDS cases occurred in women—nearly three times greater than the proportion since 1985. The median age of women who reported with AIDS was thirty-five years, and women ages fifteen to forty-four years accounted for 84 percent of cases, three times as many women as were reported in 1985 (CDC, 1995). AIDS is the number one cause of death in women ages twenty-five to forty-four in fifteen major U.S. cities and the fourth leading cause of death for women in this age range in the United States as a whole (National Institute of Allergy and Infectious Disease, 1995). In 1992, for the first time, diagnosed cases attributed to heterosexual contact exceeded those attributed to injection drug use (O'Leary and Jemmott, 1995).

African-American women are shouldering a disproportionate share of this burden. Although only 12 percent of the population in the United States is African American, 52 percent of women with AIDS are African

American (CDC, 1991). In addition, African-American women are nine times more likely to die from HIV infection than are white females (Department of Health and Human Services, 1992, as cited in O'Leary and Jemmott, 1995, p. 131). Equally, the children of African-American women are being adversely affected. Of the children with AIDS in the United States, 57 percent are African American and 23 percent are Hispanic, while these groups comprise 14 percent and 11 percent, respectively, of the population of children in the nation (Centers for Disease Control and Prevention, 1995).

The National Commission on AIDS (1992) noted that HIV infection tends to worsen already existing forms of inequality based on gender, race and ethnicity, class, sexual orientation, and ability/disability level. In short, AIDS "is a disease of the oppressed" (Scroff, 1991, p. 115). AIDS has the potential to cripple black people in a way that few other health or social forces have since slavery. This challenge is particularly poignant in 1996, when the promise of transforming HIV disease from a terminal illness to a manageable chronic disease is contingent upon having access to care and an ability to pay for the emerging and costly combination drug therapies. For African-American women who have limited access to care and financial resources for drug therapies, this transformation to a chronic disease seems unlikely.

As mental health professionals, we are ethically bound to advocate for this population and change this odious inequity. As increasing numbers of women enter HIV care, ongoing program development is necessary to respond to the unique needs of African-American women living with HIV. Only when more is known about African-American women's roles in the AIDS pandemic, with regard to their knowledge, attitudes, and beliefs, will strategies be effective to empower them to protect themselves from HIV infection and to live with AIDS.

This chapter examines issues of clinical cultural competence related to African-American women through a discussion of relevant literature and presentation of case examples from the authors' clinical experience and concludes with an exploration of critical issues that occurred in the delivery of care to African-American women living with HIV. The primary intent of this chapter is to offer our experience and our thoughts about practice implications in an effort to begin a conversation with our colleagues who are well positioned to improve services to African-American women. Programs that are more responsive to the needs of African-American women will assist the women in caring for themselves and their families.

LITERATURE REVIEW

From the onset of the HIV pandemic, the perception that AIDS is a man's disease has been widespread among health care providers as well as among the general public (Schneider and Stoller, 1995). The AIDS diagnosis was developed from the experiences of gay and bisexual men who were HIV infected. The CDC failed to include any female-specific conditions until 1993, when the gynecological manifestation of invasive cervical cancer was included as an indicator of AIDS. This is the only female-specific condition included in the definition.

Squire (1993) notes that the discourse on AIDS—medical and social policy writing, political rhetoric, media representations, and public discussion about HIV and AIDS—ignored, sidelined, or pathologized women (p. 5). Since physicians did not expect women patients to have HIV disease, they were not looking for its symptoms when treating women (Schneider and Stoller, 1995). Research supports that delays in accurate diagnosis lead to delays in treatment and missed opportunities for medical intervention early enough in the course of the disease to significantly prolong life.

Early literature regarding women primarily centered on a woman's role as mother, and women were portrayed as vectors of disease that could transmit the virus to their children. A woman's role as patient was overlooked and her role of caregiver to her infected offspring or partner was typically highlighted (Taylor-Brown, 1993). Women were frequently excluded from funding and design of HIV research, experimental protocols, and treatment (Ka'opua, 1992).

In *The Invisible Epidemic*, Gena Corea (1992) exposed the struggle of women "against the institutions that are denying them the information, resources, and care they need to prevent or treat the disease" (p. 18). Furthermore, Woodruff (1993) assessed the lack of available, accessible, and adequate treatment as the result of patriarchal society's blatant neglect and marginalization of women, particularly poor women of color, who suffered needlessly for more than a decade due to the government's reluctance to see them as a population at risk for HIV infection (p. 18).

Today, testing of pregnant women is another concern. Such testing raises issues particular not only to the race and economic status of the persons to be tested but also to how medical interventions have been directed against women (Schneider and Stoller, 1995). Even though women's gynecological needs are obviously extensive and worthy of continued study, it is important that practitioners, researchers, and policymakers avoid viewing women merely as reproductive tracts (Kurth, 1993).

Until recently, there was no significant concern expressed, even by feminists, with regard to women with HIV/AIDS. Squire (1993) suggests that perhaps this is partly because the condition disproportionately affects poor women, nonwhite women, and women drug users. Additionally, Western feminism still predominately addresses the interests of middle-class (white) women (Squire, 1993). Another reason for the paucity of literature is time related. Efforts to respond to the needs of women are comparatively recent, and it takes time to develop a program, much less to write about it. Many frontline workers are attempting diligently to design and implement programs that are underfunded, with scarce time and resources for research and writing.

Schneider and Stoller's (1995) *Women Resisting AIDS: Feminist Strategies of Empowerment* is the first text to highlight programs designed to empower women in the AIDS pandemic. The international focus and specificity of programs for target populations—for example, prevention efforts for minority women—is a promising development. The book describes the programs and offers valuable information for program development. However, a discussion of clinical issues is not included.

Although authors call for culturally competent interventions, examination of how this occurs in the client-counselor, client-psychotherapist, and client-case manager relationship and in the delivery of care is almost nonexistent. African-American women, who suffer under the triple layers of racism, gender bias, and classism, will benefit from interventions that are sensitive and responsive to these interacting layers. These interventions will be enhanced by a thorough understanding of the historical relationship between African-American women and the health care system.

THE HISTORICAL RELATIONSHIP
OF HEALTH CARE AND AFRICAN AMERICANS

For women of color and poor women, the health care relationship resonates with a history of medical interventions that included forced sterilizations and the threat of coerced contraception through such modern devices as implants (Schneider and Stoller, 1995). The Tuskeegee study with African-American men further complicates the relationship between African-American women and health care providers. Many in the African-American community still remember the Tuskeegee incident, in which African-American men were viewed as specimens in an experiment and not as valuable human beings. For forty years, African-American men with syphilis believed that they were enrolled in a treatment study, when in reality they were being denied treatment. Even after the Tuskeegee experiment's exposure, public health services officials continued to argue that little harm was done. As Jones (1981) states, "If the state of the medical art in the early 1930s had nothing better than a dangerous and less than totally effective treatment to offer, in the balance, little harm was done by leaving the men untreated" (p. 7). Not only were the men infected, but frequently, their wives and children were as well. The effect of the untreated syphilis on their health and well-being is omitted from the Tuskeegee discussion. The notation of "little harm" signals that the value of human life when considering African Americans was steeped in racism. Given this historical context, it is understandable that African-American PWAs would be skeptical about the health care system.

Additionally, African-American communities have been generally reluctant to address HIV infection and AIDS as a central health issue. Dalton (1991) sheds light on this reluctance in his article "AIDS in Blackface," in which he describes five overlapping factors that continue to influence the response of black communities to the AIDS pandemic. The first is the reluctance to acknowledge association with AIDS, as long as the larger society seems bent on blaming African Americans as a race for its origin and initial spread. Second, he reminds us of the deep-seated suspicion and mistrust many African Americans feel whenever whites express sudden interest in their well-being, which hampers progress in dealing with AIDS. Homophobia is the third factor. Fourth is the problematic relationship most black communities have with drug abuse. Last, black communities still have difficulty transcending the deep resentment of having solutions imposed once again by the construction of preventive messages without community input (Dalton, 1991). These messages are received frequently by the black community as elementary instruction on how to conduct themselves in such private and personal matters as sexual relations.

Western medical care is underutilized by people of color. When people of color interact with Western health care systems, their cultural values related to health, illness, and help seeking are often at variance with the values of the dominant system (Dalton, 1991, p. 2).

The preceding review highlights why the relationship of African-American women and mental health or other members of the team is often problematic. Despite ongoing calls for culturally competent interventions, there is limited examination of how this occurs in the client-social worker relationship and in the delivery of care. Ka'opua's (1992) curriculum provides a framework for understanding the value conflicts between providers of Western health care and patients who do not share the same assumptions. Providers frequently are oblivious to this dynamic. They must first become aware of the value conflicts and then engage in a collaborative process with patients.

Currently, the majority of infected women are women of color, while the majority of health care professionals working with them are white women. Tatum and Knaplund (1996) observe that white women who speak up against racism inevitably disturb their social relationships with other whites. By stepping outside of the circle of white privilege, they challenge those who remain inside. Another dynamic they face is being perceived by women of color as part of the dominant health care system. This barrier impedes the development of a working relationship.

The following case examples are composite profiles of women who are receiving or have received medical and psychosocial services at a community-based medical facility since 1989. As part of their medical care, women are routinely offered case management, an opportunity to participate in Making Connections, which is an open-ended support group, child care, and transportation, as well as limited outreach services for home visits. A woman can participate in the support group regardless of whether she is receiving medical care at the clinic. These cases represent some of the central challenges and rewards of working with African-American women.

CASE EXAMPLE: SHARON

Sharon, who was diagnosed HIV positive eleven years ago, is a thirty-seven-year-old mother of two sons (eighteen and ten years old) and two stepchildren (a nineteen-year-old stepdaughter with three children and an eighteen-year-old stepson) and the guardian of a nephew (three years old) and a grandniece (one year old). Her ten-year-old son, her nephew, and her grandniece live with her and her husband who has AIDS. Her eighteen-year-old is in prison. Sharon describes the mothers of her nephew and grandniece as being "on the streets." She suspects that both are HIV positive. The children have been formally placed with her by Child Protective Services (CPS). She reports that CPS does not know her HIV status, just her past drug use. No legal arrangements have been made for the children. She disclosed her diagnosis to her ten-year-old son a week ago.

Sharon came to Making Connections because "I'm afraid I will lose my sobriety if I don't take care of myself—SOON." She was diagnosed HIV positive in 1987 and her husband, in 1988, while both were incarcerated for drug-related charges. Next month she will celebrate five years of sobriety, and she openly states, "HIV saved my life. If it wasn't for HIV, I'd be dead by now from life on the streets." She is a very warm person who speaks openly about her need to connect with others to stay on the right road. She credits her higher power with helping her deal with the complexities and challenges. She doesn't believe that suffering ends until you die. She openly shared how fragile her emotional health is and how she has not taken care of her HIV disease since her husband came home three months ago. She had completely stopped her medication regimen and is just starting antiretroviral treatment again.

Sharon's husband has central nervous system (CNS) involvement, with a brain mass that is growing rapidly and affecting his ability to function independently. He was discharged from prison three months ago, when it was believed death was imminent. He is angry that he is sicker than she is. Sharon is exploring nursing home options because it is no longer possible for her to care for him at home. She reports feeling like a failure for not being able to let him pass away at home as she had promised. Her son is afraid of him and does not want to be left alone with him. Her husband has been extremely violent in the past, yet he is too incapacitated to cause harm at this time.

In this case, there are multiple issues that must be addressed. As a social worker, beginning where the client is at would mean that a plan should be developed to increase Sharon's emotional support to assist her in maintaining her sobriety. This plan might include solidifying the nursing home placement for her husband and securing child care assistance for the care of her son, grandniece, and nephew. It is apparent through this case example how interrelated the challenges are and thus how comprehensive the response must be.

CASE EXAMPLE: ADELLA

As indicated earlier in this chapter, the pursuit of adequate health care services is difficult for any person living with the HIV or AIDS. For African-American women, these issues are exacerbated, as noted by Bair and Cayleff (1993):

> . . . minority women are less likely to have personal physicians, to have quality health insurance coverage, or to be treated with respect and understanding in negotiation with health care institutions. (p. 14)

Adella talks about the frustration of trying to get adequate help as she seeks to adjust and reconcile herself to the changes that being HIV positive has brought to her life:

> Now basically my problem is that I have a lot of little health problems, little opportunistic diseases, and that is a good name for them.

Trying to get funds, trying to go to the doctor, trying to compensate for not working and acquiring transportation. [There are] special foods and things like that [that you need] and even when they give you Medicaid, it is still not enough. It is not enough with a daughter in college; it wouldn't be enough even if I didn't have her.

Securing adequate, competent, and accessible health care is the first of a series of challenges that an African-American woman must confront. This is not easy, since distrust of the health care system is not uncommon for some African-American women. This lack of trust for the providers of care and the potential loss of control over their care is also the reason some African-American women have a reluctance to enter care in the first place. Health care institutions and the African-American community have a historical relationship which at best has been problematic and at its worst, lethal.

For Adella, her decision to stop taking the medication prescribed was a way of taking care of herself:

When I did start doing the DDI, like they prescribed to me, I started getting all this pain in my arms and my feet. So, I said, no way, I am getting off this and it wasn't too long after I got off that stuff [that the pain] started going away. I said, they [are] trying to kill me. That is how I think; it is really hard for me to trust people, since so much of things that went on with me that they didn't know what it was. So, I had that doubt and thought that they may be trying to do something to me.

As mental health and social service professionals, we enter a relationship with persons, families, and communities to assist them in issues in daily living. As clinicians, one of our objectives is to provide an environment that will enhance patients' own skills and development, even if that means they reject what we believe might be best for them. This objective should be no different for African-American women living with HIV or AIDS. Once we have provided the information that they need to make informed choices, then we need to support them in their decision. Although admittedly, supporting a decision to refuse what we have to offer that would supposedly extend their lives is tricky for us.

The process of hearing the diagnosis, taking it in, reacting to it, accepting it, and finally, deciding how to contend with the ramifications that invade life, produces changes that shake a woman to her very core and leave questions that must be addressed. How will I care for my family and myself? How will I reconcile the person I am with the person I will become with the onset of illness? How will I keep on living? As workers, our aim must be to absorb how these questions and living with HIV/AIDS affects African-American women. Practitioners need to recognize that the question, impact, and response all affect African-American women in a unique, culturally based way, which in turn influences their perceptions of the services offered. Although there are a number of practice implications inherent in the questions stated, there are three that will be highlighted here: (1) clinical cultural competence issues—handling historical mistrust, (2) communication challenges, and (3) building empowering relationships.

CLINICAL CULTURAL COMPETENCE ISSUES: HANDLING HISTORICAL MISTRUST

Thomas and Quinn (1991) explore the attitudinal beliefs of African-American people as they relate to AIDS and note that "the Tuskeegee Syphilis Study's legacy [leaves] a trail of distrust and suspicion that hampers HIV education [and service] efforts in Black communities" (p. 1053). All mental health professionals working with individuals and families affected by HIV/AIDS must assist other health care professionals, the public, and the African-American community to acknowledge that HIV infection and AIDS is a significant health care problem in the African-American community. Thomas and Quinn (1991) predict the intersection of both "opportunity and danger," as we come to terms with the impact of AIDS. The opportunity is to deal comprehensively rather than haphazardly with the challenge as a whole—to see it as a social catastrophe brought on by years of economic deprivation and to meet it as other disasters are met, with adequate resources. The danger is that AIDS will be attributed to some innate weakness of black people and used to justify further neglect and to rationalize continued deprivation.

Given the negative history for African Americans and the historical lack of public services, the following five recommendations are made to assist the practitioner in establishing trust, which is the key issue that creates the core for the helping relationship:

1. Acknowledge the historical relationship between public health and social services and the African-American community. Provide the time and space for clients to discuss their ambivalent feelings about working with HIV/AIDS care services. It is helpful to clarify the scope of services that can be provided through the agency. Be prepared to revisit the issue repeatedly, without seeking to resolve the long-standing mistrust.
2. Reinforce the willingness to be supportive throughout the journey with HIV. This may mean that the practitioner could be called to

move beyond the typical boundaries of the traditional relationship. It is important for us as practitioners to keep in mind (as the case examples illustrated) that the issues presented are convoluted and complex, therefore requiring more of our time.

3. Beginning with the initial visit, emphasize consistency, joint problem solving, and a willingness to pursue alternatives and assist in obtaining resources.

4. Express a sincere desire to understand clients' value base and stress that support will not be withdrawn if their choices conflict with what the doctor or other worker feels would be the best course of treatment.

5. Work to provide greater distributive justice in the care of women; it is insufficient to provide microlevel interventions when the root of the problems is societally based. Fighting racism, sexism, and classism are inherent aspects of working with women who are HIV infected.

COMMUNICATION CHALLENGES

One of the major challenges in our work in general and in the HIV/AIDS arena in particular is communication. How do we communicate across cultures about medicines, illness, sickness, and death? How do you communicate new information in a way that is understandable and believable?

In the recent months, a significant number of patients have responded dramatically to protease inhibitors in combination with antiretrovirals. The viral load is decreasing while the T-cell count increases, carrying the promise of prolonged health. This represents a major step toward transforming HIV from a life-threatening illness to a chronic illness, resulting in reduced hospitalizations and enhanced quality of life. A barrier to the use of protease inhibitors is the need for lifelong treatment. If protease inhibitors are not taken as prescribed, drug resistance occurs. For patients who are uncomfortable taking drugs, the need to take protease inhibitors forever will be a major barrier. What will happen if people do not take their protease inhibitors? Patients risk becoming drug resistant, and providers will become frustrated with their noncompliance. Medication costs, as noted previously, are another significant barrier. This complex information must be shared in a meaningful way.

As health care professionals, we need to assist our clients in evaluating whether to take this medication by:

- developing patient education materials that help women understand the medical and financial implications of the medications;

- providing opportunities to discuss their concerns with providers and other patients;
- working to maintain the relationship regardless of who the medical provider is or was—remembering that our client is of primary concern;
- assisting the client in understanding past painful relationships or failures; and
- remembering to respect the right of the client to refuse treatment options.

BUILDING EMPOWERING RELATIONSHIPS

Empowerment means that we strive to provide our consumers with all the information we have at our disposal so that they can make informed choices about their lives. Another major piece of empowerment is how we view our clients. For those with the HIV virus, it is essential that we view them as living with a disease and not dying from it. This shift in our perception changes what services we offer and how we approach African-American women. Our responsibility is to help them enhance their lives and support them when they need our assistance. By providing them with an environment that will increase their understanding of the HIV reality, from diagnosis throughout the disease course, we can enable them to adapt and cope with this complex reality.

As programs are refined and developed for African-American women living with HIV/AIDS, it is important that they include children and are community based. Treating a woman with HIV/AIDS must be comprehensive, treating more than the complications associated with the disease. Programs and policies should offer more than mere child care services, to include emotional, physical, and financial support to both mother and child, thus allowing children to remain with their mothers for as long as they can. Woodruff (1993) notes:

> Our health and human service system appears to be polarized; its message to mothers—either you take care of your child or we will—seems to offer no middle ground, no room for cooperation or genuine assistance. (p. 22)

Additionally, we must develop approaches that promote mothers' wanting to ensure appropriate care for their children as the disease progresses, to be included in the process and have dominant power in deciding where or if a child will be placed and when, without the threat of coercion.

Other ways in which all mental health professionals can create environments that will allow an African-American woman space to connect with her own power are:

1. linking women with other women living with the virus;
2. linking women with their existing supports, e.g., church community, which they may have stopped participating in due to their fears of rejection;
3. advocating to increase availability of group interventions;
4. connecting with nontraditional alternatives such as movement therapy, acupuncture, massage, etc.;
5. networking with other services and offering a weekend retreat for families; and
6. assisting the woman in preparing a legacy of written, audiotaped, or videotaped memories for her loved ones.

CONCLUSION

Barlett and Finkebeiner (1991) notes that being diagnosed HIV positive or as having AIDS assaults our plans for the future, the principles by which we make decisions, who we think we are, and changes how we live and the relationships that support us. As health care professionals, we can help African-American women living with HIV infection or AIDS by understanding their personal fears, which are intensified by the uncertainties that this disease produces. We also must accept the very real historical relationship that African-American women have had with health care institutions and validate their feelings as they navigate through the myriad of health and social services. We must also acknowledge that biases do exist in our agencies. We must be vigilant in eradicating those biases from infecting our own practice and, when necessary, seek out consultation and critical evaluation to improve our services. African-American women are dying in great numbers. As professionals and as human beings we must critique ourselves and ask: Are we doing enough?

REFERENCES

Bair, B. and Cayleff, S. (Eds.) (1993). *Wings of gauze: Women of color and the experience of health and illness.* Detroit, MI: Wayne State University Press.
Bartlett, J. and Finkbeiner, A. (1991). *The guide to living with HIV infection.* Baltimore, MD: The John Hopkins University Press.

Centers for Disease Control and Prevention (1991). *HIV surveillance report,* June-December 1990, pp. 1-22.

Centers for Disease Control and Prevention (1995). Update: AIDS among women in the United States, 1994. *Mortality and Morbidity Weekly Report,* 41, (94-95), p. 101.

Corea, G. (1992). *The invisible epidemic: The story of women and AIDS.* New York: HarperCollins Publishers.

Dalton, H. (1991). AIDS in blackface. In N. McKenzie (Ed.), *The AIDS reader: Social, political, and ethical issues* (pp. 125-143). New York: Meridian.

Jones, J. (1981). *Bad blood: The Tuskegee syphilis experiment—A tragedy of race and medicine.* New York: The Free Press.

Ka'opua, L. (1992). Training for cultural competence in the HIV epidemic. AIDS Education Project, Hawaii Area AIDS Education and Training Center, January.

Kurth, A. (Ed.) (1993). *Until the cure: Caring for women with HIV.* New Haven, CT: Yale University Press.

McKenzie, N. F. (Ed.) (1991). *The AIDS reader: Social, political, and ethical issues.* New York: Meridian Books.

National Commission on AIDS (1992). *The challenge of HIV/AIDS in communities of color.* Washington, DC: National Commission on AIDS, December.

National Institute of Allergy and Infectious Disease (1995). *Women and HIV infection.* Bethesda, MD: U.S. Public Health Service, February.

O'Leary, A. and Jemmott, L. (Eds.) (1995). *Women at risk: Issues in the primary prevention of AIDS.* New York: Plenum Press.

Richardson, A. and Bolle, D. (Eds.) (1992). *Wise before their time: People from around the world living with AIDS and HIV tell their stories.* London: Fount.

Richie, B. (1990). AIDS: In living color. In Evelyn C. White (Ed.), *The black women's health book: Speaking for ourselves* (pp. 182-186). Seattle, WA: The Seal Press.

Schneider, B. and Stoller, N. (1995). *Women resisting AIDS: Feminist strategies of empowerment.* Philadelphia, PA: Temple University Press.

Schneider, J. and Conrad, P. (1983). *Having epilepsy: The experience and control of illness.* Philadelphia, PA: Temple University Press.

Scroff, F. (1991). The social construction of AIDS, heterosexism, racism and misogyny: The challenges facing women of color. *Resources for Feminist Research Documentation/Documentation sur la Recherche Feministe,* 24(3/4), pp. 115-123.

Squire, C. (Ed.) (1993). *Women and AIDS: Psychological perspectives.* London: Sage Publications.

Tatum, B. and Knaplund, E. (1996). Outside the circle: The relational implications for white women working against racism. Work in progress, 78. Papers from The Stone Center, Wellesley College, Wellesley, Massachusetts.

Taylor-Brown, S. (1993). HIV-positive women: Finding a voice in the AIDS pandemic. In V. Lynch, G. Lloyd, and M. Fimbres (1993), *The changing face of AIDS: Implications for social work practice* (pp. 123-151). Westport, CT: Auburn House.

Thomas, S. and Quinn, S. (1991). The Tuskeegee syphilis study, 1932 to 1972: Implications for HIV education and AIDS risk education programs in the black community. *American Journal of Public Health*, 81(11), 1498-1505.

Woodruff, G. (1993). Women and children and HIV. *Readings, A Journal of Reviews and Commentary in Mental Health, 8*(2), 18-22.

Chapter 20

Reflections from the Field: Looking Beyond the Behavior to See the Need—A Case Study

Patricia A. Stewart

Fatimah and Hassan (not their real names) are an African-American couple in their late twenties. Both were in the advanced stages of HIV disease when I first met them. That was at my last place of employment where, as intake supervisor, I received a referral for placement of their newborn son. I was told that Fatimah had been sent from another state to the Philadelphia area to live in an AIDS hospice for women. She had apparently been in an unsafe living environment. She had a history of drug abuse, had been a victim of domestic violence, and had had her other children removed from her custody. There was concern expressed by the referring agency about her ability to raise her newborn baby so we placed the baby in foster care. All involved expressed a desire to act in "the best interests of the child." I was also immediately aware of and concerned about the amount of emotional pain that would prompt Fatimah to behave in the ways described.

I got to know her well, in part, because she had weekly supervised visits with the baby at the agency. I remember the first time that I saw her. I knew intuitively that it was she: her head was bowed down, as if in shame. It was an all too familiar sight in my initial experience with people living with the virus, whose history has reached us before they do. I reached out to her. After a relatively short time of interacting with her, from the perspective of acknowledging her strengths—treating her with respect, for who she is, rather than with fear and suspicion for what she had allegedly done—she was able to raise her head, and our eyes met. She was capable of bonding.

Fatimah began to seek me out when she arrived. I was able to laugh with her, encourage her, admire the little clothes and toys she would bring to her infant son. I recall the pain that she was so clearly feeling and unable to express the day that I, in the absence of the caseworker, accompanied her to the hospital for her son's test results. I saw her denial and rationalization kick into place, as she indicated that she had not heard what the doctor had said about the ways in which they obtain an accurate diagnosis. Now he was to the point of discussing options for their next visit to the clinic, and still she acted as though she didn't hear. I saw her somehow not hear all of this and yet say to me, ". . . my other kids tested positive at first, too, and then they washed out." I watched her defense "melt" as I carefully told her what I had heard the doctor say. She walked away to get some water and came back to her seat, vowing that she would take good care of her own health so she and her son could be reunited.

She came up to me one day while visiting with her son at the agency. It was one of those rare, gratifying moments; she gave me a big hug and told me how she wished I had been around when she was sixteen. "Maybe my life would have been different," she said. I remember encouraging her to live her life as she wants it to be today; I told her I would help. I realized that I had become an integral component of her impoverished social support system. I believed in her ability to love her baby. I acknowledged her strengths. I set limits. I taught her some parenting skills. I treated her with the basic respect due any human being. She was not accustomed to this.

Some weeks after meeting Fatimah, who vowed she was not interested in reuniting with her husband, Hassan arrived in the area. Fatimah had described some of his past abuse of her. Deep sentiments of anger and dread that he had "found her" were expressed by staff both inside and outside the agency. I was able to acknowledge that I felt fear, until I met him. He was indeed an angry man, who spoke his mind about the system by which he feels oppressed. When I greeted him warmly with a smile and extended my hand, he looked at me with a mixture of curiosity and amazement. He, too, needed and accepted some of my suggestions about his parenting. Both Fatimah and Hassan had to learn how to share the visit without becoming angry with each other. I realized that regardless of how others felt about this relationship they were bonded and were resolved to be together. I advocated for intervention that would help them to be with each other safely.

When I decided to leave that job to take another, I dreaded telling them. By that time, Hassan was not coming as regularly for visits, so I could not tell him in person. Fatimah was quite disturbed when I told her. "Every time I trust someone, they walk out of my life—they leave me," she said. I took care to acknowledge her feelings, as well as my own. I felt very guilty. It was difficult for me to end my relationship with her when she still had so many needs.

Then one day, months later, I received in the office mail a large envelope with a small picture of her son. Although Fatimah had put her name and address on the envelope, she wrote no message. A note was written on the back of the picture: "From Malik [baby's name] to Miss Pat, with love." I was touched, and I sent her a note telling her so.

I heard no more, until months later, when I learned that the baby had been placed in a foster home in the agency in which I am currently working. It was then that I first learned from Hassan, who contacted me at the agency, that Fatimah had had all visiting privileges suspended indefinitely because of her "inappropriate behavior with the child." He told me she was devastated by that.

She had relapsed in her addiction to drugs. When she, who at the time was in the very progressed stages of her disease, was told that she could not see Malik, her critically ill son, infected in her womb—the pain was too great for her: she was heartbroken. Her husband says she gave up. I sent her a message through him, but she never responded.

Shortly after Malik was placed in foster care, Hassan called to say that Fatimah was in the intensive care unit of the hospital. The doctors said she was dying. He was understandably upset. The assigned social worker from our agency did a nice job of connecting with and supporting him, and he felt good about that.

I paid Fatimah a visit at the hospital. As I stood there, I thought about the time I had spent getting to know her. I wondered what kind of "inappropriate behavior" had taken place to the extent that she had been denied visits with her son. She had been so faithful in attending the four-hour visits she was allotted to see her child each week, and she did this for months; she "showed up"—she agreed to and worked toward the goals of the family service plan so that she could be "reunited" with her son, with whom she had never lived. She was a woman who had formed beginning relationships with people who were accepting of her as a person.

What happened, I wondered, that she would have become so "inappropriate"? When I arrived at the hospital, accompanied by a colleague whom he knew, Hassan, looking surprised and relieved, greeted me with a hug, which surprised me. The nurses seemed to be "tolerating" him, answering his many questions. They were moving Fatimah to another room within the ICU that day. I was impressed with the kinds of questions he was asking and took him aside to provide some support for him and to make suggestions to change his approach/attitude toward the medical team.

I noticed that his frustration with the system had heightened his mistrust and anger. By this time, he was so sure that he would be treated unfairly that his behavior was rather challenging. He was alternating between managing the pain of his impending loss and "ranting and raving" about being told by the county case manager that his visits with his son may be suspended. He responded to this with angry, threatening statements, resulting in the case manager calling him "a negative element in the environment."

His wife was dying. As he told us this, I saw in his eyes, the fear and terror, likened to that of a small child. He began to cry. He said it was too much to be losing his wife and his child, too. I do not condone threatening behavior, yet I could see he felt he had no recourse. "I'm a man," he said, "yet they treat me like I'm an animal."

He asked me for a ride to his home. I wondered how I would refuse him, given that he was so needy. However, I told him that I could not offer him that ride and why. Instead of "going off," he said, "Oh, that's the policy. Well, OK. I know that you would do it if you could. From the first time I met you, I trusted you, 'cause you treated me with respect."

I was able then to spend some time alone with Fatimah. I reflected on some memories of meaningful moments with her as I watched her half-closed, sometimes fluttering eyes, saw her frail chest rise and fall to the sounds of the ventilator, and witnessed her periodically gag and expectorate, as dozens of wires and tubes and lines surrounded her airflow mattress and bed like a giant spider web. And I thought, "What a metaphor."

The "web" symbolizes the maze of conditions associated with being poor and African American (and oppressed and abused as a child, angry, addicted, domestically abused, and HIV infected). These conditions are the result of being denied one's rights by a system that does not see the *person with the behavior,* but sees only the *behavior.* Proponents of this system think they *know the person* because they've seen the type many times before. The web becomes a trap with no way out.

The system, which includes social workers and case managers, failed this family. I would like to suggest some ways that mental health professionals can intervene to minimize the destructive elements of that web.

- We, who have the power to make decisions that significantly affect the lives of others, have also a responsibility to assess that client with a multidimensional lens, i.e., one that takes into account biopsychosocial, cultural, and spiritual aspects of the person.
- Remember basic casework principles: Start where the client is at.
- Believe in the worth of the client. If the behavior is unlovely, seek to understand the unmet needs of someone who could commit such be-

havior. Appeal to that oftentimes weak, lonely person who is behaving symptomatically. This is the humanistic approach. We can bring about the delicate balance between seeking to understand the issues underlying the behavior and developing skills in setting boundaries and limits, ensuring the emotional safety and well-being of *all* involved.

- Above all, seek to know the client, which comes with seeking to understand the behavior. That knowledge will help you to identify his or her strengths and to assist the client to build on those strengths.
- RESPECT. A simple word that means different things to people across race, culture, and class. Please find out what it means to people with whom you work—and then practice it.

Working the people living with HIV and AIDS provides an opportunity for delivering consummate social work service. The myriad social problems among the variety of those infected, many of whom are marginalized and/or disenfranchised can be addressed via many social work modalities such as clinical, advocacy, community organizing, policy development—in both micro and macro levels of practice. The impact on quality of life and the intensity of the emotional and physical pain to those affected seem to call forth passion for the work, which can be simultaneously gratifying and draining.

One thing I do realize, is that all I have learned that is specific to working with people living with HIV has complemented my basic philosophy of practice, derived from my long-standing reasons for being a social worker. I am committed to helping people reach their potential—physically, emotionally, spiritually—against all odds, by any means necessary. And when the behavior of someone placed before us is unlovely, it is important, I believe, to be mindful of the dignity and respect of which we all are worthy. When encountering someone with this disease, it is important to remember that, . . . there, but for the grace of God, go I. . . . It can keep us humble and connected.

By the time this chapter was sent to press, the young woman whom I call Fatimah crossed over into the world of the ancestors. I am hopeful that she found peace, with herself and with her Creator.

Chapter 21

Entrusted with Secrets— Working with Immigrants with HIV

Hank Flacks

Over the course of American history, immigrants to the United States have often been the targets of defamatory rhetoric and political scapegoating. Most recently, however, the intense degree of hostility and legally sanctioned discrimination directed at all our resident noncitizens is obvious to anyone exposed to the news media. Federal legislation that was recently signed into law justifiably leads immigrants to fear disclosing their immigration status since they may now be more at risk for deportation and reduction or wholesale elimination of public health and/or financial benefits if they are illegal or "out of status." There are now reports of refusal of nursing home admissions to acutely ill, legal immigrants, denial of public education to immigrant children, and more stringent rules for obtaining legal residency. Consequently, the impulse to avoid disclosure of one's immigrant status is understandable and, once revealed, entrusts the recipient of such information with a powerful secret. It is in this climate of fear and retribution that HIV-positive immigrants are desperately seeking compassionate and comprehensive medical care. This chapter will help to illustrate the special contribution of social work in one HIV-positive immigrant's search for medical treatment that engaged the staff of the HIV section at St. Vincent's Hospital and Medical Center of New York City. This remarkable staff is constantly entrusted with important private information about patients. This trust in providers is predicated on their capacity to maintain confidentiality of such "secrets," thus ensuring continuity of care and the capacity to provide lifesaving health care.

To provide such care, beginning in 1992, St. Vincent's Hospital and Medical Center's HIV section gained approval for a Ryan White CARE Act Title One grant to provide comprehensive medical care (MD, NP, RN) and social work (MSW, SWA) intervention to documented and undocumented immigrants with HIV infection. The social work component has been an integral part of the biopsychosocial care provided in this program, since the unique training of social workers equips them to address the complex clinical case management problems this population presents. Social workers play an invaluable role in assisting these patients to come out of hiding, to live with dignity and pride while fighting AIDS.

The specific components of the program are as follows: enrollment and orientation to the program (this is offered by one of the immigrant program social workers during a social work intake interview; once enrolled, the first appointment for the patient is made with a medical provider); initial outpatient medical evaluations; regularly scheduled follow-up medical appointments; psychiatric services; nutritional counseling; HIV education; laboratory and diagnostic services and screening for clinical drug research trials.

All immigrant program enrollees are offered comprehensive on-site social service case management by our multilingual social work staff, concrete services, crisis intervention, mental health services (individual, group, and family counseling), liaison to community-based organizations, referral to legal counsel, and any other social services as needed. (The program has the funding to cover the cost of medication and some diagnostic services for uninsured patients.) The immigrant program social worker also "follows" the patients if they are admitted to the hospital for acute inpatient treatment, monitoring their stay and coordinating discharge planning with the inpatient treatment team. (Uninsured patients are covered for treatment by emergency Medicaid.)

That HIV health care is challenging to patients, their caregivers and healthcare providers is obvious. HIV patients can experience stigma, isolation, fear, anger, physical pain, physical disfigurement, cognitive deterioration, and other consequences that deeply affect their lives. Yet, the additional pressures HIV-positive immigrants experience are overwhelming— economic, psychosocial, and medical problems for immigrants compound already outsized stressors.

Economically, the immigrant is at a clear disadvantage. Freedom to work and the self-esteem that might be provided by such employment is not readily available to most members of this population. If they work, it is usually "off the books," below minimum wage, and without benefits. From a meager salary, the immigrant often sends funds home to help support a significant other, children, and extended families. Illegal, undocumented immigrants and now legal immigrants can be ineligible for public assistance or medical benefits. Given the economic reality for immigrants, the social consequences are profound. With little or no money, distanced from their home and culture, unable to speak the language of most service providers, these patients often come to the immigrant program at St. Vincent's Hospital (SVH) disoriented, frightened, and deeply frustrated. They may be without housing or may live in overcrowded conditions in crime-ridden neighborhoods of the city (and this is in a country that is growing more comfortable with the notion of immigrants as enemies and pariahs).

Thus, the psychological presentation of our patients is, more often than not, crisis-ridden. The emotional effects of their status (or lack thereof) may present a wide variety of complaints, including, but not limited to, depression, anxiety, panic, fear, rage, grief, suicidal gestures or ideation, substance abuse, domestic violence, and exacerbation of any premorbid psychological disorders. The psychosocial assessment and management skills of social work case managers provide an important point of intervention to address psychological and/or social crises in a timely manner.

Early diagnosis and intervention is crucial to providing quality HIV medical care. However, an immigrant's cultural norms may prevent open discussion of safer sex and other education concerning HIV issues, which in turn presents obstacles toward the success of early HIV intervention or prevention of HIV infection altogether. The multiple stressors and isolation that immigrants may experience is clearly not beneficial to the provision of comprehensive medical care, especially for a chronic, unpredictable infection such as HIV. Undocumented immigrants can come from countries in which the reality of the HIV epidemic is a carefully guarded secret and AIDS education is nonexistent. Once beginning treatment here in the United States, if these patients find sympathetic practitioners, they often cannot keep regular appointments. Concerns about confidentiality in their community or family may cause immigrant patients to be resistant to treatment; patients may travel long distances to avoid being seen in treatment facilities closer to home, thus making appointment attendance more difficult. Sometimes they cannot provide proof of residence, or they fear receiving bills or mail at home that may identify an illness to prying eyes. Often, traditional beliefs about medical care may be at odds with Western notions of effective treatment regimens. The social case work manager is often the first to be asked to respond to a presentation of such unique stressors. How do we manage the economic, psychosocial, and medical challenges to the well-being of the immigrant with HIV infection?

In the following case, the efforts of the social work case manager, the patient, and his family to access adequate ambulatory, inpatient, and nursing home care, with necessary community entitlements, highlight the essential and invaluable assistance social workers provide to the patients enrolled in this special needs program. The unique skills of trained social work professionals make us uniquely equipped to help other health care providers understand and adapt to the cultural imperatives and psychological needs of immigrant patients, while in turn helping the patients learn the best and most effective ways to communicate their needs.

Some of the specific issues that complicated this particular immigrant's acculturation to the health care system include a diagnosis of tuberculosis, cultural mores, functional and dysfunctional denial, discharge planning crises, and countertransference reactions of the social work case manager.

In June 1985, George was referred to the immigrant program for an enrollment interview by his caseworker at the African Services Committee, a community-based organization (CBO) serving African émigrés to the United States. A major concern of the CBO was a financial problem regarding its client and a large hospital bill that was paid by his sister. An appointment was made within the week, and the patient appeared promptly on the appointed day—an impeccably dressed, tall, slim African man, who carried himself in a regal, if not haughty, manner. He spoke English very well, though his preferred language was French. He related the following personal history.

George was married in his country, the former French West Africa, and left his pregnant wife behind to obtain an advanced degree in economics in the United States, where his younger sister had emigrated and gained citizenship. He was a highly regarded government economist at home and was expected to return there with greater skills. Shortly after his arrival here, a government coup ousted his political party and made his return there inadvisable. He was threatened with serious reprisal if he were to go home to Africa. Soon thereafter, he began to suffer abdominal and dermatological problems. Assuming these were stress provoked and not serious, he visited a neighborhood MD and began a series of tests and treatments that did not improve his condition. Then, during another one of his visits, he was told he had AIDS and that his intestinal problems were HIV related. He was admitted to a local Queens, New York, hospital, where he was treated for wasting syndrome and "other problems." This was the information that George initially disclosed.

At the conclusion of his enrollment interview, he was scheduled for his first appointment for medical treatment at our clinic. He signed a release for me to discuss "some matters" with his sister, and from her, I learned what he did not disclose during our first meeting. The inpatient hospital bill that was incurred by George's HIV treatment was enormous. Since he was the "man" in the family (and culturally most important), and since his sister had invited him to the United States, she took on the responsibility for the bill and mortgaged her house to pay it. This forced her to move into the basement of the house, renting the space above to pay for the mortgage loan.

It was at this time that his sister was put in touch with the African Services Committee and asked for its help. I referred his sister to attorneys at the HIV Law Project here in New York City, with the hope that they could advocate for the return of funds she had paid. I then awaited George's return for his first medical evaluation at St. Vincent's Hospital's HIV section outpatient clinic. Shortly after he missed that appointment, I learned he had been admitted to a local hospital (in Queens) and would be in touch as soon as he was ready to come back to us. He returned to the clinic one month later, noticeably thinner, somewhat agitated, and complaining that his stomach was "acting up." He was seen by his medical provider and was scheduled for follow-up appointments.

Shortly after this, I received a call from his caseworker at the African Services Committee who expressed concern about a report from George's sister that George was "coughing a lot" and had night sweats at home. I contacted George, and once in receipt of his signed release a few days later, called the hospital in Queens where he had been admitted for treatment. George had tuberculosis. He was treated for it months before and had not been compliant with treatment. His sister was now to be prescribed prophylactic meds secondary to her own tuberculosis exposure. This was stunning news. Yet, at our next meeting, the patient denied that he ever had a TB diagnosis or any symptoms. When presented with the diagnosis obtained from the Queens hospital, he still adamantly denied the illness.

Why would he deny his tuberculosis? Did he fear a TB diagnosis would impact negatively on his pending application for political asylum? Would he be isolated from others and treated aggressively? Would his family reject him? Was his denial functioning in the service of preserving his feeling of safety and hope? Would this diagnosis prevent his travel to see his newborn son in Africa? These scenarios proved to be real.

I returned from a brief vacation to learn that George was admitted to our inpatient facility for treatment of active tuberculosis and to "rule out" multi-drug-resistant tuberculosis. He was in "isolation." The news was disturbing to me, since it was clear that I had been exposed to his TB infection during the times we met in my office. He had also exposed other staff members and patients in the waiting room. He had consistently lied about his treatment and the diagnosis received when he was previously hospitalized in Queens. At this point, my feelings were running primitive and irrational. Why was he trying to kill me? All I had done was try to engage his trust and provide him and his family with assistance previously unavailable. Also, my commitment to him still obliged me to visit him in his isolation room; all visitors were masked, and he could emerge only briefly when absolutely necessary, masked and escorted. I did not want to see him, talk to him, or oblige him in any way. This countertransference reaction was powerful. My response to him was being provoked by his own reaction to the illness and the environment in which he found himself. He did not want to oblige the staff; he felt that he was being killed by HIV and TB, and his dignity, independence, and sense of competence were all being "killed off" by his assignment to an isolation room. He certainly would feel painfully cut off from his wife and child and his former life.

However, his need for assistance and empathy was clear, as was my ethical contract with him. Understanding my countertransference feelings in this case helped to overcome the obstacles such reactions put in the way of intervening on his behalf. My colleagues at the hospital also depended on the social work contribution to encourage his compliance with treatment. He was reported as "depressed," "obstructing and refusing treatments," and "defiant" toward the staff. So this member of the treatment team donned his mask and entered the room.

George was at the foot of his bed staring blankly at the wall. Once acknowledging my presence, he wanted to know where I had been all this time (a little over a week), and why he had to be in this room. He was visibly angry with me! I had to overcome my impulse to ask him, in response to his questions, why he had lied about his diagnosis and instead asked if the doctors had informed him of what they were treating. He ignored my question and instead complained about the nurses requests and rules regarding isolation, visitors, and his meals. He did not need to take orders from women; he did not need them to tell him where he could and could not go. When I asked why he would not comply with their requests, he replied that men do not take orders from women. He was unable to eat the hospital food; it had no taste. He needed African food—his native foods were "stews" with flavor. I returned to the nurse's station, where they awaited my exit from his isolation room with anticipation. They were anxious to see my response to what they had been tolerating for the past eight days.

The nurses were exasperated with him. He was "entitled," condescending, dismissive, and insulting. In fact, he had refused to return to his room the previous day, and they had to call security to escort him back inside. (The security guard was male; they were female). When I asked about a psychiatric evaluation because of his depression, they said that he had recently had one because he sister had reported to the resident MD that he "had written on the walls" at home. That, coupled with his consistent denial of diagnosis, led them to wonder if he was becoming demented. However, my meeting with him did not convince me that dementia was the problem. I asked if his sister could bring him some food prepared at home. It was determined that he was not on a restricted diet so I informed George that his sister could provide food and called her to let her know. I asked her about the "writing on the walls." She informed me that in "her country" one would invoke the presence of spirits by writing on walls inside your house. He felt he was asking them to rid his body of the evil sickness. This was a culturally acceptable means of dealing with illness in his community but foreign to our Western notions of how to express stress or appeal for relief from deities. We "pray" in a different manner. I informed the nurses of my conversation with his sister, which educated us about their cultural style, and coupled with his clearly articulated (albeit entitled) demands and orientation to person, place, and time, the dementia diagnosis was ruled out. Cultural differences hampered his treatment up to this point, but intervention by social work helped to improve communication of his needs and to adjust treatment decisions and compliance. The presence of the social worker assisted the patient in lowering his anxiety about isolation simply by being "present" and ensuring discussion and empathy concerning cultural differences.

At this point, discharge planning was begun. I inquired whether his sister would be able to assist in George's care if he were to return home. She stated that it was not possible, as she was now providing a home for another sister who had an infant child, and she was not willing to expose the child to George's illness. I suggested that she speak with her brother's MD to determine if he was, in fact, infectious. Despite the doctor's assurances that he would be discharged in a noninfectious state, his sister refused to take him home.

On my next visit with him, I asked George if he had any thoughts about where he would live when he had recovered from this bout with tuberculosis. He quickly and confidently said, "with my sister." I pointed out that we would have to try to get him new benefits since they had expired while he received inpatient treatment. He was confident he would be returning to his sister's home; she was equally clear about the impossibility of his return and was asked to inform him of this fact. After she spoke with him about her decision, he became more profoundly depressed. Thankfully, he was released from isolation shortly thereafter, when his TB infection responded favorably to his regimen of medications, pointing to a non-MDR (multidrug resistant) TB diagnosis. As discharge approached, I explored possibilities for his placement in nursing homes, since he was too weak to care for himself. The treatment team agreed that he needed skilled nursing home placement. When he was approaching readiness for discharge, his applications for nursing homes were completed and sent out.

At this time, his sister insisted he be sent to a facility in a nice neighborhood, since she now realized, having been in the United States for a few years, how poorly people of color were treated. She worried about the quality of his care and her ability to travel to the area where he would be placed. She also wanted me to know about their family: her mother was a psychiatrist; her father was in government. They were proud of their heritage and well-educated. I assured her that I would do my best to "place" George according to her request, within the limits of what was available. I also assured her that all my patients were treated without regard to national origin, color, or creed, and I believed that to be true about my colleagues as well. There might, however, be limits on the choice since George was considered to be "pending status" in the eyes of INS (Immigration and Naturalization Service). Consequently, to entitlement analysts in the nursing homes to which we had applied, he might be a risky admission. His hospital Medicaid at SVH was covering his inpatient stay on an "emergency basis," but his entitlement was provisional on his voluntary departure status being approved by INS. (Voluntary departure is an immigration status that entitles persons with acute serious illnesses to remain in the United States for treatment on a humanitarian basis and, within this status, to receive benefits for treatment while a decision on this status is pending. Immigrants are "PRUCOL," or protected under the color of the law while awaiting decision.) He actually had applied for voluntary departure but was considering political asylum as well. Yet his protection was provisional since a decision on his case was pending. On the basis of his PRUCOL status, his application to a nursing home in Upper Manhattan was fortunately accepted. His transportation was arranged and his sister informed of his transfer. He agreed to the transfer understanding that, once in this skilled nursing facility, it was expected that he would improve and then get his own apartment. However, hours before his discharge, the nursing home administration decided that because of his immigration status they would not accept him. His admission was rescinded because he was not an American citizen, and they might be "stuck" with his charges for treatment if he died before his status was approved. (Current litigation is challenging such decisions by nursing homes, holding that such patients' treatment should be considered "acute care" equal to that provided in hospitals.)

George was finally admitted to Goldwater Hospital on New York City's Roosevelt Island for his medical rehabilitation. The day following his transfer, the Blizzard of '96 arrived, leaving him isolated from family for three long days. However, within two weeks of his admission, he was walking to the patient lounge in the facility, eating, gaining weight, and growing more responsive to his sister and staff. Unfortunately, he died two months later, awaiting approval of a transfer to scattered-site housing.

This brief outline of the care afforded George only minimally describes the enormous responsibility that rests on the social work staff of the immigrant program (and in the HIV section in general) at St. Vincent's Hospital and Medical Center in New York City. Our impact is profound. This patient was helped in his struggle to gain treatment and social assistance when his pride made it very difficult to accept such help. With the intervention of the legal referral by this social worker, his sister has thus far received a reimbursement of 75 percent of the monies she paid on her brother's behalf. (She is hoping to receive the balance as well.) Many of the complications of this case were managed to the benefit of the patient and his family. The social work, medical, nursing, and ancillary staff at the hospital provided comprehensive care to this patient, affording him dignity and some sense of control in negotiating his care. Without the intervention of the social work component of this grant program, this beneficial outcome might not have occurred. Obviously, the current political climate is not encouraging with regard to entitlements for this special needs population. However, the immigrants with HIV program is staffed by a community of health care professionals who believe that health care is a basic right for all people—not a special privilege for some.

Chapter 22

Couples of Mixed HIV Status: Therapeutic and Policy Issues

Robert H. Remien
Raymond A. Smith

INTRODUCTION

The situation in which one member of a couple is HIV seropositive and the other is HIV seronegative (mixed HIV status or "serodiscordant") is a relatively new phenomenon confronting mental health workers their clinical practice. As new HIV infections continue to occur in both the heterosexual and homosexual populations, coupled with the phenomenon of people living longer and healthier with HIV than before, the likelihood of such couples presenting for treatment is increasing. Therapists must increase their skills to enable work at the dyadic level with the many challenges these couples face, to reduce distress and strengthen the partnership rather than referring each to his or her separate support group or individual therapy. This chapter will focus on therapy and policy considerations for the couple (heterosexual, homosexual, married, and unmarried) as a unit.

PSYCHOLOGICAL DISTRESS WITHIN COUPLES

Although some studies have shown that people with HIV/AIDS have higher levels of psychological morbidity and greater sexual difficulties than both the general population and their HIV-negative counterparts (Catalan, Klimes, Bond et al., 1992; Atkinson et al., 1988), other studies

This chapter has been adapted with permission from "Couples of Mixed HIV Status: Challenges and Strategies for Intervention with Couples," by Robert H. Remien, in *Psychotherapy and AIDS: The Human Dimension,* edited by Lucy A. Wicks, pp. 165-178. Copyright 1997 by Taylor and Francis, Washington, DC.

found rates of current depressive disorders among HIV-positive men and women to be more or less equal to rates for HIV-negative men and women and general population samples (Klimes et al., 1992; Williams et al., 1991; Perry et al., 1990). However, HIV-positive samples compared to HIV-negative controls consistently express more symptoms of distress on both clinician-administered and self-rated scales.

Furthermore, studies of psychiatric morbidity in HIV-infected people rarely, if ever, consider the relationship status of the participants. One systematic study that assessed psychological distress in male couples of mixed HIV status found significantly elevated levels of self-reported depression, anxiety, and hopelessness in both members of the couple, as compared to couples in which both members share the same HIV status (Remien, Carballo-Dieguez, and Wagner, 1995). Other studies have revealed an increased vulnerability for psychological distress among heterosexual couples of mixed HIV status, particularly, soon after notification of HIV-seropositive status. Studies have also found psychological distress to be a factor associated with risky sexual behavior (Kennedy et al., 1993). It is believed that the issues faced by individuals in mixed-status partnerships pose unique and difficult challenges to maintaining positive mental health in each member of the dyad.

CHALLENGES FOR THE COUPLE

HIV serodiscordance makes the issues that typically confront any couple particularly complex and multifaceted. Barriers to open communication that can be challenging for all couples are exacerbated due to the often overwhelming fear of HIV transmission, illness progression, and future loss. Avoidance of the topic is common in these couples because of the powerful emotions associated with HIV-related concerns. Major issues that typically arise include difficulties associated with future planning, fear of HIV transmission, lack of sexual spontaneity and satisfaction, decisions about pregnancy and child rearing, fantasies of fleeing, fear of abandonment, fear of increased intimacy in the context of potential loss, caretaking concerns, and feelings of sadness, guilt, and rage.

Avoidance

It is common for mixed-status couples to avoid talking about HIV-related topics, including all of their fears and concerns about many issues. Anything that is related to the topic can become emotionally charged. It is fairly safe to assume that every person who is aware of his or her HIV-positive serostatus, and every person who is the partner of an HIV-positive person, entertains, in his or her own mind, a range of fantasies about the future possibility of severe illness, physical dependence, cognitive decline, and premature death. It can be difficult to verbalize these fears to oneself and to one's partner, thus individuals often endure these fantasies in isolation. Both members of the couple will typically express the need to "protect" their partner from these thoughts and feelings. The seronegative partner typically does not want to express his or her sadness and fear to avoid burdening the partner with "something else to worry about" or making the partner "feel bad," since, after all, the partner is infected, and he or she is not. This may lead the seronegative partner to think that his or her emotional needs are less valid. The seropositive partner, likewise, feels that he or she needs to protect the partner from worrying about him or her and may feel guilty for bringing HIV infection into the relationship, whether he or she already knew their seropositive status before or after forming the relationship. Eventually, it is realized that both share similar concerns and that, to a large degree, they are attempting to protect themselves from confronting the potential reality of what may lie ahead.

SEXUAL RISK BEHAVIOR

Since one partner is HIV-positive and the other is not, the fear of transmission is ever present, and difficulties emerge concerning the need to *always* engage in *protected* sex and achievement of satisfaction with safer sex. Research has shown that consistent use of condoms for vaginal intercourse is highly effective in preventing the transmission of HIV (Vincenzi, 1994). Among couples not using condoms regularly, the risk of HIV transmission varies widely and is influenced by several factors, including stage of HIV illness in the seropositive partner, other genital infections in the seronegative partner, bleeding as a result of intercourse, and participation in anal intercourse (Vincenzi, 1994; Seidlin et al., 1993; Anderson, O'Brien, and Politch, 1992).

Consistent maintenance of protected sex is difficult to achieve in ongoing intimate relationships (Remien, Carballo-Dieguez, and Wagner, 1995; Padian et al., 1993). Condoms can be perceived to be a barrier to intimacy or a constant reminder of HIV infection and, therefore, can interfere with the spontaneity and pleasure of sexual expression. Many couples say that using condoms is like "bringing death into the bedroom" because of all of the cognitive and emotional associations attached to the necessity of their use. Not using condoms, or engaging in sex behavior that may be risky, can be perceived as exciting, passionate, and a "true" expression of love and commitment.

Many couples do not think that unprotected oral sex is extremely risky for transmission of HIV and are willing to engage in this behavior with each other on a regular basis. Nevertheless, there is often fear and discomfort associated with the behavior that interferes with pleasure and satisfaction. Some even have concerns about body fluids (e.g., saliva, ejaculate, vaginal secretions) being on the uninfected partner's skin, particularly if there are cuts or sores anywhere on the body. Often, these concerns, as with other HIV-related issues, go unexpressed and are avoided. These intrusive, and at times irrational, thoughts and fears may be felt by either the HIV-positive or HIV-negative partner or, at times, by both of them.

CARETAKING CONCERNS

Fear about such issues as illness, loss of functioning, and dependency can be persistent, even when the infected partner is entirely asymptomatic. Distress about these concerns may be intermittent or chronic in one or both members of the couple. When illness is manifested in the HIV-positive partner, the challenge and associated distress created by illness move from being hypothetical to being real. Studies of chronically ill patients and their families have shown that the lack of control over symptoms and the debilitating effects and unpredictability of the disease contribute to the stress of caregiving (Cohen and Lazarus, 1979; Jessop and Stein, 1985; Moos and Tsu, 1977; Zarit and Zarit, 1986). These effects can be most pronounced in spouses and partners of the person with chronic illness (Revenson, 1994; Rolland, 1994; Chowanec and Binik, 1989; Badger, 1990; Webster, 1992; Wright, 1991). Being part of a couple affected by HIV/AIDS is perceived as a major life transition, as both partners are confronted by multiple losses including the possible death of the person with AIDS, dissolution of the relationship, health, independence, intimacy, and privacy (Powell-Cope, 1995).

HIV presents couples with several unique challenges. Most of the literature concerning chronic illness and couples does not deal with communicable diseases. The transmissibility of HIV adds another major dimension of stress. Further, for gay couples or couples with a history of IV drug use, living a lifestyle seen as "deviant" by many, the intensity of this experience is magnified tremendously when facing another highly stigmatized condition such as AIDS (Rolland, 1994). As a result of these stressors, the primary partners of people with HIV/AIDS are not always able to provide adequate support. Although support of various types is usually available for persons who are ill, the needs of their partners are less often addressed. Spouses occupy a dual role in the coping process, as primary provider of support to the ill person and as a family member who needs support in coping with the illness-related stresses he or she is experiencing (Revenson, 1994).

FUTURE PLANNING

Planning for the future is an activity usually shared by two people in intimate relationships, particularly as relationships grow and solidify over time. In mixed-HIV-status relationships, such planning is typically fraught with mixed emotions and, as a result, often avoided. Coping with future uncertainty may be one of the most difficult psychological challenges for anyone living with HIV. For the mixed-status couple, it is especially difficult because of the perception that they have very different health and life expectancies. The often stated comment that "either one of us could get sick with something else . . . or hit by a bus" usually does not help because of the very present and "real" potential for illness and death associated with HIV infection.

The perception that the couple cannot engage in long-term future planning, as do other couples not living with HIV, is experienced as a significant loss by the couple. This loss can impede the development of intimacy in the relationship. Further, unexpressed and unexamined feelings of loss can hinder normal developmental tasks of the couple. When couples recognize their avoidance of discussing the future, they may express feelings of rage and despair, believing that "it just isn't fair" that they must live with this overwhelming uncertainty and dread of the future. Members of the couples may find that they have disparate views of optimism and hope for the future (i.e., regarding improved treatments for HIV illness), and this itself can become a significant source of conflict within the couple.

Future planning and thoughts about the future can include an array of topics, including career, savings and retirement, housing, living location, vacations, and children. Mixed-HIV-status couples may already have children (who may or may not be infected themselves), or they may want to have children, biologically or via adoption. This can hold equally true for homosexual as well as heterosexual couples. Having and raising children is an extremely important life goal and activity for many people. Feeling that this possibility is either taken away from them or significantly impaired can be a difficult loss with which to cope.

ISOLATION

Many couples of mixed-HIV status feel alone and isolated. Disclosure of HIV status is a very personal matter. Generally, people with HIV are encouraged, by counselors, to disclose their HIV status to some people (e.g., close friends, some family members, a confidante) so that they are not so alone and can receive support. They are also, however, advised to be clear about their reasons and desire to disclose, to consider potential negative consequences of such disclosure (e.g., discrimination, rejection, hostility, etc.), and to be selective about disclosure and not disclose to others indiscriminately. Decisions about disclosure in mixed-status couples are complicated by the fact that there are two people involved. There may be significant differences within the dyad regarding desire to disclose, reasons for wanting to disclose, to whom to disclose, when to disclose, and how to disclose. Often the HIV-negative partner believes that it is up to the HIV-positive partner to make decisions about disclosure because it is his or her seropositive status that is the significant information being shared. As a result, the HIV-negative partner may deny his or her own need for others to know and to seek desired support out of deference to his or her partner. Often, when asked, the HIV-positive partner does not agree with this position. It is striking how often incorrect assumptions are made, by both partners, regarding their perceptions about each other's thoughts and feelings regarding disclosure.

Members of mixed-status relationships often experience the lack of support and validation of their relationship from significant others in their lives. This can be true for either or both members of the couple. The seronegative partner may find that his or her friends and family do not think they should allow themselves to get involved or remain involved with someone who is infected because of the possibility of transmission of the virus, potential illness and need for caretaking, and early loss and death. Similarly, the HIV-positive partner may be advised that he or she is placing too much burden on himself or herself by being involved with someone who does not share his or her HIV status. Mixed-status couples often do not know many, or any, other couples in the same situation. They often question the viability and validity of their relationship. Because of these many challenges, there may be an ever-present fear that "I (or my partner) will not be able to handle it, and may walk out at any time."

THE THERAPEUTIC PROCESS

Working with mixed-HIV-status couples can be an extremely rewarding, as well as challenging, experience. One must believe in the couple's ability to confront the issues and in the power and advantage of working with the couple as a unit rather than seeing their needs as distinct and different, and thus only treating them individually or in separate groups.

Working with the couple can facilitate the emotional and behavioral processes necessary for them to meet the challenges they face while achieving and maintaining optimal mental health and well-being.

Creating a Safe Space

It is essential that the therapist be able to create a safe environment in which all of the difficult issues may be confronted. Often there is a buildup of many unexpressed feelings, concerns, and conflicts by the time the couple presents for treatment. It is useful to establish a commitment to the therapy process, whereby the couple agrees to work with the therapist for a specified period of time. This commitment may be outlined as a number of sessions or as a specific length of time, after which the process will be evaluated. This helps to establish that, although the work may be difficult, each member of this working alliance (both partners and the therapist) is agreeing to be there (return for each subsequent session) regardless of what may be expressed in the therapy room. The therapist should also consider and then discuss with the couple how they will conduct planned sessions if one of the members of the couple is unable to attend (e.g., due to illness). Although there are no definitive solutions applicable to all situations (e.g., meeting with one member of the couple, meeting at home, in hospital rooms, canceling), it is important that expectations be clarified prior to such events occurring.

For a period of time, the therapy room may be a container for tremendous fear, rage, and despair that is too frightening or overwhelming to be communicated outside of the room. In the beginning of treatment, many couples find it useful to be told by the therapist that they may want to *avoid* talking about some of the issues at home, now that they have a place where they know these things will be discussed. This helps to establish the therapy room as the place where they can confront difficult feelings that do not necessarily have to spill over and interfere with their everyday functioning. By "normalizing" the emotional impact of HIV infection on the couple, therapy can also address many of the other issues encountered in relationships.

SESSION CONTENT

Although couple dynamics (e.g., ways that couples communicate, express their needs, their emotions, etc.) is the important focus of most couples therapy, the content of the sessions is also important when working with mixed-HIV-status couples. The therapist may need to be the one who raises unexpressed issues such as concerns about HIV transmission, future illness, potential death, etc. This direct approach is often necessary to facilitate discussion of otherwise avoided topics. This will involve a careful balancing of HIV-related and "other" issues within the relationship. Although HIV concerns are often avoided, it is also common for couples to "blame" HIV for all of their interpersonal and life difficulties. The therapist must pay attention and articulate this when excessive focus on HIV is observed. Although HIV cannot and should not be the sole focus of the therapy, at some time during the treatment the key HIV-related challenges must be addressed. The timing of these particular discussions will vary across couples and is up to the clinical judgment of the therapist.

Sexual Behavior

When discussing sex, it is important to speak about it frankly and directly, including frequency of sex, sexual satisfaction (what feels good and what does not), and knowledge and thoughts (rational and irrational) about HIV risk attached to specific behaviors. Each member of the couple needs to be able, from time to time, to express what may seem to be irrational concerns about possible transmission of HIV, if it is something that enters their mind. These intrusive thoughts will interfere with sexual satisfaction and desire for sexual contact.

If the couple finds themselves engaging in nonreciprocal behaviors with each other (e.g., positive partner performing oral sex, but the negative not, or negative partner penetrating, while the positive does not), they need to voice their feelings about this. The HIV-positive partner may feel disempowered or less worthy to voice his or her feelings of disagreement with the "default" mode of sexual behavior they have adopted. The couple may have found themselves behaving in this nonreciprocal fashion without ever discussing it, and it is important to share their feelings about it, to clear up incorrect assumptions they each may have, and to discuss any possible desired change in their sexual encounters.

Anxiety and fear (e.g., about HIV or other sexually transmitted diseases) is a hindrance to sexual satisfaction and pleasure. With time, couples usually can find ways to alleviate their fears while maintaining spontaneity and pleasure. It may, however, take time and considerable discussion and experimentation for this to happen. The therapist should not assume that both partners understand viral transmission and the levels of risk associated with specific behaviors. Either one or both of them may be reluctant to admit their lack of knowledge or may have some serious misunderstanding of basic facts. The therapist can normalize the confusion that many people have and encourage a discussion of the "basic facts" as well as the more ambiguous areas of risk perception. If the couple can agree on what they believe to be risky and what they feel is okay for them, then they will each know what the limits are, and they can relax and be creative within those bounds. When couples are successful at this negotiation, their sex becomes less "cognitive" and more natural.

For heterosexual couples, pregnancy or the desire for pregnancy can be an important and challenging topic. Clearly a couple cannot become pregnant while engaging in "fully" protected sex. Nevertheless, wanting to have children and having both members of the couple be the "biological" parents may be a priority for some couples. Both "individual" and "couple" desires need to be fully articulated. All options regarding having children need to be considered, including sperm donation, arranging for a surrogate mother, adoption, and strategies for reducing risk of HIV transmission if sex between the couple is the chosen method of achieving pregnancy. Other issues to consider are the age and current health of each member of the couple, consequences for other children or members of the family, financial resources, custody concerns, and risks to health and medical treatment options for the woman, if she is the HIV-positive partner.

Sex outside of the relationship may or may not be an accepted aspect to the relationship. Some couples may desire and strive for monogamy, while others may agree to "not discuss it." There may be concerns and unresolved feelings about source and time of infection of HIV in the infected partner, as well as the potential for other sexually transmitted diseases, substance use history, bisexual behavior, etc. If such topics are avoided, lack of mutual trust will continue to interfere with intimacy and growth within the relationship. If the HIV-positive partner is feeling less desirable, like "damaged goods," or experiencing sexual dysfunction due to illness or medication side effects, he or she will be seeking reassurance from the uninfected partner. The therapist can facilitate discussion of these challenging issues. It may be useful for the therapist to normalize many of these feelings and concerns by stating, "It is common in couples of mixed HIV status for one or both partners to feel . . . ," as a way of introducing some of the feelings that are difficult to express. Also, standard sex therapy techniques, such as sensate focus or paradoxical interventions (e.g., prohibiting certain sex acts) can be useful clinical interventions to help the couple overcome some of their difficulties.

Caretaking Concerns

Typically, a strong resistance manifests toward discussing fears and concerns about illness and caretaking, whether HIV illness is already in progression or is anticipated, because of the couple's desire to "protect each other" from these thoughts. When illness develops, it is fairly common for couples to feel some relief, realizing that they *can* handle it and that it is not as overwhelming and awful as they had feared. Talking about their fears can be very reassuring and can increase feelings of intimacy and caring, particularly when each member recognizes that they both have been having many of the same thoughts and fantasies but hiding them from each other.

The couple needs to voice their expectations of each other and discuss limitations they think they have. It is very useful and important to have the couple note and discuss ways that they currently take care of each other. The therapist may need to note that there are many ways of caring for each other and that this is bidirectional, lest the HIV-negative partner gets automatically labeled as "the caretaker" in the relationship. Couples may need help realizing that the HIV-positive partner can help and nurture his or her HIV-negative partner, even in the context of illness progression. A very simple and concrete example is teaching the HIV-positive partner to inquire as to how the HIV-negative partner is coping with new physical symptoms or new health care demands being placed on him or her. This can help maintain "emotional equality" in the relationship, even when there is not "physical equality" in terms of health status.

Often there can be conflict in the relationship about the degree of involvement in each other's health care, particularly when it comes to health care for the HIV-positive partner. The negative partner may "nag" his or her partner about taking better care of himself or herself, treatment adherence, etc. Positive partners may feel that they want a "lover, not a nurse" in their relationship. Resentment can build and it is important that their expectations of each other in this regard be clarified. This discussion may need to be concrete, such as discussing whether they will accompany each other for doctor visits or for HIV tests. More important, the therapist may need to facilitate a discussion of the feelings behind their behavior with, and expectations of, each other. One of the ways that the couple may need to address their caretaking concerns and behavior with each other is to involve others (e.g., family, close friends) in their plans.

Future Planning

The distress of the uncertainty of the future must be acknowledged, while effective strategies to cope with this distress need to be supported. Nobody can decide the appropriateness of making many long-range plans for the future for people living with HIV. It has been shown that having meaningful goals and a "sense" of future is associated with psychological resilience for AIDS long-term survivors (Remien et al., 1992). If the couple has clearly avoided thinking about the future and having any long-range goals as a couple, the recognition of that fact can lead to a discussion of each of their perspectives regarding the future. This avoidance may be associated with a degree of hopelessness about their future as a couple or because of HIV. Although "living for today" or "living in the moment" is a useful coping strategy for people living with HIV (including couples), thinking about and discussing the future is a part of intimacy that can be important to couples. This includes discussing their dreams, hopes, and wishes and setting priorities in their lives. Simply sharing these thoughts with each other can have a very positive effect on feelings of intimacy for the couple.

It is also true that many people (and couples) may deny the potential for significant health problems in the future. This may be detrimental to the relationship, if absolutely no thought is given to the possibility for HIV-illness progression. The therapy room may be a good place to facilitate such a discussion. Getting issues about planning for the future on the table for discussion can be difficult but will have a positive emotional effect in the end. To make plans for the possibility of illness progression does not mean that the couple needs to feel hopeless about the future. On the contrary, having these affairs in order allows them to go about the business of living their lives, including making plans for the future. In the wake of emerging new combination treatments for HIV disease, there is a renewed hopefulness for the potential for a closer-to-normal life span for people with HIV. Such hopefulness needs to be supported, provided the couple does not ignore the realities of HIV disease and the necessary medical care.

Social Supports and Disclosure

In therapy, the couple can examine their social support network and evaluate the extent to which it meets their needs as individuals and as a couple. They also need to explore and check out each other's assumptions about who does and who does not know about their situation and who they want to know. The therapist may need to legitimize both the desire for and the fear of disclosure for both members of the couple. Merely framing it as a "couples" issue generally has a powerful therapeutic effect. At the same time, each member of the couple may have a need for a personal confidante, and this can be legitimized as well.

There may be times when one or both members of the couple may withdraw from each other or from their social network. This is normal for all couples at different times in the relationship. It may be more pronounced at times because of HIV, such as at the time of serostatus notification or with the onset of physical symptoms or the occurrence of an opportunistic infection. Normalizing such responses is important, as is noting whether such emotional states are persistent or perhaps severe (i.e., indicative of a clinical depression), necessitating referral for other psychological or psychiatric intervention.

THEMES THROUGHOUT THERAPY

Therapy needs to validate the emotional concerns of both partners and help the couple see that neither member's concerns are more or less valid, but rather, both have legitimate emotional needs. By "normalizing" the emotional impact of HIV infection on the couple, therapy can also address many of the other issues that most relationships face. Too often, couples, and even the therapist, may blame HIV for every conflict in the relationship, since communication in general may be severely restricted. Throughout therapy, these couples must be supported and their existence as a couple validated.

It is important to *keep HIV in its place*. To avoid blaming each other and to make it easier to work on a common enemy, couples are encouraged to reframe their situation, perceiving HIV as an intruder in their lives. By objectifying and extruding HIV, the couple can achieve some distance from the virus and then work together to repair the disruptiveness of its impact. In this way, the couple can also avoid blaming each other and focus on dealing with the demands of the illness. One way couples can gain strength to work against the impact of HIV is by increasing their sense of identity as a couple. It is useful to facilitate a discussion of who they are as a couple, what makes them special, and what their strengths are as a couple.

There is often a fear that discussing all of the HIV-related concerns will make those events come true or make matters worse. There can also be a fear that once they begin talking about these things, they will not be able to "forget about them" or focus on other aspects of their lives. The therapist, through both verbalization and modeling, can help the couple recognize that there is room for both direct discussion of HIV-related fears and for living their lives with some sense of "normalcy," focusing on the many other facets of their lives. HIV is just one of many identifying characteristics of their relationship, and that fact will probably need to be stated in many different ways, in many different contexts.

Assessment of Psychopathology

The couples therapist should always be attentive to individual psycho-pathology, identifying its presence and understanding its effect on couple functioning. The most common mental disorders seen in this population are mood, anxiety, and substance use disorders. These need to be acknowledged and discussed in the couple's therapy but should not be treated in that modality. If the therapist does not feel confident in his or her own assessment of the psychopathology, he or she may need to refer the couple for evaluation. It is probably good practice, however, to refer for treatment in most cases rather than treat one of the members of the couple individually.

Special Role of Groups

Multiple-couple groups can be a highly effective intervention for couples of mixed HIV status (Livingston, 1966). All of what has been outlined in this chapter can take place in a group setting. A group, however, has the potential to enhance several therapeutic processes. Bringing mixed-HIV-status couples together can quickly reduce isolation and the resulting feeling that "they are the only ones." Couples find their worries and concerns legitimized by seeing them occur in other couples. Often, the raising of particular issues by other couples will trigger discussions within dyads that have never occurred before. Couples also have the opportunity to share effective, and often creative, coping strategies with one another. Modeling of affection and intimate behaviors by some couples can greatly influence couples who are struggling with their own expression of these feelings and behavior. Most important, couples can offer one another support and validate one another's existence and viability as they struggle to meet all of the challenges that being mixed-HIV-status couples entails.

POLICY IMPLICATIONS

A wide range of issues affected by policy exist when a couple is of mixed HIV status, but most of them can be organized into three distinct clusters: medical decision making, emotional and practical support for the caretaking partner, and survivorship. The therapist can play an important role in helping the couple first to identity and then to address many of these issues. In fact, the role of the therapist can be crucial, given the characteristics of mixed-status couples cited previously, including a tendency toward avoidance of difficult issues, a lack of support sources, and difficulty with future planning.

It should be noted that for homosexual couples or unmarried heterosexual couples, whose relationships are not recognized by legal authorities, policy-related issues can become particularly complicated. It is also crucial to emphasize that the flow of concern and support between the partners needs to be *bidirectional*. An excessively rigid conception of the seronegative partner as the "care provider" and the seropositive partner as the "care recipient" can undermine each person's identity as an equal member of a relationship and also overlooks the fact that seronegative partners have important needs of their own. All seronegative individuals will develop personal needs, often entirely unrelated to HIV, and will naturally turn to their partners for comfort, guidance, and care.

Medical Decision Making

As discussed earlier, it is important that the members of a mixed-status couple prepare for the eventuality of serious illness before it arrives. Although either partner can become ill, HIV-positive partners obviously face a chance of developing AIDS, which encompasses an extraordinary number of different opportunistic infections and cancers—each of which has their own unique symptomatology, treatment, and prognosis. Medical decision making in this context can be extremely complex, and the best course of action is not always clear. When an individual with HIV or AIDS moves out of the home setting and is admitted to a hospital or other public facility, medical decision making is no longer a matter for the couple to resolve between themselves but becomes embedded in an institutional setting that may be impersonal, indifferent, or even hostile. Unfortunately, at the same time, the ill partner's ability to make decisions may be diminished by physical and/or cognitive impairment.

All of these factors make it particularly important that partners have discussions about the difficult but very real health decisions that they may face before they arise. The therapist can help with this process by identifying some of these medical questions and providing couples with a structured environment in which to explore them. In this way, the couple can reach more reasoned and fully informed decisions, increasing the likelihood that the ill partner will receive the types of treatment which he or she desires rather than those decided upon by health care providers. The inherent stress concerning illness, hospitalization, and treatment can be reduced if both partners know that the wishes of the ill partner are clearly understood.

One important issue to be considered is medical directives or "living wills," indicating whether the ill partner wishes to have "heroic measures" used to sustain life or, alternatively, wishes to create a standing "do not resuscitate" (DNR) order. Even before such end-stage considerations come to bear, couples will need the communication skills to work together to make decisions about the often bewildering range of treatment issues with which people with AIDS must contend. If the couple has already had discussions in which ethical, religious, and other concerns have been addressed, the well partner will have a better sense of how to make medical decisions that can often be difficult and complicated.

For couples whose relationships are not recognized by law, special legal steps, such as the assignment of medical power of attorney, need to be taken to ensure that medical decision making remains in the hands of the partner rather than some other legal next of kin. Particularly in the case of homosexual relationships, it is not uncommon for institutions to disregard the wishes of a partner when they conflict with those of a biological family member; in some extreme cases, partners are even denied hospital visitation rights. The rights of same-sex partners have been more widely recognized in recent years, particularly in the larger cities of the United States. Nonetheless, in the absence of a marriage certificate, proof of the wishes of the ill partner and of the significance of the relationship (such as registration as domestic partners) can be helpful.

Support for the Caretaking Partner

Issues such as medical decision making highlight the strains put upon caretaking partners in mixed-status relationships. Beyond the emotional and psychological needs of such partners, a number of practical policy issues also emerge concerning caretaking. One example is the ability of the caretaking partner to get time off from work—or even simply the understanding and cooperation of co-workers and employers—when his or her partner is ill. If the couple has not disclosed either their status as a couple or their mixed HIV status in the workplace, either out of a desire for privacy or out of fear of discrimination, the well partner may be forced to act as though nothing is going on or to make up excuses for missed time or a drop in job productivity.

If, conversely, the ill partner was the primary income provider, the couple may be faced with serious financial problems, particularly if adequate provisions for insurance or disability allowance have not been made. Further, among unmarried couples, the well partner may not be eligible for all the benefits accorded to married couples. Couples with children may also face practical difficulties with child care, when the home situation changes from having two adults to one adult whose attentions must be largely refocused to the ill partner. Therapists can facilitate discussions about these complex challenges and help couples develop possible solutions. This process may include holding sessions with other family members or making referrals to private or governmental social service agencies.

The issue of social support is one in which, ironically, homosexual couples may sometimes actually be better situated than heterosexual couples. Many community-based organizations offer services for which all may be eligible but from which heterosexuals may feel excluded. Heterosexual couples may also be less aware of AIDS-related support services and may have fewer people in their social networks who can empathize with them and offer support. Therapists can be helpful in highlighting the question of support sources for the caretaking partner, clarifying that it is not "selfish" for the caretaker to be concerned with his or her own well-being. It should perhaps be reemphasized, however, that there are many cases in which, perhaps unexpectedly, the HIV-positive partner is called upon to care for the physical or emotional well-being of the HIV-negative partner.

Survivorship

A final policy area of major concern involves the full range of survivorship issues. As with medical decision making, it is crucial for the couple to plan for the possible death of one partner. Yet death and widowhood can be even harder to discuss and easier to avoid or deny. Once death is near or has occurred, however, it is obviously too late to provide for such basic needs as life insurance policies, inheritance, and in some cities, apartment succession rights. Although it may seem to couples that it is petty to discuss "practical" issues in the face of impending death, the abrupt loss of income, property rights, or housing will greatly worsen the already difficult situation of the survivor. Therapists can help by validating the importance of pragmatic concerns and providing an opportunity for couples to address them; the earlier this process occurs, the better.

Custody of children also requires significant planning. The surviving partner may be unable or unwilling to care for children alone, particularly if the children are not his or her own but were from the partner's prior relationship. Alternatively, a surviving partner may very much wish to continue caring for a child who is not a blood relative but may lose custody rights to a biological parent or other family member. Some courts in the United States have been increasingly willing to recognize the rights of same-sex "co-parents," but this remains a contentious area. Careful planning and discussion with biological relatives prior to a death may clarify the wishes of the deceased and smooth the way for the best child custody arrangement. It can also assist with the disposition of any inheritance or property rights of the surviving spouse. Legally married couples have the protection of the law in this regard, but among unmarried partners, families of origin may retain considerable legal rights, which they may use in ways which contradict the will of the deceased. Even when survivors have a good relationship with their partner's biological family, the heightened emotions surrounding a death can create tense situations. An officially notarized, unambiguous will may be the best way to avoid such difficulties.

SUMMARY

Working with mixed-HIV-status couples can be both a challenging and rewarding process. It is essential for the therapist to feel comfortable working with the couple as a unit rather than only treating and/or referring each to his or her separate therapy. The challenges that these couples face are many and include issues related to sex behavior, future planning, illness and caretaking, social supports, and disclosure. It is common for couples to avoid topics related to HIV as a way of "protecting" each other from the powerful emotions associated with HIV and all of its uncertainty. This avoidance serves to impede the continued growth of intimacy necessary for positive couple functioning and mutual satisfaction.

The therapy needs to validate the emotional concerns of both partners and normalize the emotional impact of HIV infection on the couple, while helping to keep HIV in perspective. Working at the dyadic level can facilitate the emotional and behavioral processes necessary for the partners to meet the challenges they face, to reinforce their viability as a couple, and to help them achieve and maintain optimal mental health and well-being. Therapists can also play a helpful role in enabling the couple to reach agreements about sensitive policy areas such as medical decision making, support for the caretaking partner, and survivorship.

REFERENCES

Anderson, D. J., O'Brien, T. R., and Politch, J. A. (1992). Effects of disease stage and zidovudine therapy on the detection of human immunodeficiency virus type 1 in semen. *Journal of the American Medical Association* (November 18), *19*:2651-2652.
Atkinson, J. H., Grant, I., Kennedy, C. J., Richman, D., Spector, S., and McCutchan, J. A. (1988). Prevalence of psychiatric disorders among men with HIV virus: A controlled study. *Archives of General Psychiatry, 45*:859-864.
Badger, T. (1990). Men with cardiovascular disease and their spouses: Coping, health, and marital adjustment. *Archives of Psychiatric Nursing, 4*(5):319-324.

Catalan, J., Klimes, I., Bond, A., Day, A., Garrod, J., and Rizza, C. (1992). The psychosocial impact of HIV infection in men with hemophilia: Controlled investigation and factors associated with psychiatric morbidity, *Journal of Psychosomatic Research, 36*(5):409-416.

Chowanec, G. and Binik, Y. M. (1989). End stage renal disease and the marital dyad: An empirical investigation. *Social Science Medicine, 28*(9):971-983.

Cohen, F. and Lazarus, R. S. (1979). Coping with the stresses of illness. In Stone, G. C., Cohen, F., and Adler, N. E., (Eds.), *Health Psychology.* San Francisco: Jossey Bass, pp. 217-254.

Jessop, D. J. and Stein, R. E. K. (1985). Uncertainty and its relation to the psychological and social correlates of chronic illness in children. *Social Science and Medicine, 20*(10):993-999.

Kennedy, C. A., Skurnick, J., Wan, J. Y., Quattrone, G., Sheffet, A., Quinones, M., Wang, W., and Louria, D. B. (1993). Psychological distress, drug and alcohol use as correlates of condom use in HIV-serodiscordant heterosexual couples. *AIDS, 7*(11):1493-1499.

Klimes, I., Catalan, J., Garrod, A., Day, A., Bond, A., and Rizza, C. (1992). Partners of men with HIV infection and hemophilia: Controlled investigation of factors associated with psychological morbidity. *AIDS Care, 4*(2):149-156.

Livingston, D. (1966). A systems approach to AIDS counseling for gay couples. In Shernoff, M. (Ed.), *Human Services for Gay People: Clinical and Community Practice.* Binghamton, NY: Harrington Park Press, pp. 83-94.

Moos, R. H. and Tsu, V. D. (1977). The crisis of physical illness: An overview. In Moos, R. H. (Ed.), *Coping with Physical Illness.* New York: Plenum, pp. 1-22.

Padian, N. S., O'Brien, T. R., Chang, Y. C., Glass, S., and Francis, D. P. (1993). Prevention of heterosexual transmission of human immunodeficiency virus through couple counseling. *Journal of Acquired Immune Deficiency Syndrome, 6*(9):1043-1048.

Perry, S. W., Jacobsberg, L. B., Fishman, B., Frances, A., Bobo, J., and Jacobsberg, B. K. (1990). Psychiatric diagnosis before serological testing for HIV virus. *American Journal of Psychiatry, 147*(1):89-93.

Powell-Cope, G. M. (1995). The experiences of gay couples affected by HIV infection. *Qualitative Health Research, 5*(1):36-62.

Remien, R. H., Carballo-Dieguez, A., and Wagner, G. (1995). Intimacy and sexual risk behavior in serodiscordant male couples. *AIDS Care, 7*(4):429-438.

Remien, R. H., Rabkin, J. G., Katoff, L., and Williams, J. B. W. (1992). Coping strategies and health beliefs of AIDS long term survivors. *Psychology and Health, 6*(4):335-345.

Revenson, T. (1994). Social support and marital coping with chronic illness. *Annals of Behavioral Medicine, 16*(2):122-130.

Rolland, J. (1994). In sickness and in health: The impact of illness on couples' relationships. *Journal of Marital and Family Therapy, 20*(4):327-347.

Seidlin, M., Vogler, M., Lee, E., Lee, Y. S., and Dubin, N. (1993). Heterosexual transmission of HIV in a cohort of couples in New York City. *AIDS, 7*(9):1247-1254.

Vincenzi, I. (1994). A longitudinal study of human immunodeficiency virus transmission by heterosexual partners. *The New England Journal of Medicine, 331*(6):341-346.

Webster, L. (1992). Working with couples in a diabetes clinic: The role of the therapist in a medical setting. *Sexual and Marital Therapy, 7*(2):189-196.

Williams, J. B. W., Rabkin, J. G., Remien, R. H., Gorman, J., and Ehrhardt, A. (1991). Multidisciplinary baseline assessment of homosexual men with and without HIV infection. II Standardized clinical assessment of current and lifetime psychopathology. *Archives of General Psychiatry, 48*(2):124-130.

Wright, L. (1991). The impact of Alzheimer's disease on the marital relationship. *The Gerontologist, 31*(2):224-237.

Zarit, S. H. and Zarit, J. M. (1986). Dementia and the family: A stress management approach. *Clinical Psychologist, 39*(4):103-105.

Chapter 23

HIV-Associated Cognitive/Motor Complex: Early Detection, Diagnosis, and Intervention

Stephan L. Buckingham
Wilfred G. Van Gorp

Clinicians who work with HIV-infected individuals quickly learn that these clients may evidence a variety of neuropsychiatric difficulties during the course of their illness. These neuropsychiatric complications may be the result of a psychological reaction to the trauma of learning of one's HIV seropositivity, with the associated psychosocial stress throughout the course of the illness, and/or HIV-related changes to the central nervous system. Evidence of the presence of HIV can be found in the central nervous system of over half of asymptomatic but infected (seropositive) individuals, and at death, 90 percent of persons with AIDS have neuropathological evidence of central nervous system abnormalities (Navia et al., 1986).

This chapter will provide an overview of the various organic mental disorders found in HIV-infected individuals and how they can be detected and differentiated from other neuropsychiatric illnesses. HIV-associated cognitive/motor disorder will be the central focus of this chapter since it represents one of the most common neuropsychiatric illnesses experienced by HIV-infected individuals. This chapter will equip clinicians with the information needed for early detection of HIV-associated cognitive/motor disorder to determine when a referral for further workup is indicated, to make a differential diagnosis, and to provide the most effective mental health treatment services for these individuals.

BRIEF HISTORY

Two years after the initial case reports of what later came to be known as acquired immune deficiency syndrome (AIDS) (Gottlieb et al., 1981), descriptions of significant changes in the mental status of these patients appeared (Snider et al., 1983). Early studies reported that up to one half or more of these patients exhibited "subacute encephalitis," "encephalopathy," or "altered mental status." These early observations suggest that these patients must have demonstrated clinically significant levels of cognitive, emotional, and/or motor impairment since the symptoms were detected by mostly nonpsychiatric or neurologic physicians who were not expecting to find dementia in predominantly young adults.

Shortly after HIV was identified as the agent responsible for AIDS, it was learned that HIV could be isolated in the brains of demented, seropositive individuals (Ho et al., 1985) and that, in fact, HIV could even be found in the cerebrospinal fluid in half or more of asymptomatic, HIV-seropositive persons (Resnick et al., 1985; Resnick et al., 1988).

Although much work has since been done to identify the effects of HIV on the central nervous system, the exact mechanism by which this happens is still not fully known. Nevertheless, we do know which brain regions tend to be most affected and, as a corollary, which neuropsychiatric syndromes secondary to these brain changes most frequently result. Although pathologic studies at autopsy have found that virtually all brain regions can be affected, there is a consensus that the structures beneath the cortex—the subcortical regions—are those which are most significantly affected (Navia, Jordan, and Price, 1986; Rottenberg et al., 1987; Aylward et al., 1993).

Developments in Nomenclature

Navia, Jordan, and Price (1986) observed psychomotor slowing, slowed thinking, and flat affect in two-thirds of their patients with AIDS. They termed this condition the AIDS dementia complex to highlight this triad of cognitive, motor, and behavioral abnormalities. In 1987, the Centers for Disease Control published diagnostic criteria for HIV encephalopathy (Centers for Disease Control, 1987), which was somewhat similar to Navia and colleagues' description of the AIDS dementia complex.

More recently, the American Academy of Neurology AIDS Task Force (1991) published diagnostic criteria for HIV-associated cognitive/motor complex (see Appendix). For less severe cases, in which all but the most demanding activities of daily living can be performed but neuropsychological abnormalities are present, the diagnosis of HIV-associated minor cognitive/motor disorder is given. In more severe cases, individuals with more serious cognitive impairment and encroachment on activities of daily living are diagnosed with HIV-associated dementia complex. In all cases, *other* causes of cognitive, motor, or behavioral impairment must first be ruled out by medical history (such as history of severe alcoholism, head injury, etc.), brain imaging, and analysis of cerebrospinal fluid, since lesions from toxoplasmosis, progressive multifocal leukoencephalopathy, stroke, or tumor can all produce significant cognitive impairment. According to the American Academy of Neurology AIDS Task Force recommendations, neuropsychological testing should be performed whenever possible to assist in making this diagnosis and assessing severity of disability.

INCIDENCE/PREVALENCE OF HIV-ASSOCIATED COGNITIVE/MOTOR COMPLEX

As stated earlier, approximately 90 percent of patients who die with AIDS have evidence of neuropathologic abnormalities, and approximately half have evidence of a clinical dementia by the time of death. Up to two-thirds of patients with advanced HIV disease demonstrate significant neuropsychological abnormalities (though not necessarily severe enough to receive a diagnosis of dementia). One study (McArthur et al., 1993) has reported an annual incidence of HIV-associated cognitive/motor complex as 7 percent for those patients diagnosed with AIDS (this refers to the number of *new* cases diagnosed per year). Although the exact prevalence of HIV-related neuropsychological impairment is not known, there is agreement that it is highest in patients who are symptomatic.

What does the cumulative research show regarding the nature, incidence, and prevalence of HIV-related neuropsychological impairment or dementia in asymptomatic individuals? In a large study on neuropsychological status in seropositive and seronegative men (Multicenter AIDS Cohort Study, MACS), the seropositive individuals who were symptomatic demonstrated poorer performance on several traditional neuropsychological tests than did the seronegative control subjects. In contrast, this was *not* found to be true for those with asymptomatic infection, who, as a group, did not perform worse than the seronegative control subjects on any neuropsychological test (Miller et al., 1990). Several subsequent studies have tended to confirm this: on traditional, clinical, neuropsychological measures, those with asymptomatic HIV infection tend to perform no worse than seronegative controls with similar levels of age and education. Symptomatic individuals do tend to perform worse, as a group, on measures of psychomotor speed, memory, and reaction time (see Van Gorp et al., 1993).

More sensitive measures of information, processing speed (typically assessing reaction time via a computer) have confirmed subtle slowing in reaction time and decision-making speed in asymptomatic HIV-infected individuals relative to their seronegative peers (Martin et al., 1992; Wilkie et al., 1990). These results suggest that HIV infection is associated with *subtle* slowing of information processing in some individuals, but in all but a small subset, these changes are not typically severe enough to be considered clinically significant, until the individual evidences other symptoms of serious immunosuppression (e.g., night sweats, weight loss, fever of unknown origin, Kaposi's sarcoma, etc.).

NEUROANATOMIC AND CLINICAL FEATURES
OF HIV-ASSOCIATED COGNITIVE/MOTOR COMPLEX

An understanding of brain-behavior relationships will help the mental health clinician comprehend the relationship between HIV-related central nervous system changes and the neuropsychiatric manifestations that result from these changes.

The subcortical structures that have frequently been implicated in HIV-related neurologic disease, such as the basal ganglia and thalamus, are known to mediate specific cognitive and motor functions. Fine motor imprecision, psychomotor slowing, hypophonia (lowered volume of speaking), bradyphrenia (slowed information processing), a forgetful pattern of memory impairment, and difficulty on complex cognitive tasks, such as shifting of mental set and planning/strategy formation, have all been documented in diseases differentially implicating subcortical structures, including their rich connection to the frontal lobes of the brain. This produces a similar pattern of cognitive and motor impairment to that found in patients with other dementias resulting from predominantly subcortical pathology, such as Parkinson's disease and Huntington's disease. Damage to some subcortical structures has also been reported to result in delusions, mania, and depression (Cummings, 1990).

HIV-associated cognitive/motor complex as a "subcortical dementia," resembles other subcortical dementias and can be sharply contrasted with cortical dementias, such as Alzheimer's disease, by several key neuropsychological features. Psychomotor slowing, a "forgetful" pattern of memory disturbance, and difficulty on cognitive tasks requiring "executive" functions (such as mental set shifting, planning, and coping with novel situations), mediated by the frontal/subcortical connections, are the hallmark characteristics of subcortical dementia. Unlike the profound memory impairment in Alzheimer's disease, which produces an inability to learn new information, memory impairment in HIV-associated cognitive/motor complex is characterized by a relative preservation in the ability to learn new information, although *recall* of the information is often impaired. When testing memory, a patient with an HIV-associated cognitive/motor complex may exhibit impaired recall of a list of words he or she has been shown or in recalling complex medication instructions from a physician or nurse; however, when asked to *recognize* the correct information from multiple choices, the patient will often be able to perform correctly, indicating that the material has been learned, but the patient has difficulty with spontaneous, accurate retrieval of that information. This "forgetful" pattern of memory disturbance often leads to the incorrect assumption by some caregivers or hospital staff that the patient is merely being manipulative and that they "can recall it when they want to."

On formal neuropsychological testing, multiple cognitive domains should be assessed. The domain in which patients with an HIV-associated dementia have the greatest difficulty is psychomotor speed. HIV-related neurocognitive deficits are most pronounced on timed tasks in which thought is tied to action. In contrast to deficits in psychomotor speed and memory, language function (including naming items and generating word lists) and overall intellectual function, as measured by traditional IQ tests, are typically preserved until moderate or severe stages of dementia are reached.

When the patient with an HIV-associated cognitive/motor complex suffers severe immunosupression and the dementia advances, more serious memory problems become apparent and worsening visuospatial problems may place the patient at risk for wandering and becoming lost. The patient may forget to take medications or forget to turn off the stove. In the end stage, the demented patient may be bedridden, mute, or grossly aphasic and exhibit hallucinations or delusions. In the final or terminal state, the patient may be mute and in a fetal position.

DIFFERENTIAL DIAGNOSIS: HIV-ASSOCIATED COGNITIVE/MOTOR IMPAIRMENT VERSUS OTHER HIV-RELATED NEUROPSYCHIATRIC DISORDERS

Dementia, delirium, psychosis (including delusions), depression, and mania have all been identified in association with infectious illnesses producing central nervous system disease (Cummings, 1985). Although many psychological disorders and emotional changes occur in individuals who have experienced a traumatic life situation, changes in mood and affect can also be the manifestation of central nervous system disease. Such a relationship was first demonstrated in the early case descriptions of syphilis (dementia praecox). It has also been shown that the frequency of depression is elevated in patients with various illnesses involving subcortical structures (Cummings, 1990) or in which focal lesions involving the left or right frontal brain regions are present (Robinson et al., 1984; Bolla-Wilson et al., 1989).

Delirium

Delirium, also known as a confusional state, may be acute or chronic and is characterized by a dramatic disruption of attention and concentration. It may be caused by a number of medical abnormalities, such as toxicity secondary to medications, metabolic disturbance (such as an electrolyte imbalance related to fluid loss), or an undiagnosed infection (such as a urinary tract infection). Because a high rate of morbidity is associated with delirium, patients identified as having a delirium must be promptly referred for a full medical workup so the underlying medical problem causing the delirium can be identified and treated, thereby reducing the risk of death. Delirium has been reported in up to 43 percent of hospitalized, HIV-infected patients. Because the many ongoing medical illnesses in HIV-infected individuals can often lead to a delirium, any clinician evaluating an HIV-infected patient with an altered mental status must be vigilant to the possibility that a confusional state may be present and responsible for that alteration.

The primary differential diagnosis for an HIV-infected patient with a confusional state is between an HIV-associated cognitive/motor complex versus a delirium, although other secondary focal illnesses such as toxoplasmosis should be ruled out first by means of brain imaging. In contrast to an HIV-associated cognitive/motor complex, the patient with a confusional state will typically present with an *abrupt onset* of confusion, have dramatic attentional difficulties, and will often demonstrate a language impairment characterized by rambling, incoherent speech and agraphia (impaired writing). In contrast, the patient with an HIV-associated cognitive/motor complex will usually have *intact* basic attention, experiencing difficulty with only the more complex measures of divided and sustained attention. Neuroimaging and lumbar puncture will be most helpful in ruling out a secondary neurologic process accounting for mental status changes, and laboratory blood analysis will assist in identifying the underlying cause of a delirium.

Psychosis

Psychosis is often among the first symptoms of mental status changes that can present in an HIV-infected individual, although this is still a relatively rare occurrence in these patients. More often, psychosis is associated with an acute delirium or end-stage dementia. Nevertheless, some HIV-infected individuals evidence delusions or hallucinations unrelated to a delirium at some point during their illness.

It is likely that the high prevalence of psychosis in HIV-infected persons (relative to the population at large) represents primary psychiatric illness or, instead, a primary manifestation of central nervous system involvement. Delusions and hallucinations have been shown to be higher than expected in other subcortical dementias and other disorders of the central nervous system (see Cummings, 1990). Thus, given the differential involvement of subcortical structures affected in HIV-related central nervous system changes, it appears reasonable to conclude that psychosis, at least in some of those experiencing such symptoms, is a reflection of altered function of the central nervous system.

For an HIV-infected individual presenting with a psychosis, the clinician must make a distinction among an organic delusional disorder or organic hallucinosis; a delirium, possibly secondary to medication toxicity or metabolic disturbance; coincident schizophrenia or schizophreniform disorder; a brief reactive psychosis to a severe life stressor; or major depression with psychotic features. A pessimistic, morbid outlook will often assist in determining if a depression with psychotic features is present, and a positive family history of psychosis may make a diagnosis of a coincident schizophrenic disorder more likely. Careful review of all medications and laboratory studies on a psychotic patient should be done any time a patient presents with a new onset of psychosis.

Depression

Not surprisingly, depressed mood (but not necessarily diagnosable clinical depression) has been reported in up to 76 percent of HIV-infected individuals, with the prevalence of major depression in HIV-infected individuals being 10 to 15 percent (Boccellari, Dilley, and Shore, 1988; Dilley et al., 1985; Perry and Tross, 1984).

Elevated levels of depression (relative to the general population and to medically ill patients in general) have been noted in patients with several neurologic disorders, especially those differentially affecting subcortical structures. For instance, it is known that, as a group, patients diagnosed with Parkinson's disease, Huntington's disease, and progressive supranuclear palsy—all of which differentially affect subcortical structures—have higher levels of depression than medically ill patients with severe movement abnormalities not caused by central nervous system disease (e.g., severe rheumatoid arthritis). Hence, the mood disorder in patients with subcortical brain involvement may, at least in part, relate to actual central nervous system changes rather than being solely a reaction to their illness.

The dementia syndrome of depression, sometimes called pseudodementia, has been reported in HIV disease. This condition can occur when a severe depression is thought to be responsible for cognitive deficits present in affected patients. The majority of cases of the dementia syndrome of depression have been older adults, and it has been shown that the majority of depressed HIV-infected individuals do not sustain neuropsychological deficits related to their depression (Hinkin et al., 1992). However, in a small subgroup of HIV-infected patients, the dementia syndrome of depression can occur and produce the appearance of an HIV-associated cognitive/motor complex complex. Thus, when examining any patient with suspected HIV-associated cognitive/motor complex, the effects of a significant depression must first be ruled out.

The clinical symptoms associated with a diagnosed depression may mimic those of a patient with an HIV-associated cognitive/motor complex such as psychomotor slowing, fatigue, irritability, difficulty concentrating, weight loss, and insomnia. Whenever there is evidence of a subjective mood disturbance, marked by sad affect, crying, hopelessness, guilt, and self-loathing, the clinician should first treat the probable depression and *then* reevaluate the patient for residual cognitive deficits to determine if these symptoms were the result of the depression, a dementia, or, in some cases, both. Careful assessment over time will often demonstrate the correlation between changes in mood state and resulting improvement in neuropsychological performance when a dementia syndrome of depression is evident.

The depressive effect of medications—including steroids or antineoplastic drugs—must also be taken into consideration when determining the etiology of a possible depressive disorder.

Mania

Symptoms of mania—including pressured speech, spending sprees, and sleeplessness—occur in patients with various neurologic disorders, especially those following focal brain injury to the frontal lobes. Mania may also occur in response to various pharmacologic agents—licit and illicit—and the clinician should be aware of the possibility of a secondary mania related to the effect of various medications. Focal central nervous system disorders in HIV-infected individuals, including progressive multifocal leukoencephalopathy, toxoplasmosis, or neoplasm, can all produce a secondary mania, especially if the frontal lobes are involved.

SCREENING FOR COGNITIVE IMPAIRMENT IN HIV DISEASE

HIV-infected individuals' self-report of everyday cognitive failures and memory problems is—contrary to expectations—related more to their mood state than to their actual neuropsychological test performance. This is especially true of patients in the asymptomatic stage. In one study, patients with asymptomatic HIV infection who were depressed had more complaints about everyday cognitive failures than their nondepressed peers, regardless of their actual level of neuropsychological functioning. These findings indicate that it is essential to obtain an independent, objective assessment of a patient's cognitive functioning rather than relying solely on the patient's assertion of cognitive deficits, particularly if the patient is experiencing a clinical depression.

How may the clinician screen for cognitive impairment in an HIV-infected individual? Brief tests of gross mental status, such as the Mini-Mental State Exam, have been shown to be remarkably *insensitive* to HIV-related neurocognitive impairment, and as such, they are not appropriate for screening of cognitive function in this population. Standard neuropsychological tests administered and interpreted by a trained neuropsychologist are the most sensitive measures to detect subtle, HIV-related cognitive dysfunction. Although a multihour, comprehensive neuropsychological evaluation may be necessary to elicit subtle cognitive impairment or to assist in making a differential diagnosis among other complex conditions such as depression, prior heavy substance abuse, or learning disability, the nonneuropsychologist mental health clinician can nevertheless carefully evaluate patients' mental status to discern key signs of HIV-related neurocognitive impairment.

Because psychomotor speed is the domain most frequently affected in HIV-related cognitive impairment, tasks that require timed psychomotor performance—in which thought is tied to action—will be particularly sensitive as early markers of impairment. Evidence of slowed movement or driving difficulties (a "real life" test of psychomotor speed and reaction time) may represent early signs of neurocognitive compromise. Patient or caregiver reports of psychomotor slowing—including driving difficulties or one or more automobile accidents—will provide important diagnostic information regarding the presence of this condition. Psychological tests such as the Trail Making Test A and B and the Digit Symbol Subtest of the Wechsler Adult Intelligence Scale—Revised may also be useful tools for the psychologist to use for clinical screening. Assessment of a patient's memory functioning is also important in evaluating a patient with a possible HIV-associated dementia. Requiring the patient to learn a list of several words and recall them following a twenty-minute delay may be sufficient to detect clinically significant memory problems. Questioning the patient about details of *recent* (rather than remote, which will be much less impaired memory retrieval) news events or movies he or she has seen may also prove useful as screening tools. Patient or caregiver reports of significant memory problems (such as double booking appointments at work) may be key diagnostic markers. If a memory impairment is suspected, it is important to refer the patient to a neuropsychologist for formal memory assessment, using such measures as the California Verbal Learning Test, the Rey Auditory Verbal Learning Test, and the Wechsler Memory Scale—Revised.

Assessment of other cognitive domains, such as attention, visuospatial function, language, and judgment are also important. Because the normal digit-span memory is seven, plus or minus two, it is important to ask the patient to repeat back a series of digits—spoken at the rate of one digit per second—presented first by the clinician. The clinician should start with four digits forward, and as the patient successfully repeats back each string, the examiner can increase the next string by one (five, six, seven, and so forth). Patients with attentional difficulties will often repeat fewer than five digits in a sequence. Spatial functioning can be tested by asking the patient to describe a route through the city to go from point A to point B. Since language function is typically normal in HIV-associated cognitive/motor complex, any patients exhibiting serious language problems, such as word substitution, should be referred for neurologic or neuropsychologic workup. Formal measures of attention, spatial function, judgment, and other cognitive abilities can also be assessed by the Neurobehavior Cognitive Status Exam, a relatively brief (approximately thirty minutes) test of many of these cognitive functions. If deficits are present, a complete neuropsychological evaluation should be requested. We recommend a patient be referred for neuropsychological evaluation when any of the following conditions exist:

1. The patient reports changes in cognitive functioning.
2. Another person observes cognitive difficulties in a patient.
3. There is an abrupt change in a patient's personality or cognitive abilities.
4. The clinician is attempting to differentiate between dementia versus depression.
5. Evidence is needed to support an application for disability.
6. The clinician is trying to determine the effect of a medication on cognitive functioning.
7. There is a need to document a patient's competency to make or amend a will.
8. The clinician is trying to differentiate between the effects of substance abuse versus HIV on cognitive functioning.

If neuropsychological deficits are suspected, the neuropsychologist will likely administer a measure of general intelligence, such as the Wechsler

Adult Intelligence Scale-III. Other measures will include the Trail Making Test (psychomotor speed); Digit Span and/or the Paced Auditory Serial Addition Test (attention/concentration); Wechsler Memory Scale-III and/or the Rey or California Auditory Verbal Learning Test (verbal and nonverbal memory); the Rey Osterrieth Complex Figure Test (visuospatial function); the Category Test or Wisconsin Card Sorting Test and/or the Stroop Color Interference Test (frontal lobe functioning); Finger Tapping Test and/or Grooved Pegboard Test (motor speed); and the Minnesota Multiphasic Personality Inventory-2 (MMPI-2) or the Beck Depression Inventory (as a measure of mood).

CLINICAL INTERVENTION WITH HIV-ASSOCIATED COGNITIVE/MOTOR COMPLEX

Once clinicians have a basic understanding of the various neuropsychiatric illnesses frequently seen in HIV-related disease, they can begin the process of making a differential diagnosis. Several important implications emerge for practice that can guide appropriate treatment and assist the affected individual. We will focus this section on clinical intervention for patients with HIV-associated cognitive/motor complex, since it is the most common neurologic illness seen in this patient population.

Practical Considerations

Many patients state that it is the simple things which create the most frustration for them. As the following lists (Buckingham and Van Gorp, 1988) indicate, there are several practical recommendations that can greatly assist the person struggling with cognitive changes and the limitations these changes represent. These include the conspicuous placement of a large calendar near the bed or living space so that the individual may remain oriented to the month, day, and year. In less impaired patients, heavy reliance on an appointment book—in which reminders and notes to oneself are carefully recorded and reviewed—may allow an impaired patient to retain employment or independent functioning longer than he or she could without such a device. In the home, the liberal use of Post-It notes, which serve as reminders to do such household essentials as turning off the stove or coffee pot or feeding the pet, can allow the person to retain independent living status longer. Reliance on a "medication log" to help keep track of a complex medication regimen may prevent forgetting to take medications or retaking medications already consumed. Because the memory impairment in HIV-associated cognitive/motor complex is characterized by impaired retrieval in the presence of preserved recognition, these notes will usually serve as effective reminders, since the information can be effectively recognized if cues are present. The following lists offer practical recommendations for helping patients overcome problems associated with HIV-associated cognitive motor complex:

Forgetfulness

1. Use calendars and appointment books.
2. Place Post-It notes in conspicuous places as reminders.
3. Make lists (questions for your physician, grocery needs, people to call, etc.).
4. Develop a list for important things to check when leaving the residence (stove, lights, etc.).
5. Use an alarm clock as a reminder for medications.
6. Keep a list of medications with dosages and times taken.
7. Ask for help if medications must be taken at different times and dosages.
8. Keep a journal detailing complex projects.
9. Use a tape recorder to dictate thoughts and questions.
10. Purchase a noise-activated key chain.
11. Keep a telephone log and important numbers by the phone.

Slowed Speech

1. Allow more time to collect your thoughts and for conversations.
2. Do not hurry; give yourself permission to take your time.
3. Keep talking. Good conversation is good practice.

Visuospatial Problems

1. Do not drive if unable to do so.
2. If able to drive, plan routes in advance, allow plenty of time, and take a friend along when you can.
3. Use verbal directions instead of maps.

Depression and Social Withdrawal

1. Plan recreational activities.
2. Be an active participant.
3. Rekindle old hobbies and interests or create new ones.

Concentration Problems, Inattentiveness, or Distractibility

1. Try to limit distractions by confining your activities to a single task.
2. Meet with people one at a time.
3. Break large tasks down into more manageable jobs.
4. Turn the TV off when conversing or needing to concentrate.
5. Do not drive in heavy traffic.

Problems with Sequential Reasoning or Multistep Tasks

1. Do not take on new or unfamiliar job responsibilities.
2. Avoid tasks in which speed of performance is important.
3. Simplify such things as meal preparation.
4. Plan activities when you are at your best (e.g., a "morning person").

Because motor and gait problems are prominent in HIV-associated cognitive/motor complex, living arrangements which are one story or which avoid many steps will allow for easier mobility. The psychomotor slowing experienced by many patients makes it difficult for them to function effectively in situations that require quick decisions and action. Working in a busy office where quick decisions—often on the spot—are required (such as in a management meeting) or where quick actions are needed (such as a busy switchboard receiving multiple calls almost simultaneously) will likely produce considerable frustration and a sense of failure for even the mildly impaired patient. Similarly, driving on crowded streets or freeways should be avoided by any patient with psychomotor slowing.

Because cognitively impaired patients do not adapt easily to novel situations or work demands, providing structure and a familiar environment will facilitate greater independence in activities of daily living. Whenever possible, demented patients should be in familiar environments that have considerable structure and support. Unfamiliar environments without adequate assistance for activities of daily living may promote increased confusion in a patient with only mild dementia, and the patient may temporarily appear more demented in these settings than is actually the case, until the environment no longer seems unfamiliar to the patient.

Patients with HIV-associated cognitive/motor complex may have sufficient *motivation* to undertake activities or tasks but may lack the necessary *initiation* to actually begin the activity. This is common to other subcortical disturbances (such as Parkinson's disease), and assistance with initiating desired activities and tasks by family members or loved ones may provide the crucial impetus for actually starting a desired activity.

Educational Considerations

Understandably, family members and significant others are often frustrated by the physical and mental deterioration their loved one may have experienced. In these circumstances, this frustration or anger may provide fertile ground for a "need to blame," so that they may unconsciously act out their anger by attributing a patient's forgetfulness to willful stubbornness or manipulation. This is a common pattern, and the skillful clinician must educate those close to the demented patient as to what actual limitations exist for their loved one. Slowing, confusion and forgetfulness are all characteristics of HIV-associated cognitive/motor complex and, when present, are not usually intentional manipulation by the patient but rather symptoms of central nervous system involvement related to HIV infection.

Providing information and educational resources to patients diagnosed with the more severe HIV-associated cognitive/motor complex or the less severe HIV-associated minor cognitive/motor disorder is another important component of HIV-related mental health care. Many patients have little or no understanding of neurological functioning or the diseases that can affect cognition. Most patients, when first presented with the term dementia, may think of severe mental deterioration, such as that seen in Alzheimer's disease, including complete memory loss and a vegetative-like existence. Helping patients to better understand the neurocognitive components of the disease—when present—and the types of changes associated with subcortical disease will greatly reduce the fears and worries of those affected.

Clinical Considerations

Careful clinical assessment of depression is important in any patient with HIV infection, but this is especially true when questions arise regarding the patient's mental functioning. When psychomotor slowing, forgetfulness, and concentration problems are present, the clinician must attempt to differentiate the effects of depression from early signs of HIV-associated cognitive/motor complex. This is best done by inquiring into the mood state of the individual and by being alert to atypical signs of pessimism, feelings of worthlessness, and suicidality. Since most patients diagnosed with an HIV-associated cognitive/motor complex are aware of their declining mental capabilities, they may be understandably depressed. This, coupled with the well established and broad range of psychosocial assaults associated with HIV infection itself, creates a high-risk situation for depression in patients who are also experiencing cognitive impairment. If signs of depression are present, the depressive condition should be appropriately and promptly treated because depression can further encroach upon the cognitive capabilities of an already impaired individual.

Assessment of potential for suicide is also important in these patients, in light of the increased frequency of depression in patients with subcortical disease (such as in Parkinson's disease or Huntington's disease) (Dewhurst et al., 1970). Crisis resources should be available to the clinician working with this population in case an impaired patient exhibits suicidal intent. The unique mix of psychosocial assaults with a probable biological contribution to depression creates fertile ground for suicidal intent and planning (Saunders and Buckingham, 1988). The clinician must be vigilant and resourceful when signs of suicidality are present.

Psychotherapy may be an appropriate treatment approach for a patient with HIV-associated cognitive/motor complex, particularly in the earlier stages. Clinicians are unfortunately hesitant to use psychotherapeutic interventions with patients who are experiencing central nervous system compromise since, for many conditions (e.g., Alzheimer's disease), psychotherapy with the impaired individual may not be appropriate. For this disorder, however, psychotherapy provides an opportunity for patients to vent their frustration with declining capacities and other issues unique to AIDS itself. Psychotherapy may serve to assist with problem solving, to educate the patient and his or her significant others regarding the problems associated with this condition, and to set limits regarding activities that may create potential problems in light of their slowed thinking and motor difficulties. Appropriate planning may make the difference between success and failure and prevent further assaults on the self-concept of an individual already beset by limitations, frustration, and failure on many fronts. Psychotherapy may also serve as a supportive environment for patients wishing to discuss estate planning. Because wills and other legal documents are sometimes contested after death, based upon allegations of diminished mental capacity, referral for neuropsychological evaluation may establish the patient's level of competency prior to death. It should be noted that compromised neuropsychological performance alone does not necessarily render a patient incompetent.

In some cases, countertransference issues arise for therapists. Professionals who work with cognitively impaired patients frequently experience countertransference problems. This dynamic is particularly important for clinicians who work with HIV-associated cognitive/motor complex because HIV is still a relatively new, lethal, and predominantly sexually transmitted disease that was first identified in socially stigmatized groups. Identification and acknowledgment of countertransference issues are crucial and require the clinician to have adequate self-awareness to respond effectively.

CONCLUSION

Since the earliest documented cases of AIDS, there have been reports of neuropsychological disturbances and cognitive changes that have challenged both those infected with HIV and the health and mental health professionals who serve them. The neuropsychological complications associated with HIV remain some of the most common problems faced by those infected with the disease. With little hope for a curative treatment that is effective in the battle against HIV-associated cognitive/motor complex or HIV disease, it becomes clear how important understanding the complexities of HIV-related cognitive compromise is to effectively assist this population with intervention and treatment. The mandate is clear: clinicians must arm themselves with the knowledge, skills, and resources necessary to respond to the wide range of problems that HIV-associated cognitive/motor complex presents a population already beset by multiple losses and compromises. Through solid clinical consideration and intervention, clinicians offer the greatest hope and real assistance for those affected by HIV-associated cognitive/motor complex. Mental health professionals can make an important and critical difference in the care and management of those experiencing cognitive compromise. Through early detection, accurate differential diagnosis, and sound clinical intervention, practitioners can increase the quality of life and the care available to those affected by HIV-associated cognitive/motor complex.

APPENDIX: CRITERIA FOR CLINICAL DIAGNOSIS OF CENTRAL NERVOUS SYSTEM DISORDERS IN ADULTS AND ADOLESCENTS

HIV-1-Associated Cognitive/Motor Complex

All of the following diagnoses require laboratory evidence for systemic HIV-1 infection (ELISA test confirmed by Western blot, polymerase chain reaction, or culture).

Sufficient for Diagnosis of AIDS

A. HIV-associated dementia complex[1]

Probable (must have each of the following):

1. Acquired abnormality in at least two of the following cognitive abilities (present for at least one month): attention/concentration,

speed of information processing, abstraction/reasoning, visuospatial skills, memory/learning, and speech/language. The decline should be verified by reliable history and mental status examination. In all cases, when possible, history should be obtained from an informant, and examination should be supplemented by neuropsychological testing.

Cognitive dysfunction causing impairment of work or activities of daily living (objectively verifiable or by report of a key informant). This impairment should not be attributable solely to severe systemic illness.

2. At least one of the following:

   a. Acquired abnormality in motor function or performance verified by clinical examination (e.g., slowed rapid movement, abnormal gait, limb incoordination, hypertonia, or weakness), neuropsychological tests (e.g., fine motor speed, manual dexterity, perceptual motor skills), or both.
   b. Decline in motivation or emotional control or change in social behavior. This may be characterized by any of the following: change in personality, with apathy, inertia, irritability, emotional lability, or new onset of impaired judgment characterized by socially inappropriate behavior or disinhibition.

3. Absence of clouding of consciousness during a period long enough to establish the presence of number 1.

4. Evidence of another etiology, including active CNS opportunistic infection or malignancy, psychiatric disorders (e.g., depressive disorder), active alcohol or substance use, or acute or chronic substance withdrawal, must be sought from medical history, physical and psychiatric examination, and appropriate laboratory and radiologic investigation (e.g., lumbar puncture, neuroimaging). If another potential etiology (e.g., major depression) is present, it is not the cause of the previous cognitive, motor, or behavioral symptoms and signs.

Possible (must have one of the following):

1. Other potential etiology present (must have each of the following):

   a. See *Probable,* numbers 1, 2, and 3.
   b. Other potential etiology is present but the cause of number 1 (*Probable*) is uncertain.

2. Incomplete clinical evaluation (must have each of the following):

   a. See *Probable,* numbers 1, 2, and 3.
   b. Etiology cannot be determined (appropriate laboratory or radiologic investigations not performed).

B. HIV-1-associated myelopathy

Probable (must have each of the following):

1. Acquired abnormality in lower-extremity neurologic function disproportionate to upper-extremity abnormality verified by reliable history (lower-extremity weakness, incoordination, and/or urinary incontinence) and neurologic examination (paraparesis, lower-extremity spasticity, hyperreflexia, or the presence of Babinski signs, with or without sensory loss).

2. Myelopathic disturbance (see number 1) is severe enough to require constant unilateral support for walking.

3. Although mild cognitive impairment may be present, criteria for HIV-1-associated dementia complex are not fulfilled.

4. Evidence of another etiology, including neoplasm, compressive lesion, or multiple sclerosis, must be sought from medical history, physical examination, and appropriate laboratory and radiologic investigations (e.g., lumbar puncture, neuroimaging, myelography). If another potential etiology is present, it is not the cause of the myelopathy. This diagnosis cannot be made in a patient infected with both HIV-1 and HTLV-I; such a patient should be classified as having possible HIV-1-associated myelopathy.

Possible (must have one of the following):

1. Other potential etiology present (must have each of the following):

   a. See *Probable,* numbers 1, 2, and 3.
   b. Other potential etiology is present but the cause of the myelopathy is uncertain.

2. Incomplete clinical evaluation (must have each of the following):

   a. See *Probable,* numbers 1, 2, and 3.
   b. Etiology cannot be determined (appropriate laboratory or radiologic investigation not performed).

Not Sufficient for Diagnosis of AIDS

A. HIV-1-associated minor cognitive/motor disorder

Probable (must have each of the following):

1. Cognitive/motor/behavioral abnormalities (must have each of the following):

   a. At least two of the following acquired cognitive, motor, or behavioral symptoms (present for at least one month), verified by reliable history (when possible, from an informant):

      1. Impaired attention or concentration
      2. Mental slowing
      3. Impaired memory
      4. Slowed movements
      5. Incoordination
      6. Personality change or irritability or emotional lability.

   b. Acquired cognitive/motor abnormalities verified by clinical neurological examination or neuropsychological testing (e.g., fine motor speed, manual dexterity, perceptual motor skills, attention/concentration, speed of information processing, abstraction/reasoning, visuospatial skills, memory/learning, or speech/language).

2. Disturbance from cognitive/motor/behavioral abnormalities (see number 1) causes mild impairment of work or activities of daily living (objectively verifiable or by report of a key informant).

3. Does not meet criteria for HIV-1-associated dementia complex or HIV-1-associated myelopathy.

4. No evidence of another etiology, including active CNS opportunistic infection or malignancy, or severe systemic illness, determined by appropriate history, physical examination, and laboratory and radiologic investigation (e.g., lumbar puncture, neuroimaging). These features should not be attributable solely to the effects of active alcohol or substance use, acute or chronic substance withdrawal, adjustment disorder, or other psychiatric disorders.

Possible (must have one of the following):

1. Other potential etiology present (must have each of the following):

    a. See *Probable,* numbers 1, 2, and 3.
    b. Other potential etiology is present and the cause of the cognitive/motor/behavioral abnormalities is uncertain.

2. Incomplete clinical evaluation (must have each of the following):

    a. See *Probable,* numbers 1, 2, and 3.
    b. Etiology cannot be determined (appropriate laboratory or radiologic investigations not performed).

NOTES

1. For research purposes, HIV-1-associated dementia complex can be coded to describe the major features:

HIV-1-associated dementia complex requires criteria 1, 2a, 3, and 4.

HIV-1-associated dementia complex (motor) requires criteria 1, 2a, 3, and 4.

HIV-1-associated dementia complex (behavior) requires criteria 1, 2b, 3, and 4.

The level of impairment due to cognitive dysfunction should be assessed as follows:

Mild: Decline in performance at work, including work in the home, that is conspicuous to others. Unable to work at usual job, although may be able to work at a much less demanding job. Activities of daily living or social activities are impaired but not to a degree making the person completely dependent on others. More complicated daily tasks or recreational activities cannot be undertaken. Capable of basic self-care, such as feeding, dressing, and maintaining personal hygiene, but activities such as handling money, shopping, using public transportation, driving a car, or keeping track of appointments or medications is impaired.

Moderate: Unable to work, including work in the home. Unable to function without some assistance of another in daily living, including dressing, maintaining personal hygiene, eating, shopping, handling money, and walking, but able to communicate basic needs.

Severe: Unable to perform any activities of daily living without assistance. Requires continual supervision. Unable to maintain personal hygiene, nearly or absolutely mute.

2. The severity of HIV-1-associated myelopathy should be graded as follows:

Mild: Ambulatory, but requires constant unilateral support (e.g., cane) for walking.

Moderate: Requires constant bilateral support (e.g., walker) for walking.

Severe: Unable to walk even with assistance, confined to bed or wheelchair.

3. Able to perform all but the most demanding aspects of work or activities of daily living. Performance at work is mildly impaired but able to maintain usual

job; social activities may be mildly impaired, but person is not dependent on others. Can feed self, dress, and maintain personal hygiene, handle money, shop, use public transportation, or drive a car, but complex daily tasks, such as keeping track of appointments or medications, may be occasionally impaired.

REFERENCES

American Academy of Neurology AIDS Task Force (1991). Nomenclature and research case definitions for neurologic manifestations of human immunodeficiency virus-type 1 (HIV-1) infection. *Neurology, 41*, 778-785.

Aylward, E. H., Henderer, J. D., McArthur, J. C., Brettschneider, P. D., Harris, G. J., Barta, P. E., and Pearlson, G. D. (1993). Reduced basal ganglia volume in HIV-1-associated dementia: Results from quantitative neuroimaging. *Neurology, 43*, 2099-2104.

Boccellari, A., Dilley, J. W., and Shore, M. D. (1988). Neuropsychiatric aspects of AIDS dementia complex: A report on a clinical series. *Neurotoxicology, 9*, 381-390.

Bolla-Wilson, K., Robinson, R. G., Starkstein, S. E., Boston, J., and Price, T. R. (1989). Lateralization of dementia of depression in stroke patients. *American Journal of Psychiatry, 146*, 627-634.

Buckingham, S. L. and Van Gorp, W. (1988). AIDS-dementia complex: Implications for practice. *Social Casework: The Journal of Contemporary Social Work, 69*, 371-375.

Centers for Disease Control (1987). Revision of the CDC surveillance case definition for acquired immunodeficiency syndrome. *Morbidity and Mortality Weekly Report* (Supplement 1S), 3-15.

Cummings, J. (1985). *Clinical neuropsychiatry*. New York: Oxford University Press.

Cummings, J. (1990). *Subcortical dementia*. New York: Oxford University Press.

Dewhurst, K., Oliver, J., Trick, K. L. K., and McKnight, A. L. (1970). Sociopsychiatric consequences of Huntington's disease. *British Journal of Psychiatry, 116*, 255-258.

Dilley, J. W., Ochitill, H. N., Perl, M., and Volberding, P. (1985). Findings in psychiatric consultation with patients with acquired immune deficiency syndrome. *American Journal of Psychiatry, 142*, 82-86.

Gottlieb, M., Schroff, R., Schanker, H., Weisman, J., Fan, P., Wolf, R., and Saxon, A. (1981). Pneumocystis carinii pneumonia and mucosal candidiasis in previously healthy homosexual men: Evidence of a newly acquired cellular immunodeficiency. *New England Journal of Medicine, 305*, 1425-1430.

Hinkin, C., Van Gorp, W., Satz, P., Weisman, J., Thommes, J., and Buckingham, S. (1992). Depressed mood and its relationship to neuropsychological test performance in HIV-1 seropositive individuals. *Journal of Clinical and Experimental Neuropsychology, 14*, 289-297.

Ho, D., Rota, D., Schooley, R., Kaplan, J., Allan, J., Groopman, J., Resnick, L., Felenstein, D., Andrews, C., and Hirsch, M. (1985). Isolation of HTLV-III from cerebrospinal fluid and neural tissue of patients with neurologic syndromes related to the acquired immunodeficiency syndrome. *New England Journal of Medicine, 313,* 1493-1497.

Martin, E. M., Sorensen, D. J., Edelstein, H. E., and Robertson, L. C. (1992). Decision-making speed in HIV-1 infection. *AIDS, 6,* 109-113.

McArthur, J. C., Hoover, D. R., Bacellar, H., Miller, E. N., Cohen, B. A., Becker, J. T., Graham, N. M. H., McArthur, J. H., Selnes, O. A., Jacobson, L. P. et al. (1993). Dementia in AIDS patients: Incidence and risk factors. *Neurology, 43,* 2245-2252.

Miller, E., Selnes, O., McArthur, J., Satz, P., Becker, J., Cohen, B., Sheridan, K., Machado, A., Van Gorp, W., and Visscher, B. (1990). Neuropsychological performance in HIV-1 infected homosexual men: The Multicenter AIDS Cohort Study (MACS). *Neurology, 40,* 197-203.

Navia, B., Jordan, B., and Price, R. (1986). The AIDS dementia complex: I. Clinical features. *Annals of Neurology, 19,* 517-524.

Navia, B., Cho, E. S., Petito, C., and Price, R. (1986). The AIDS dementia complex: II. Neuropathology. *Annals of Neurology, 19,* 525-535.

Perry, S. and Tross, S. (1984). Psychiatric problems of AIDS patients at the New York Hospital: Preliminary report. *Public Health Reports, 39,* 200-205.

Resnick, L., Berger, J. R., Shapshak, P., and Tourtellotte, W. W. (1988). Early penetration of the blood-brain-barrier by HIV. *Neurology, 38,* 9-14.

Resnick, L., deMarzio-Veronese, F., Schupbach, J., Tourtellotte, W., Ho, D., Muller, F., Shapshak, P., Vogt, M., Groopman, J., Markham, P., and Gallo, R. (1985). Intra-blood-brain-barrier synthesis of HTLV-III specific IgG in patients with neurological symptoms associated with AIDS or ARC. *New England Journal of Medicine, 313,* 1498-1504.

Robinson, R., Kubos, K., Starr, L., Rao, K., and Price, T. (1984). Mood disorders in stroke patients: Importance of location of lesion. *Brain, 107,* 81-93.

Rottenberg, D., Moeller, J., Strother, L., Sidtis, J., Navia, B., Dhawan, V., Ginos, Z., and Price, R. (1987). The metabolic pathology of the AIDS dementia complex. *Annals of Neurology, 22,* 700-706.

Saunders, J. M. and Buckingham, S. L. (1988). Suicidal AIDS patient: When the depression turns deadly. *Nursing, 18,* 59-64.

Snider, W., Simpson, D., Nielsen, S., Gold, J., Metroka, C., and Posner, J. (1983). Neurological complications of acquired immune deficiency syndrome: Analysis of 50 patients. *Annals of Neurology, 14,* 403-418.

Van Gorp, W., Hinkin, C., Satz, P., Miller, E., and D'Elia, L. F. (1993). Neuropsychological findings in HIV infection, encephalopathy, and dementia. In R. Parks, R. Lee, and R. Wilson (Eds.), *Neurosychology of Alzheimer's disease and other dementias.* New York: Oxford University Press, pp. 153-185.

Wilkie, F., Eisdorfer, C., Morgan, R., Loewenstein, D., and Szapocznik, J. (1990). Cognition in early HIV infection. *Archives of Neurology, 47,* 433-440.

POLICY ISSUES

Chapter 24

Identifying and Confronting Racism in AIDS Service Organizations

Larry M. Gant

As the demographics of AIDS shift in the United States to reflect increasing numbers of individuals and families of color, dealing with racism in AIDS service organizations (ASOs) is crucial in terms of not barring clients from access due to overt and covert racism. In addition, many ASOs that began as gay white male organizations serving largely gay white males now also serve people of color (some of which are gay; some of which are not).

However, when it comes to discussing racism and multicultural issues, ASOs, in particular, and the social work profession, in general, face three large, badly kept secrets—one societal, one professional, and one empirical.

Societal secret—U.S. society is tired of hearing about multiculturalism. Despite the many books, articles, and workshops addressing the topic, hate crimes continue to increase, racial tolerance is eroding, and racial antipathy is increasing.

Professional secret—even as more books and trainings on diversity emerge, predominantly white social workers' attitudes toward their multicultural peers will not change much at all in the coming years. Liberal attitudes and expressions to the contrary, paternalism, condescension, and ambivalence will remain.

Empirical secret—despite the insistence that ethnic sensitivity results in improved personal relationships and better service delivery, little published empirical support exists for this belief (see, however, Gant, 1996, and Gant and Gutierrez, 1996, for work corroborating this finding—finally).

The reality—particularly for AIDS service organizations—is that clientele and staff are simply going to become more, not less, ethnically diverse. AIDS service organizations, fragile as many of them are, cannot afford the luxury of either racist behavior or attitudes (overt and covert varieties), nor can the issues simply be ignored under the falsely unifying guise of "E pluribus unum," not seeing color (how terribly offensive!), or otherwise denying that "race matters" (apologies to Cornell West, 1993).

This chapter is written for those of us who feel we do not need to read another article on confronting and identifying racism. This chapter is written because, despite the mass of publications and workshops, many of us do not know or do not care to know how to transact business and communicate with diverse populations. This chapter is full of direct, unvarnished strategies for taking care of business in our AIDS service organizations. First, I am going to provide some simple assessment tools for identifying and assessing personal and organizational responses to racism. Second, I will provide a series of practical suggestions for confronting racism at both personal and organizational levels. I wish to point out that in the last two years a literature has emerged which challenges the contemporary conventional readings on cultural sensitivity and diversity. Termed "antiracism," this literature directs "well-meaning white people [and others] to understand and address their unique brands of unintentional, unconscious racism" (Burton, 1995, p. 34). The literature further "identifies and confronts the racism practiced by people who claim to know better" (Burton, 1995, p. 53). This literature is a direct challenge and outgrowth of prior work on ethnic competence, sensitivity, and practice, some of which was wonderful, but some (too much) of which characterized racism and cultural issues with "Racism 101," "Ethnicities of the month," or "food and fiestas" orientations that provided a celebration of dance, music, and the food of diverse populations, while dealing only timidly (if at all) with the social and political contexts and economies of racism and oppression.

IDENTIFYING PERSONAL AND ORGANIZATIONAL RESPONSES TO RACISM

Personal Responses

Randall-David (1989) has ten of the best pages anywhere in the literature on assessing personal responses to racism. Those seriously interested in analyzing their personal responses to racism are urged to access her work.[1] I have incorporated many of her ideas in the Personal Cultural Sophistication Scale (PCS) (Gant, 1995). The scale (see Table 24.1) is meant to detect attitudes toward clients, but there are also items relating to staff-staff relationships. The scale has strong reliability (Cronbach's alpha = .86), and validation studies are currently ongoing. (Basically, this means that the scale is a good one, so feel free to use it.)

TABLE 24.1. Personal Cultural Sophistication Scale

Item	Response Categories 1=Strongly agree 5=Strongly disagree
I can easily understand how my clients of color feel about things.	1 2 3 4 5
I can easily understand how my white colleagues feel about things.	1 2 3 4 5
I can easily understand how my colleagues of color feel about things.	1 2 3 4 5
I deal very effectively with the problems of my clients of color.	1 2 3 4 5
I feel I deal less effectively with the problems of my clients of color.*	1 2 3 4 5
Color is unimportant in interpersonal relations.*	1 2 3 4 5
My co-workers are generally unaware of minority-organized community programs.*	1 2 3 4 5
I think "liberals" are free of racism.*	1 2 3 4 5
I think people of color are often oversensitive.*	1 2 3 4 5
I really think that culture and ethnicity are differences but not the basis on which to determine behavior.	1 2 3 4 5
I think that negotiation and collaboration are possible strategies between whites and people of color.	1 2 3 4 5
The only way to gain attention with whites or people of color is through confrontation.*	1 2 3 4 5

*Reverse score these items (1=5, 2=4, 3=3)
Range = 12-60
12-24 = Strong Personal Cultural Sophistication
24-36 = Moderately Strong Personal Cultural Sophistication
36-48 = Moderately Weak Personal Cultural Sophistication
48-60 = Weak Personal Cultural Sophistication

Organizational Responses

To assess your organization's response to racism, nothing beats a cultural audit—period. Many corporations have developed cultural audits for their organization. Audits have also been developed for human service organizations. I recommend two; both are helpful; both have similar lineage, but are somewhat different in the final product. The first is the Cultural Competence Self-Assessment Instrument (Child Welfare League of America, 1993). It is a very simple checklist that allows participating staff and board members to rate the organization's response to racism in the areas of service delivery, policies and procedures, governance, procurement, and personnel. The instrument is proscriptive in that it embeds ameliorative strategies in the self-assessment items. There is no cumulative score and no assignation of a label. Participants have three responses (no progress, some progress, progress complete) for each of the items. Organizations interested in undergoing a self-study without becoming shell-shocked should consider this audit.

The second audit pulls no punches. Developed jointly by the National Child Welfare Leadership Center and the Child Welfare League of America in 1989, the Cultural Competency Agency Self-Assessment (Cross et al., 1989) was the predecessor measure to the Cultural Competence Self-Assessment Instrument. In addition to a similar inventory of organizational domains (with "yes" and "no" responses for each item), this assessment required participants to provide a summary evaluation of agency performance in each domain by categorizing the extent to which agency policies and procedures reflected diversity on the following six-point continuum:

1. Cultural destructiveness
2. Cultural incapacity
3. Cultural blindness
4. Cultural precompetence
5. Cultural competence
6. Cultural proficiency

The continuum had no psychometric properties per se, but the descriptions of each category and the attempts of agencies to rate themselves in the pilot process were memorable (Cross et al., 1989). Interestingly, many of the agencies participating in the pilot process, held in May 1990, in Las Vegas, Nevada, scored in categories 1-3; the ratings so discouraged the agencies that they requested the categories be removed from later versions of the survey (CWLA National Task Force on Cultural Responsiveness, 1990).[2] This measure also reflects proscriptive strategies embedded in their questions.

Ultimately, it comes down to a matter of style. One strategy that a colleague found useful was to first present the Cross inventory to her agency. As the members of the audit team grumbled, winced, and shook their heads, she then suggested the CWLA manual as an alternate format. The audit team used the latter measure and moved effectively to institute changes in the organization.

CONFRONTING RACISM IN THE AGENCY AND AMONG COLLEAGUES

It is a counterintuitive assertion, but confronting and transforming racist agency or organizational practices is much easier than confronting personal racist practices among work colleagues. So, let us look at implementing agency change first.

Implementing Agency Change

Neither measure mentioned previously provides strategies for implementing change or securing required information or resources. Fortunately, Randall-David (1989) has very detailed and explicit procedures for conducting community needs assessments and obtaining required resources and contacts. More recently, Kretzmann and McKnight (1993) provide an extensive discussion of ways to conduct community gap analyses and community asset assessments and to solidify relationships between organizations and ethnic communities. Either Randall-David or Kretzmann and McKnight provide a good complement to the cultural audit process.

Agencies that cannot implement the recommendations generated by the audit probably should not be in business—or will probably self-destruct on their own in due time. Finally, agency leadership that cannot implement at least some of the recommendations coming from audits all but defines their agency as racist and in the best interests of *no one*.

Despite the titles of many best-selling books, there are no "real secrets to successful organizational change"; most texts in the area find the following four principles classic, yet among the most effective:

- Mandates for change must be declared, confirmed, and implemented by agency leadership first, then by staff.
- Timetables for change must be clearly indicated and understood.
- Parties for change efforts must be clearly identified and held accountable.

- Change must be shown to enhance, not burden, the mission of the agency.

In summary, to identify and confront organizational racist practices, consider (1) an organizational cultural audit or self-study, using either the Cultural Competence Self-Assessment Instrument or the Cultural Competency Agency Self-Assessment, and (2) using the techniques available in Randall-David (1989) or Kretzmann and McKnight (1993) to fill organizational gaps and omissions and implement changes to intentional and unintentional organizational racism.

Implementing Personal Change

Clyde Ford may have given his book a naive-sounding title, but *We Can All Get Along: Fifty Steps You Can Take to Help End Racism at Home, at Work, and in Your Community* (Ford, 1994) describes very direct steps toward confronting and implementing antiracist behavior and practices. Some examples:

- End any denial you have about the existence of racism; racism is alive and prevalent in America, and throughout the world, today.
- Share your awareness with others about the new face of racism.
- Replace the word "race" in your vocabulary with another term, such as "ethnic group, human variation, our cultural background" . . . the term race is loaded with a history of friction, conflict, violence, and racism. Defuse racism by discarding this outmoded term.
- Avoid qualifiers when referring to people of different ethnic groups. For example, "We're looking for a qualified black to fill this position." The natural assumption is that everyone considered for a position should be qualified.
- If you do not know how persons of color wish to be referred to, ask them.
- Acknowledge your stereotypical views. In private, verbalize your stereotypes (out loud or silently). What is it like to hear yourself verbalize those views? Transpose each statement by saying, "This belief about [stereotypical view] comes from an attitude I have about myself." What is it like to realize your stereotypes stem from beliefs you have about yourself?
- Release the stereotypes you have of yourself.
- Learn to confront a racist remark. When you hear a bigoted remark, say something as simple as, "I find what you're saying offensive [or disgusting]. Please keep your views to yourself."

- Racist remarks in the workplace are forbidden under civil rights laws. If racist remarks continue in the workplace, keep a record and report them to a supervisor or the equal opportunity office. If need be, contact your state human rights commission to report workplace racism.

  Report racist incidents, regardless of how inconsequential, to appropriate local authorities such as the police or human rights commission. Filing a complaint may help to strengthen a pending legal case against an individual or organization accused of racist activities.
- Build mutual understanding rather than trying to understand where another is "coming from." No one is really able to "walk in another person's shoes."
- Bridge differences rather than insist on similarity of views.
- Learn to hold the parties you communicate with in the highest positive regard. That is, accept and respect whatever is communicated without trying to change, control, or alter that communication.
- Develop a personal vision for eliminating racism.

PEOPLE RECOVERING FROM RACISM

Part I: How People of Color Aid and Abet Racism

It is not politically correct to suggest that African Americans, Latinos, and other people of color use racism to self-advantage, but it is the case more than people would care to admit.[3] Historically, instead of confronting the source of community pain and racism, people of color have sometimes turned feelings of anger, frustration, and depression inward. These feelings emerge in self-destructive attitudes and behaviors, and many times, these are observed by our white colleagues. A partial list, taken from Burton (1995), is suggestive:

- exploiting and oppressing one another—evident in the increasing rate of drive-by shootings, gang wars, illegal drug trade perpetuated by African Americans on African Americans, the growing number of black men who refuse to be financially and emotionally responsible to lovers, spouses, and children, and black parents who abuse their children;
- dating or marrying white people as a status symbol because one believes white is "better than" (*Whose* ice is colder?);
- using racist and other epithets to refer to one another;

- using racial epithets against white people or against other people of color;
- denying or being shamed by one's own racial identity, either by surgery or assertion;
- sniping at one another in the workplace, tattling to the boss about one another, and vying for white supervisors' attention and approval, instead of helping one another become better and stronger;
- buying into negative stereotypes about black people's professionalism and competence; and
- publicly bashing collective efforts to redress racial wrongs.

Elsewhere, Randall-David (1989, pp. 12-14) lists forty assumptions and behaviors made by both blacks and whites that block authentic relations—and lists forty assumptions and behaviors that facilitate authentic relations as well. The eighty collective assumptions and behaviors are too numerous to mention here, but they are well worth the time spent in acquisition and study.

In battling racism in service organizations, people of color must acknowledge their own contributions to the maintenance of racist structures. The struggle belongs to all of us, not only the ascribed beneficiaries of racism.

Part II: The Rights of Sincere and Recovering Racists

> ... Many white liberals are looking for praise for being liberal and at least trying [to deal with racism]. . . . If you think *you're* tired of being called racist, think how weary *we* are of dealing with it. . . . If you're sincerely making an effort to understand . . . racism, and endeavoring to root it out, starting with yourself, then you understand there's a lot more to be done before we hand out Nobel Prizes. Still, as a human being and recovering racist who is truly trying, you are justified in expecting some understanding and consideration from African Americans and other people of color. (Burton, 1995, pp. 71-72)

Challenging and confronting racism is difficult. Even for those of us who do so as a daily part of life, it is normal to feel frustrated, annoyed, bemused, and "pissed off." People of color are very, very tired of teaching white people about the dos and don'ts of racism, and white people are tired, very tired of being categorized as "white" people and as racists. Given these realities, there is a genuine case to be made for placing the challenges of racist practices in some perspective. In *Never Say Nigger*

Again, Burton (1995) lists some very intelligent and realistic provisos, or "rights" of recovering racists. Although the title invokes a disease model, some of the suggestions are liberating. Consider:

- Don't feel guilty when you inadvertently do or say something racist. (do not feel guilty—feel compelled to change.)
- Don't be accused of racism when racism is clearly not in play.
- Take a hard line with African Americans, Latinos, or persons of color who deserve a hard line.
- Don't be angry or annoyed when confronted about your racism. (Be open to criticism, even though the manner in which you are criticized may bug you. You may learn something, and instead of pretending to be open, the next time you really will be.)
- Don't disagree with someone's assessment of your behavior or speech as "racist." (Reexamine your own behavior. Check with another person of color for their opinion. If you truly disagree with that person, say so, but be sensitive to his or her individual concern.)
- Ask questions on unclear issues of white racism and race relations. (Be aware that people of color have the right to be suspicious or annoyed about your asking.)

CONCLUSION

This chapter began on a grim note but ends on one of guarded pragmatism. Yes, racism exists and often seems intractable in U.S. society and in AIDS service organizations. Many people wonder aloud what can be done, if anything. In a rather direct mode, I have identified several resources and provided some very direct and effective strategies for identifying and confronting racism in organizations and personally. These materials are easy to implement, but they admittedly can cause pain and discomfort in some people and for some organizations. Despite this, these tools are effective and can be used by nearly anyone and any agency.

In the final analysis, the presence and availability of these tools lead me to believe that any AIDS service agency which claims incredible problems with racism should try these tools. If they refuse to do so, or say, "We've tried these things before," my response would be twofold: (1) I would seriously doubt it, since I have found most people in either academia or AIDS-related practice *do not* know about these resources, and (2) I would paraphrase the sentiments of one of the most profound griots of our time, Gator (Flipper's brother in Spike Lee's *Jungle Fever*), and wonder if such organizations were not "seriously perpetratin' on the green."

NOTES

1. If anyone experiences difficulty in obtaining her work, contact the author of this chapter for further information.

2. This scale, with the categories intact, was published for several years by the CASSP Technical Assistance Center, Georgetown University Child Development Center, in Washington, DC.

3. Oh, no! Another secret escapes from the closet! Sincere apologies to those offended.

REFERENCES

Burton, M. G. (1995). *Never say nigger again: An anti-racism guide for white liberals.* Nashville, TN: Winston Publishing Company.

Child Welfare League of America (1993). Cultural competence self-assessment instrument. Washington, DC: Child Welfare League of America.

Cross, T. L., Bazron, B. J., Dennis, K. W., Isaacs, M. R., and Benjamin, M. P. (1989). Towards a culturally competent system of care. Washington, DC: CASSP Technical Assistance Center, Georgetown University Child Development Center.

CWLA National Task Force on Cultural Responsiveness (1990). Pilot cultural competence self-assessment process, May 1-2, 1990, Las Vegas, Nevada. Washington, DC: Child Welfare League of America and National Child Welfare Leadership Center.

Ford, C. W. (1994). *We can all get along: Fifty steps you can take to help end racism at home, at work, and in your community.* New York: Dell Publishing.

Gant, L. (1995). *The personal cultural sophistication scale: Psychometric properties.* Manuscript under review.

Gant, L. (1996). "Are culturally sophisticated agencies better workplaces for social work staff and administrators?" *Social Work, 41*(2), 163-171.

Gant, L. and Gutierrez, L. (1996). Effects of culturally sophisticated agencies upon Latino social workers. *Social Work, 41*(6), 624-632.

Kretzmann, J. P. and McKnight, J. L. (1993). *Building communities from the inside out: A path toward finding and mobilizing a community's assets.* Chicago, IL: ACTA Publications.

Randall-David, E. (1989). *Strategies for working with culturally diverse communities and clients.* Washington, DC: Association for the Care of Children's Health.

West, Cornell (1993). The new cultural politics of difference. In Charles Lemert (Ed.), *Society Theory: The multicultural and classic readings.* Boulder, CO: Westview Press.

Chapter 25

The Challenges of HIV/AIDS Education and Training for Social Workers and Other Mental Health Professionals

Arnold H. Grossman

In working with people infected and affected by HIV/AIDS, social workers and other mental health professionals simultaneously confront a growing diversity of population groups, unprecedented psychosocial and health issues, and personal and professional challenges in an expanding HIV/AIDS pandemic. Through 1995, a cumulative total of 513,586 persons with AIDS was reported to the Centers for Disease Control and Prevention (CDC), with 62 percent having died. Although the number of cases reported during 1995 (74,180) was lower than the numbers reported for the years 1993 and 1994, reflecting the waning of the expanded 1993 AIDS surveillance case definition, it was 56 percent higher than in 1992, before the case definition was expanded (CDC, 1995). In addition to diagnosed AIDS cases, one million Americans are estimated to be infected with HIV (CDC, 1992).

The 1995 AIDS cases indicate that the demographic characteristics, behavioral risks, and geographic distribution of persons with AIDS are changing. Blacks and Hispanics represented the majority among men (54 percent)

The author gratefully acknowledges the professional services of the following individuals who contribute to the effectiveness and quality of education and training provided by the NYU AIDS/SIDA Mental Hygiene Project: Doneley Meris, Project Administrator; Dr. Robert Malgady, Director of Evaluation; Steven Henle, graduate assistant; and the many consultants who offer their expertise to educate mental health providers about HIV/AIDS. The ongoing support and guidance of Angela Christofides, Frank Machlica, and Debra Groger of the NYC Department of Mental Health's Mental Retardation and Alcoholism Services, enhances effectiveness and efficiency of the education and training activities.

and women (76 percent); and for the first time, the proportion of persons who were black was equal to the proportion who were white (40 percent). Among men, male-to-male sexual contact continued to account for the largest proportion of cases (51 percent), followed by injection drug use (24 percent). Among women, injection drug use or sexual contact with a man with or at risk for HIV infection accounted for the greatest proportions (both 38 percent), and women accounted for 19 percent of the 1995 adult/ adolescent cases, the highest proportion reported in any year (CDC, 1995).

The 1995 AIDS incidence rates per 100,000 population remained the highest in Puerto Rico, New York, Florida, New Jersey, Maryland, and Connecticut and in heavily populated metropolitan areas (many of which are in these same states): Jersey City, New York City, San Francisco, San Juan, and Miami (CDC, 1995). These 1995 descriptive statistics provide a contextual framework for examining the purpose, goals, and activities of the education and training program for mental health professionals working with people with HIV disease in New York City, which continues to be the epicenter of the U.S. epidemic, with 16 percent of the cumulative cases of AIDS.

THE AIDS PROFESSIONAL EDUCATION/TRAINING PROGRAM

In 1984, three years after the first cases of AIDS were diagnosed in Los Angeles and New York City, Dr. Sara Kellerman, then commissioner of the New York City Department of Mental Health, Mental Retardation, and Alcoholism Services (DMHMRAS), "ordered city-wide training and mandated services for people with and at risk for HIV (sic) as a prerequisite to qualify for the hundreds of millions of dollars of city, state and federal money routinely poured into hundreds of institutions throughout New York [City]" (McFarlane, 1996, pp. 2-3). Rodger McFarlane was appointed to direct the two education and training contracts that were awarded to Memorial Sloan-Kettering Cancer Center and Gay Men's Health Crisis (McFarlane, 1996).

In response to two competitive requests for proposals sponsored by DMHMRAS, two contracts for HIV/AIDS education and training were awarded for the periods 1992-1994 and 1994-1997. The first was issued to New York University's School of Education (NYU AIDS/SIDA Mental Hygiene Project), to provide education and training for providers working in the areas of mental health and alcoholism/substance abuse services, directed by Arnold H. Grossman. The second was issued to the Young Adult Institute (APEP: AIDS Professional Educational Program), to provide HIV/AIDS education and training for providers working with people who are mentally retarded or have other developmental disabilities, initially founded and directed by the late Raymond Jacobs. This chapter focuses on the work of the NYU AIDS/SIDA Mental Hygiene Project.

ASSESSING HIV/AIDS EDUCATION NEEDS

McFarlane (1996) reports that the initial measurement of education and training needs revealed that knowledge about AIDS was substantial across all disciplines. However, four major barriers were identified in the realm of attitudes and beliefs: (1) realistic and unrealistic fears of contagion, (2) confrontation with mortality, (3) feelings of helplessness and hopelessness, and (4) social barriers to information and services resulting from differences in class, race, gender, sexual orientation, and psychiatric histories.

Two assessments were conducted by the NYU AIDS/SIDA Mental Hygiene Project. The initial assessment, conducted in January 1992, was based on a random sample of mental health agencies under contract with DMHMRAS. The six content areas that received the highest ratings in terms of training needs, based on 204 responses, were (1) death, dying, and bereavement; (2) HIV prevention with a multicultural client base; (3) community services/resources for people with HIV/AIDS; (4) crisis intervention; (5) mental health issues of long-term HIV/AIDS survivors; and (6) confidentiality issues and HIV/AIDS.

A recent assessment was conducted in June 1996, through a survey mailed to 1,000 providers working in 200 institutions and community-based organizations (i.e., five to each agency) from the DMHMRAS list of contractors providing mental health and alcoholism/substance abuse services. Surveys were returned by 250 individuals, of which 243 were usable, for a 24.3 percent response rate. The questionnaire asked research participants to rate the importance of education/training for themselves and/or their staff members in thirty-three enumerated HIV/AIDS content areas, with space provided for other topics. Ratings were on a five-point Likert-type scale, with 1 = not important to 5 = very important. A second part of the questionnaire asked the participants to rate the types of education/training activities and/or materials that most assist in their learning (e.g., conferences, workshops, small group sessions, newsletters), with space provided for other activities to be listed. Ratings were again requested on a five-point Likert-type scale, with 1 = not effective for me to 5 = very effective for me.

Descriptive statistics were used to analyze the data, and those reported here are the percentages combined from categories 6 and 5 of each section of the survey, i.e., very important and important, and very effective for me and effective for me, respectively.

The ten content areas and the respective percentages that received the highest ratings were as follows:

1. HIV/AIDS keeping current—91.0 percent
2. Women and HIV/AIDS (including women of color and women who partner with women)—87.9 percent
3. Mentally ill chemical abusers (MICA) and HIV/AIDS—85.7 percent
4. HIV/AIDS prevention education with specific groups (those specified most frequently were adolescents, mentally ill, substance abusers)—85.2 percent
5. Death and dying, bereavement, and loss—84.9 percent
6. Suicide risk assessment and prevention—84.2 percent
7. HIV/AIDS and people with severe and persistent mental illness—84.1 percent
8. HIV/AIDS prevention education (community)—84.1 percent
9. Men and HIV/AIDS (including men of color and men who have sex with men)—84.0 percent
10. Issues related to HIV/AIDS disclosure (including significant others, children, family, work)—84.0 percent

Other content areas that received ratings of 75 percent or more were confidentiality issues, psychotherapeutic intervention strategies, families and children (including orphans), countertransference issues, and HIV testing and counseling.

It is apparent that educational needs related to the issues of (1) confidentiality and (2) death, dying, and bereavement continue to be primary among many mental health providers. Both of these content areas raise questions related to personal, professional, and ethical issues with which individuals continue to struggle, and they are central to the psychological distress experienced by many in working with people with HIV disease (e.g., loss, grief, and dealing with people who continue to engage in behaviors potentially dangerous to themselves and others).

With regard to education/training activities, the analysis indicated that more than 50 percent of the participants found all the activities effective in assisting their learning; however, there was a decided preference for smaller group learning experiences (small groups at their own facilities—87.3 percent; seminars of twenty-five to fifty people—78.0 percent) to larger group activities (workshops of fifty to seventy-five people—61.7 percent; conferences of seventy-five people or more—50.2 percent). Almost two-thirds of the participants also found the eight-page newsletter and "HIV/AIDS Focus" (a four- to eight-page newsletter insert on a specific topic) as effective or very effective for their learning.

PROGRAM GOALS AND ACTIVITIES

The overall goal of the NYU AIDS/SIDA Mental Hygiene Project is to provide educational forums and other training programs to mental hygiene professionals serving mental health and alcoholism/substance abuse clients in New York City on approaches and strategies to prevent the spread of HIV infection and to improve the quality of mental health care and rehabilitation of people with HIV disease, their significant others, families, and communities. Current information is provided about the neuropsychiatric aspects of HIV, the psychosocial sequelae, and the diverse cultural contexts within which HIV disease is experienced. Further, the Project assists professionals in coping with emotional stresses of the epidemic through facilitating support group services (Grossman, 1994).

The Project achieves its goals through a variety of activities. These include curriculum development, workshops, conferences, technical assistance, support group services, publications, and evaluation.

Curriculum Development Committees

Based on the outcome of the needs assessment(s), four curriculum committees, with expertise in specific content areas and representing diverse constituencies, are convened each year. Committee members decide on the content to be included in each curriculum guide and assume responsibility for developing specific modules. The committees are chaired by the project director, who also serves as editor of the curriculum guides. The guides provide the content for workshops; however, time does not permit all modules in each guide to be addressed at each workshop, and some variability by leaders/facilitators relates to the expressed needs of those present. Curriculum guides are distributed at workshops, and it is suggested that the guides be shared with colleagues who were unable to attend the workshops.

Workshops

Two three-hour workshops are provided on five days (one in each borough of New York City) every six months. Participants are recruited through the mailing of brochures, announcements in the Project's newsletter, listings in the NYU and DMHMRAS monthly calendars of education and/or service activities, special flyers for distribution in agencies in and around the site for the workshop, and verbal announcements at technical assistance seminars and support groups. Modes of instruction vary; they include lecture/discussion, small group exercises, case studies, and use of videotapes and role-plays. Some of the topics of recent workshops include the following: "The Challenge of Counseling Women on HIV/AIDS-Related Issues," "The Challenge of Counseling Men on HIV/AIDS-Related Issues," "Families and Children: The Challenge of HIV/AIDS," "HIV/AIDS and People with Severe and Persistent Mental Illness," and "Mental Health Issues of Long-Term Survivors of HIV Disease."[1]

Conferences

One-day conferences are offered during each six-month period. These focus on communicating new information to a large audience (e.g., "HIV/AIDS: Keeping Current") or on a topic of interest to many mental hygiene providers (e.g., "Caregivers in the Presence of Death" or "Psychotherapeutic Intervention Strategies in Working with people with HIV/AIDS").

Technical Assistance

The technical assistance component allows the Project to meet specific education, training, and guidance needs of administrators and personnel in institutions and community-based organizations who have contracts with DMHMRAS. Expert consultants first assess, over the telephone, the training and educational needs expressed by the organization's contact person. Needs are also assessed with those in attendance on the day(s) that the assistance is provided. Not only does the assessment on each day help to clarify the training needs, but the process enables the group members to communicate what they expect from the educational experience in their own words and helps them take part in determining the group's learning objectives. Experience indicates that the areas to be marketed for technical assistance (i.e., ones that stimulate personnel to think of their specific needs) include death, dying, and bereavement; developing and implementing policy and procedures regarding HIV/AIDS confidentiality; providing culturally diverse and sensitive services to clients with HIV disease; and working with gay and lesbian youth and adults.

Support Group Services

These services are provided by expert facilitators in response to requests from groups of personnel in institutions and community-based organizations who have contracts with DMHMRAS. They are closed group sessions that range from two weeks to ten weeks. The issues that are typically the focus of shorter-term groups include time management (including budgeting time for establishing and using support networks), stress management, death and dying, and motivational change (i.e., changing environmental factors to enhance self-motivation in prevention of burnout and staff turnover). Longer-term support groups focus on awareness, shared experiences, supportive and helping relationships, and emotional consequences of working with people with AIDS. They also assist social workers and other mental health professionals in managing stress and enhancing their capacity and effectiveness to work with people with HIV disease by helping participants feel less isolated and by sharing feelings regarding difficult issues such as anger, helplessness, and loss.[2]

Publications

The two publications that are referred to earlier are published quarterly. The newsletter "HIV/AIDS and Mental Hygiene" has a lead article on a current topic related to HIV disease and has regular columns such as "Update," "News Briefs," "Coming Events," "From the Desk of the Commissioner" (of DMHMRAS), and an article focusing on issues related to HIV/AIDS and people who are mentally retarded or have other developmental disabilities, written by the staff of the HIV/AIDS program at the Young Adult Institute.

The second publication, "HIV/AIDS Focus," concentrates on a specific topic. Recent issues were devoted to "Counseling End-Stage Clients with AIDS," "AIDS Dementia Complex," and "The Moral Challenges for Professionals in AIDS Care."

Evaluation

Integral to all activities of the Project is the process of evaluation, which is managed by a Director of Evaluation. Approaches range from informal discussions held with workshop leaders and curriculum committee members to formal and anonymous evaluative instruments completed by participants at the conclusion of workshops, conferences, technical assistance seminars, and support group sessions. Information gathered is used to improve and adjust ongoing and future education activities, including issues of relevance, effectiveness, outcomes, and accessibility.

The current evaluative instruments focus on satisfaction with the various types of education and training in terms of the participants' goals and expectations for the learning experiences. They also include items related to the quality of training, amount of knowledge gained, degree of involvement of the participant in the learning processes, and usefulness of the training in enhancing the effectiveness of work. Evaluation instruments used previously measured the amount of specific knowledge gained and attitudinal changes through the use of pretests and posttests. After findings indicated that the educational activities were effective in increasing knowledge and in changing attitudes, these tests were discontinued and replaced at the suggestion of the Director of Evaluation.

CONCLUSIONS AND IMPLICATIONS FOR FURTHER TRAINING

Demographic information collected from those individuals who participate in the Project's education and training activities indicate that they are mostly women, members of diverse ethnic minority groups, and professionals who are providing direct client services, followed by health education. By profession, they are predominantly counselors, case managers, social workers, and nurses.

Although many individual social workers and nurses have been exemplary in their responses to the challenges of the HIV/AIDS epidemic, others continue to make moral judgments about the behaviors that transmit the virus and those who practice those behaviors. Therefore, members of those two professions and others continue to struggle with many psychosocial issues, including homophobia, negative attitudes toward injection drug users and homeless people, discomfort with death and dying, and fear of contagion (Shernoff, 1990; Ungvarski, 1995). Education and training are effective in assisting many social workers, nurses, and other health care professionals in confronting and coping with these issues.

Peterson's (1991) study found that social workers felt they did not have professional reasons for being knowledgeable about AIDS, and during the 1980s, nurses in New York and California had to be reminded of "their responsibilities to provide nursing care to all patients including people with HIV disease" (Ungvarski, 1995). Much of this professional distancing has been and continues to be mitigated by effective training regarding psychosocial and countertransference issues related to fear of contagion, fear of the unknown, stigmatization of gay people and injection drug users, feelings related to powerlessness and helplessness, fear of working with difficult patients, and fear of working with people who are likely to experience untimely deaths (Dunkel and Hatfield, 1986).

Observations and conversations with participants at the Project's education and training events, along with requests for names to be added to and deleted from mailing lists, indicate that new people are continually entering the field of HIV/AIDS work to meet the needs of the growing epidemic as well as to replace professionals leaving the areas of HIV/AIDS work. As indicated in support group sessions, many professionals are presenting issues related to burnout, such as emotional exhaustion, work overload, not being able to meet professional expectations, complexity and uncertainty inherent in the HIV/AIDS epidemic, coping with death and dying, and the emotional impact of HIV/AIDS on their lives and families (Grossman and Silverstein, 1993).

Although the nature and composition of HIV/AIDS service delivery units and the shifting of the health system response to managed care influence burnout, educational and support activities are effective in assisting mental health providers to examine their own feelings, to acknowledge that personal attitudes affect professional work, and to look at ethical and cultural issues (e.g., duty to warn, confidentiality, testing and counseling, cultural competency).

The introduction of new treatments, such as protease inhibitors, means that many people with HIV disease will be living for more years with a manageable chronic disease than was previously expected. Although this may be considered good news by most people infected and affected by HIV, it raises many psychosocial issues with which mental health professionals must cope. For example, providers may have to assist some individuals who thought they were living with a terminal illness to adjust to the fact that they now have a chronic disease and to assist individuals who cannot benefit from these new medications to cope with that outcome. Not only do these changes and future developments affect the psychological well-being of clients and their significant others, but they also simultaneously impact the mental health of the providers. Competent and effective education and support services help social workers and other mental health providers to meet the ongoing new challenges of the pandemic as well as to continue high standards of practice. Their roles in controlling the epidemic and enhancing the quality of lives of people with HIV disease must be recognized by administrators and subscribed by funding sources, and those providing direct services should advocate for the establishment or continuation of HIV/AIDS education, training, and support programs.

From the experiences of the Project's directors and trainers in educational programs at the local, national, and international levels, we have learned that the majority of HIV/AIDS mental hygiene and psychosocial issues are similar, regardless of geographic location. Although cultural and religious diversity may influence strategies, knowledge of the psycho-social sequelae of HIV/AIDS has general applicability to a variety of situations. Therefore, the educational model and materials that we have developed and evaluated in New York City are well suited to meeting the training needs of professionals, volunteers, and nonprofessionals in other localities. In addition, the curriculum guides used for the workshops and some technical assistance seminars are available at a nominal cost through the author. In other words, we want to give away knowledge to assist social workers and other mental health professionals in enhancing their art of helping people with HIV/AIDS and themselves during this pandemic.

NOTES

1. A listing of curriculum guides available for purchase can be obtained by writing to the author.
2. For a more complete discussion of these types of support groups, see: Grossman, A. H., and Silverstein, C. (1993).

REFERENCES

Centers for Disease Control and Prevention (1992). Projections of the number of persons diagnosed with AIDS and the number of immunosuppressed HIV-infected persons—United States, 1992-1994, *Morbidity and Mortality Weekly Report, 41*(RR-16), 1-29.

Centers for Disease Control and Prevention (1995). *HIV/AIDS Surveillance Report, 7*(2), 5-9.

Dunkel, J. and Hatfield, S. (1986). Countertransference issues in working with persons with AIDS. *Social Work, 31*(2), 114-117.

Grossman, A. H. (1994). HIV/AIDS education/training for mental hygiene professionals. Program proposal. New York: New York University, School of Education.

Grossman, A. H. and Silverstein, C. (1993). Facilitating support groups for professionals working with persons with AIDS. *Social Work, 38*(2), 144-151.

McFarlane, R. (1996). The moral challenges for professionals in AIDS care. *HIV/AIDS Focus,* March, 1-8.

Peterson, K. J. (1991). Social workers' knowledge about AIDS: A national survey. *Social Work, 36*(1), 31-37.

Shernoff, M. (1990). Why every social worker should be challenged by AIDS. *Social Work, 35*(1), 5-8.

Ungvarski, P. J. (1995). Meeting the challenge of HIV/AIDS. *Imprint,* September/October, 51-54.

Chapter 26

Models Created in Response to the HIV/AIDS Pandemic: The New York Peer AIDS Education Coalition

Edith Springer

The Chinese word for crisis is also the word for opportunity. What can we learn about service delivery from the HIV/AIDS crisis? The models that have come out of this pandemic are extremely creative, effective, less expensive, and more empowering to the participants than the old charity/dependency models. These are community models which have benefits beyond the tasks that are performed in the service of the consumers: they empower the community to develop the necessary expertise to take care of itself.

MODELS CREATED IN RESPONSE TO AIDS

Because of a lack of response on the part of government, private agencies, and community-based organizations to the onset of the HIV/AIDS pandemic in the early 1980s, a small group of gay men conceived of a model of care by which gay men would volunteer to take care of other gay men who had this new debilitating illness and, at the same time, create and implement prevention-oriented interventions and programs. This was a radical notion in the social services world. When Diego Lopez told his social work professor about this new idea for the gay community to take care of itself, the professor was discouraging. He could not believe that gay men who came from all different professions, many of them not in the social and medical service delivery worlds, would give up their time and energy to care for the sick and the lonely. Today, the organization that this handful of gay men founded, the Gay Men's Health Crisis (GMHC), is a mainstay in prevention and care for people living with HIV. Through their volunteer programs, people take care of people living with HIV and AIDS by serving as buddies, volunteer trainers, case managers, masseurs, hairdressers, cooks, and almost any role one can imagine. Their unique prevention interventions, including workshops, "bar zaps," education at "drag balls," etc., are vital and effective because they were created by a population for itself. Today, GMHC is so much a part of the service delivery system and the philosophies of care of all HIV/AIDS organizations, that we can hardly remember a time when it did not exist. "Buddy" and volunteer programs now exist in almost every HIV/AIDS organization and project in the United States, not only for gay and lesbian people, but for all people. Also, significantly, many of the caregivers who started as volunteers have become paid workers in HIV/AIDS work, outreach work, and other areas of service delivery.

With the help of professionals and paid staff, the HIV community takes care of itself. Who could do it better? The cost efficiency and cost containment evinced in these delivery systems are attractive to everyone since so much more can be done with the resources available. Agencies can get the highest quality work because they do not have to pay for it and the people who do it are committed to the cause and to the people they serve.

Another model that developed as a result of the HIV/AIDS pandemic is the harm reduction model, which grew out of needle exchange programs. Most needle exchange programs in the United States began as illegal outreach interventions run by activists, many of whom were ACT UP members or people in recovery from drug dependency. Risking arrest and worse, they put clean injection equipment into the hands of users and collected the used equipment to keep it from being reused. Even today's funded legal programs operate with minimal staff and use the consumers of the programs as volunteer workers. Unlike the Gay Men's Health Crisis, however, needle exchange programs are scandalously underfunded. Often there is only one paid staff member, constant shortages of supplies, and logistical problems caused by inclement weather, police harassment, and the NIMBY (not in my backyard) syndrome—and still they continue to place clean injection equipment in the hands of thousands of users and collect thousands of used syringes regularly each week. Many of the participants in these programs request referrals to drug treatment, housing, and other services, all of which can help them improve their lives. Many of the exchange volunteers, similar to buddies and other HIV/AIDS volunteers, go on to paying jobs that utilize the skills they have learned in their volunteer capacities. Even those who do not go on to paying jobs use the skills and knowledge they gain within their communities.

COMMUNITY EMPOWERMENT MODELS

The types of programs that HIV has spawned, such as the Gay Men's Health Crisis and the needle exchange and other harm reduction programs, in which consumers serve as volunteer (and later, paid) workers, fit right into current cost-containment/cost-efficiency themes. Social work as a field has no choice but to look at its community organizing traditions and to work to develop structures and interventions that prioritize community development rather than apply individual Band-Aids to community problems.

Communities need to be given information, taught skills, and encouraged to create the interventions and structures that will help them to heal themselves and thus progress. They cannot rely on charity model programs that provide services but neglect to engage the community in service provision. What harm reduction programs do is give communities the tools they need to assume their own care and engage the consumers in the service provision itself, similar to the Gay Men's Health Crisis and needle exchange programs. The problems professionals often encounter in trying to make interventions culturally relevant to people whose cultures they do not share are vastly reduced when the consumers assist in creating the interventions. The services are more "user-friendly" because they are designed by the users for themselves rather than by people from another community. Community empowerment is not an abstract idea; it flows from the increased power of the consumers and a consequent reduction in the power of professionals. Hiring fewer highly educated and credentialed professionals reduces costs without reducing the effectiveness of the interventions. Still, there will be a need for social workers, but their role needs to change from that of a service provider to that of a consultant who helps the community create its own interventions and build its own agencies, eventually reducing the need for the consultant in that role. The community organizing model allows the values, norms, habits, and practices of the community in question to be incorporated into real and practical interventions rather than asking communities to change to the values, norms, and practices of the workers and agencies to obtain service.

Traditionally, social service agencies have been set up in ways that are more comfortable for the workers and the administrators than for the consumers. Thus, they are often "user-unfriendly." The array of services offered, the hours services are provided, the qualifications and documentation required to entitle consumers to receive services have generally been established without consumer input. Thus, only consumers who are able to conform to the way the services are provided and who can get their needs met by the continuum of services selected for delivery will be served. Many agencies push more consumers out of their offices than they entice.

With some agencies, this result may be intentional, since they are seeking a particular type of consumer, namely that segment of the population in need of services who are most like the providers and with whom the providers feel more comfortable. In the case of public assistance and other such entitlements, the services appear to be designed to reduce the number of consumers by making the process so daunting, difficult, and humiliating that potential clients give up. Still other agencies may unintentionally discourage people from seeking their services by failing to recognize the differences in values, culture, practices, and needs between consumers and providers. How can agencies better address the needs of their consumers?

THE NEW YORK PEER AIDS EDUCATION COALITION

The New York Peer AIDS Education Coalition (NYPAEC) is an example of a harm-reduction, community-organizing model designed to respond to the needs of its consumers and implemented by a social worker. NYPAEC began as the Clinton Peer AIDS Education Coalition, named for its location, the Clinton neighborhood in the old Hell's Kitchen community in New York City. It was created by an Episcopal church, St. Clement's, a youth outreach agency, Streetwork Project of Victims Services, and a battered women's shelter, Sanctuary for Families. It hoped to address the HIV-prevention needs of the many street youths in the Times Square area of New York City who survived economically through prostitution and other sex industry work and who survived psychologically through the chronic and compulsive use of drugs, particularly crack cocaine, alcohol, heroin, and marijuana.

As is still true today, many of the street youths were gay, lesbian, bisexual, and transgendered. The staff, including a social worker, an Episcopal priest, an AIDS coordinator, and a seminarian, served as volunteers. How could we provide HIV information, condoms, bleach kits, skill instruction, and referrals to some of the ten to twenty thousand street youths in New York City? It was clear that street youths would not respond well to a direct intervention by the staff, since past efforts by staff to reach the most marginalized street youth had failed. The staff were too old, they did not know the proper vernacular, and they were seen as untrustworthy to the youths, who had suffered much pain at the hands of adults. Street youths are largely nonwhite, from poor and often single-parented families, overrepresented by gay, lesbian, bisexual, and transgendered youths and a majority have suffered from trauma: physical abuse, sexual abuse, emotional abuse, and deprivation. The transgendered youths, in particular, are difficult to engage and are often unknown to social workers and other professionals since they avoid agencies and tend to stay in their own worlds where they feel accepted.

One of the group of professionals trying to determine how to serve this population suggested a peer model. Thus, we recruited street youths with the promise of money to be earned, a hot meal if they came to a meeting, and the plea to help stop AIDS in their community. A flier was created and distributed to youths through the Streetwork Project, announcing the first meeting of the project. Over thirty youths attended the first meeting in the church and twelve signed up to become peer AIDS educators. Next, they were trained in HIV/AIDS, harm-reduction, risk-reduction, and outreach work. The courses were designed to be relevant to their lifestyles. They were nonjudgmental, practical, sex positive, and did not tout drug abstinence as the be-all and end-all of life. They were also short, preparing the youths to go out and do outreach work immediately.

The newly trained peer educators were sent out into the streets with condoms, bleach kits, literature, newly mastered skills, and enthusiasm. They were told to do their outreach wherever they happened to be in their daily lives: on prostitution strolls, in drug purchasing and using venues, on the streets, in agencies, in hospitals and medical centers, in their neighborhoods. The peer educators were the same as the population they were trying to reach. Many were involved in the sex industry, and all were using drugs. Most were homeless and had no legal sources of income. A weekly meeting, during which they would discuss their outreach work, have a meeting and support group, eat a hot meal, and receive a twenty-dollar "stipend" for expenses in outreach, was the basic structure of the project, in addition to their outreach. They had to educate, counsel, or give risk-reduction supplies (condoms, dental dams, finger cots, latex gloves, bleach kits, lubricants) to a minimum of seven street youths each week. The meetings were held at Streetwork for a time and then at St. Clement's Church. The budget was donated by the church for the first couple of years. Condoms, bleach kits, and other outreach supplies were donated by other agencies.

As time went on, it became apparent that the intervention was working. Peer educators were seeing scores of people each week despite the ups and downs of their chaotic lives. Peers became expert at their work and wrote their own brochure specifically targeted to other street youths. The project learned to deal with hospitalizations, incarcerations, emotional breakdowns, anger, drug problems, and to manage itself in new ways—primarily, that the peer educators had maximum input into all decisions. It became clear that the way to help people was to give them information, show them the array of choices they could make, and then support them in their decisions. Staff did not tell peer educators to stop prostituting or to give up drugs. They showed them how to do both more safely and explained the harms and risks involved without judgment, moralizing, or coercion. This harm-reduction approach is the most successful with marginalized people. Over time, a contract was developed between the staff and the peer educators that spelled out each one's obligations and rewards. After a year, it became clear that the work was not only successful in putting HIV-prevention messages and materials into the street life of youths it was also helping to change the lives of the peer educators. All had become housed, and most were now receiving legal income, mostly public assistance and SSI. Most were practicing safer sex regularly and all had been HIV tested. Peers were starting to talk about education, vocational training, employment, and goals for themselves. Some opened up spiritually and religiously; and two peers were baptized; one had her baby baptized in our host church. Peers spoke frequently about the positive impact of the project on their lives and their feelings about themselves. Many peers stated that they finally felt like "somebody in life."

Of interest to the staff was that the peer educators could perform social work, outreach, and counseling. Certainly their skills are not at the same level as a graduate-level social worker with experience; however, their skills were adequate to help the people they encountered in outreach, and when they were not up to the task or when the problems they encountered were beyond their abilities, they learned to make referrals and even take their "clients" to agencies and advocate for them until they got what they needed. In many cases, they were reaching people who would not have accessed professional help and would never have received any HIV-prevention or harm-reduction services without their presence in the street community.

The project began to solicit grant funds and received a three-year grant from the Trinity Foundation. It recruited more peer educators to establish a second outreach team, which had to meet in a second church due to spatial limitations. St. Clement's Church became its fiscal sponsor and managed the grant funds for the project. Over time, staff changed and new peers came on, negotiating new, longer, and more detailed contracts and adding new components, such as presentations, trainings, and other speaking engagements. Soon the peers and the staff felt the need to create a separate agency for the project. The name was changed to New York Peer AIDS Education Coalition to emphasize that outreach was being done all over the city and not just in the original Times Square area; the project became incorporated, set up a board of directors, and obtained more grant funds. It was set up as a membership organization to ensure that peer educators would always have a prominent voice in the organization and retain their power. In fact, according to the bylaws of the organization, one-third of the board must be composed of peer educators before outside directors can be added. Finally, enough money was raised to rent an office, and another peer expansion took place.

Today, NYPAEC has twenty-seven peer educators and four staff members. Peer educator workers are also employed as office help, data entry clerks, office cleaners, supply clerks, etc. This prevocational sheltered workshop program helps those with no work history to become employable and those with work histories to increase and perfect their skills and abilities to work "in the straight world." All policy and program decisions are made with peer educator input, and all hiring decisions are made with peer participation. The contract is now renegotiated once a year, with representatives from each outreach team conducting the negotiations with the two clinical staff members.

Over the six years the project has been in existence, many peer educators have left NYPAEC; some have died. Of those who have left, several are now employed elsewhere, including in AIDS organizations. Several have given up drugs and prostitution. One is raising a family and going to school. Most of the peers who have left and moved to other states still keep in touch with NYPAEC, particularly during holidays. Several of the peers have decided to strive to assume staff jobs in NYPAEC, which staff have encouraged, suggesting they start by getting an education.

Annually NYPAEC makes 20,000 outreach contacts with street youths involved in risk behavior for HIV infection and drug-related harm, while also developing its peer educators to take over the organization and to continue serving their communities. All this is done with a fraction of the cost it would take professional workers to do the same job and with more effectiveness because it is totally culturally appropriate. In time, there will be minimal need for outside experts and professionals, as NYPAEC trains its consumers and peer educators to run the organization. NYPAEC is putting the expertise in the community, empowering the community to care for itself. Even when peer educators are incarcerated in Riker's Island and Upstate they continue their HIV-prevention education. The prison health educators who are supposed to give HIV-prevention lectures rarely show up, and when they do, they present inaccurate information, according to the peers. NYPAEC's peer educators fill the gap and often ask for literature to be sent to them in jail. There have already been several replications of NYPAEC's model: in Edinburgh, Scotland; in Santa Fe, Mexico; and within the United States.

Funding is NYPAEC's greatest stress, as foundations and government prefer to fund "safer," more traditional agencies that retain power while providing "charity" to clients. If NYPAEC fails to survive, it will not be because the work is not proceeding well—it is. If it folds, it will be because NYPAEC's focus on changing the balance of power between agencies and those whom they serve is too revolutionary for most funders to invest in at this time.

CONCLUSION

Times are changing. AIDS has seen to that. The old charity/dependency models of the past, in which people are "taken care of" by service providers, are giving way to community-empowerment models that are constructed to teach consumers how to take care of themselves and their communities. This ushers in a new era for social workers, an era of organizing communities, helping to set up new structures, and training the customers to become the providers. Let us look forward to this new work, which does not eliminate society's need for our skills but allows us to take people to a higher level of accomplishment and success and multiplies the effects of our labor.

Chapter 27

HIV, Suicide, and Hastened Death

Michael E. Holtby

INTRODUCTION

The year is 2020. The AIDS pandemic is over, leaving a legacy that has changed the demographics of the world. Large numbers of baby boomers are just beginning to die of heart disease and an array of cancers, which are apparently on the rise due to decades of ozone depletion and other assaults on our environment. Medical science is now so advanced that doctors can keep our bodies alive for months, even years, beyond what used to be considered a "natural" death, in part because of the knowledge gained during the AIDS epidemic. However, they have not been able to restore health to the degree that these patients can leave their beds and return to normal lives. Patients are too often a mass of tubes and catheters, hooked to ventilators and dialysis machines. For decades, the right-to-life movement has successfully blocked physician-assisted suicide in the political arena, after the Supreme Court's ruling in the summer of 1997 that it was a matter for the state legislatures to decide. Despite concerns about terminal patients being coerced to end their lives, physician-assisted suicide has finally become legal in most states, facilitated by the collision between medical advances and the population's increase in disease due to the aging baby boomer population. Managed health care has begun to ration medical interventions, viewing the indefinite prolongation of bedridden patients' lives as pointless. Despite a loud right-to-life outcry, the general population is in agreement with these changes. At the forefront of the right-to-die movement is AARP, now run by the post–World War II babies, who are concerned with not ending their lives as helpless invalids with no quality of life left. Mental health practitioners have taken on the role of assessing competence, helping to differentiate between those patients with terminal, irreversible conditions wanting a "hastened death" and those who are suicidal due to depression or some other psychiatric disorder. Social workers have developed a specialization as mortal midwives. In the history books, there is a footnote about the PWAs, infectious disease doctors, and mental health clinicians in the era of AIDS, pioneering standards for what, in the year 2020, is called "final transition interventions."

If this scenario strikes you as science fiction, think again. As clinicians, we are closer to being "mortal midwives" than you may realize, and the AIDS epidemic has been "the fast-forward factor," as observed by physician Frederick R. Abrahms, associate medical director for the Colorado Foundation for Medical Care and a former clinical ethics professor (Martin, 1997).[1] Many factors have conspired within the AIDS community to make this happen.

The ingredients of cultural change were sown in an epidemic affecting young gay men. These men, as a group, were affluent, well educated, and activist. Gay men had already been forced to confront themselves, their families, and society with their homosexuality. As such, they now approached being sick in a whole new way: they were proactive. They questioned. They did not accept authoritarian edicts. They expected their doctors to be collaborators with them, whereas many of the elderly allow their doctors to be paternalistic and tell them what to do. In fact, a now classic study of long-term survivors found that PWAs had fired at least one doctor (Solomon and Temoshok, 1987). The majority took it upon themselves to be educated about the virus, the immune system, and the myriad of treatments out there from which to choose. This attitude carried over into the dying process: they want more control over when and how they die.

In addition, these men were gaining extensive experience with dying. Some have been the primary care takers for more than one partner who has died of AIDS. A San Francisco study, published in 1991, found that the average PWA had lost nine close friends (Hedge, 1991). One of my clients knows 103 people who have died. Another talks of traditional Thanksgiving gatherings of forty men at a Mexican resort, which has now dwindled down to less than a half dozen. Another man shows me a photo of his motorcycle club, with all but a few faces blacked out. As of June 1996, the CDC has reported 319,849 deaths nationwide since the onset of the epidemic (CDC, 1997). For many within the AIDS community, the number of personal losses has been likened to living in a war zone.

These men have an extraordinarily intimate and immediate knowledge of what it means to die and what the process involves. They do not necessarily accept the hospice view that all pain is controllable. In fact, a recent *JAMA* article talks about how AIDS pain is often undertreated (Stephenson, 1996; Passik et al., 1996). They also know that dying with dignity is not about pain; it is about suffering, and suffering can take many forms that compromise quality of life.

One of the defendants (who, by the time of the appeal, was deceased) in the New York, *Vacco v. Quill* case, which went before the U.S. Supreme Court in January of 1997, was Willy Barth. Barth was a patient of another defendant, Dr. Howard Grossman, whose caseload is 50 percent HIV related. Willy was not depressed and was not in pain. He had his family around him and had reached a comfortable closure with them. Yet he lay bedridden with Kaposi's sarcoma (KS), cryptosporidum, and cytomeglia virus (CMV) for eight weeks waiting to die. He kept asking Dr. Grossman, "How much longer is it going to take?"(Span, 1996, p. B101).

The case of *Dennis C. Vacco, Attorney General of New York et al. v. Timothy Quill, MD et al. (95-1858)* involves three doctors and the patients asserting their right to have a physician-assisted, hastened death. This won on appeal to the second U.S. Circuit Court of Appeals which found New York Laws on assisted suicide violated the equal protection clause of the 14th Amendment, saying that those patients on respirators have the right to die while those without life support do not. In January 1997 this case was argued before the U.S. Supreme Court along with another related case, the *State of Washington v. Harold D. Glucksberg MD et al. (96-110)*. The Supreme Court ultimately ruled against sanctioning assisted dying, but left the door open for the matter to be reviewed again in the future, depending upon any state laws enacted addressing the matter.

The Medical Director of San Francisco General's AIDS Clinic, Dr. John Stansell, has been quoted as saying, "The simple fact is that there are some patients for whom we cannot make death a tolerable process" (Guthrie, 1996).[2] He admitted writing prescriptions for opiates and barbiturates for several patients who were near death, until admonished by his superiors for going public.

Now we have three ingredients for cultural change: (1) a large number of young, affluent, educated individuals (2) who are assertive and proactive and (3) who have a great deal of experience with death. Now add a fourth ingredient—a sense of community. The AIDS community is, in fact, a *community*. It has a wealth of local and national newsletters as well as two national magazines. It has support groups and a plethora of professionals and agencies catering to the needs of PWAs. In addition, there are empowered groups such as ACT UP, the Gay Men's Health Crisis, and in my state, Denver's PWA Coalition. Also, in the age of cyberspace, there is a community connected by the information highway. Those who are isolated have not searched very far for resources. That same study about long-term survivors also found that the people who did the best healthwise had models for how to do it, through knowing others who are infected and further along than themselves (Solomon and Temoshok, 1987). This community developed its own values and protocol regarding suicide, which became so much a part of the common experience that a movie was made about it last year—*It's My Party.*

THE EXTENT OF AIDS SUICIDE

It is difficult to assess the extent of hastened and aided death among the PWA population. A 1988 study in New York City found the suicide rate among PWAs was sixty-six times higher than for the general population (Marzuk et al., 1988), and a more recent study in Louisiana found the suicide rate to be 134.6 times higher (Moncoske et al., 1995). However, many of these deaths do not constitute a "rational" suicide. For instance, many in the New York study killed themselves within the first nine months of diagnosis. I have, in my own clinical practice, seen many men depressed and suicidal when they are asymptomatic, which is a reversible condition. This is in contrast to the man who is close to his inevitable demise from multiple infections, who wants to control how death occurs.

How many of these suicides are actually similar to this last scenario? An indication is how many are assisted. Most aided deaths involve loved ones or physicians and take place when the PWA can no longer do the deed without help. In a San Francisco study of 136 couples, one out of nine reported giving drugs to their ill partners to accelerate death (Leiser et al., 1996). San Francisco has an extensive underground of physicians, pharmacists, and activists who will help, and it is common for men to bequeath stockpiled lethal drugs to others after they are gone. Randy Shilts, the late author of *And the Band Played On,* once said, "Gay men facing AIDS exchanged formulas for suicide as casually as housewives swap recipes for chocolate chip cookies" (Stolberg, 1996, p. 1).[3] San Francisco psychologist Peter Bradley, whose practice is primarily with gay PWAs, was quoted in the *Family Therapy Networker* as saying, "Nearly everybody hurries it along" (Henry, 1997, p. 14).[4] The *San Francisco Chronicle* reported one man who had attended over fifty assisted deaths (Stolberg, 1996).[5] On the other hand, the hinterland is not without its underground. I have spoken with a man here in Denver who claims to have attended at least a dozen. In a sample of PWAs in Vancouver, British Columbia, Russel Ogden found 83.3 percent were considering rational or assisted suicide (Ogden, 1994).

If it was legalized, how many PWAs would choose assistance? The Netherlands is some indication. Although it remains a crime there, assisted suicide has been an accepted practice for over twenty years. The Royal

Dutch Medical Association issued guidelines for the practice of euthanasia in 1984, and they were endorsed by a government-appointed commission. Doctors who follow the guidelines are rarely prosecuted. In Amsterdam, the most common cause of death among men between the ages of twenty and forty years of age is AIDS. Of those with AIDS, 26 percent choose physician-assisted suicide (Laane, 1995).

IMPACT ON HEALTH PROFESSIONALS

The cultural shift within the AIDS community has also affected those professionals who work with PWAs. As reported at the Eleventh International Conference on AIDS, in Vancouver in 1996, 35 percent of the AIDS physicians in San Francisco in 1990 reported they would help a PWA who was adamant in his or her request for aid in dying. By 1995, the percentage had risen to 51 percent. Indeed, the study found that 53 percent admitted having given lethal medication or otherwise helping PWAs to hasten their deaths an average (mean) of 4.2 times, with a total of up to 100 patients. The more AIDS patients a doctor had, the more likely he or she was to be inclined to help (Slome et al., 1997).

Traditionally, among psychotherapists, suicide has been viewed as a sign of mental illness, and there has been an obligation to hospitalize anyone who is an "imminent danger to himself or herself or others." The protocol was to give them a choice: either they went to the hospital on their own accord, or the therapist could impose a *seventy-two-hour hold,* or involuntary hospitalization. This, however, became impractical with someone who was bedridden and close to dying anyway. It made little common sense, and the trend began to change among therapists whose client specialization was HIV related. An interim *don't ask—don't tell* policy ensued, in which a client would be advised that if he or she was serious about committing suicide, he or she was not to discuss it further, or the therapist would interpret the client's bringing it up as a desire to be prevented. This approach was undesirable as well, as it left the client isolated, without professional support for a very important decision.

In 1993, the National Association of Social Workers (NASW) issued a policy statement that permitted their clinicians "to participate or not participate in assisted suicide matters or other discussions concerning end-of-life decisions depending on their beliefs, attitudes, and value systems." The statement also noted that if the professional could not do so, he or she had *an obligation* to refer the client to someone who could (NASW, 1994, p. 60).

In 1996 James Werth published his book, *AIDS and Rational Suicide?*, which outlined criteria that the majority of mental health professionals could accept as indeed "rational":

> The results demonstrate that the criteria outlined may be acceptable to a majority of ethicists, suicidologists, and psychologist-attorneys. This is important for it is these individuals who will be deciding about ethical violations, establishing the standard of care, and providing legal consultation for and against cases of rational suicide. (Werth, 1996, p. 69)

These criteria were used by a psychiatrist to evaluate one of Kevorkian's patients and are becoming the gold standard for such evaluations.

ESTABLISHING ASSESSMENT STANDARDS

Dr. Werth is a principal author of the amicus *curiae* (friend of the court) brief submitted to the U.S. Supreme Court on behalf of the Washington State Psychological Association, the American Counseling Association, the Association for Gay, Lesbian, and Bisexual Issues in Counseling, and a Coalition for Mental Health Professionals (Supreme Court, 1996). The brief addresses the question of whether mental competence can adequately be assessed. Can motivations for assisted suicide be differentiated between that which is "rational" and other clinical conditions such as depression, dementia, psychosis, or post-traumatic stress disorder? We believe the answer is "yes."

To reframe the manner in which we think about this subject, we need to change the semantics. There is a need to separate the act of "suicide" from a "hastened" or "assisted" death.

Criteria of Hastened or Assisted Dying

1. The person has an irreversible, terminal condition close to the end stages of the disease (Werth, 1996, p. 62).[6] The guidelines of the Seattle Compassion in Dying organization include confirmation of the patient's condition by two physicians, attesting it is terminal within six months. They also state "the patient's condition must cause severe, unrelenting suffering which the patient finds unacceptable and intolerable" (Preston and Mero, 1996, p. 185).
2. The person is making a free choice without coercion or pressure from others. Compassion in Dying states, "The request for assistance

must originate with the patient. The request must be made in writing or on videotape on three occasions, with an interval of at least 48 hours between the second and third requests. Requests for our involvement may not be made through advance directives or by a health-care surrogate, attorney-in-fact, or any other person. We will not provide assistance if there is expressed disapproval by any member of the immediate family" (Preston and Mero, 1996, p. 185).

3. The person is mentally competent to make such a decision, as opposed to having their judgment impaired by dementia, clinical depression, psychosis, etc.
4. The person engages in a sound decision-making process, considering all the alternatives. As Preston and Mero (1996) state, "the patient must understand the medical condition, prognosis, and types of comfort care which are available as alternatives to suicide" (Preston and Mero, 1996, p. 185).

Assessing Capacity to Make Reasoned Decisions

The appropriate standard would require that a terminally ill patient (Werth, 1996, p. 94):

1. understand and remember information relevant to an end-of-life decision;
2. appreciate the consequences of the decision;
3. indicate a clearly held and consistent underlying set of values that provides some guidance in making the decision; and
4. communicate the decision and explain the process used for making it.

Assessing the Rationality of a Decision

The person should engage in a sound decision-making process that includes the following (Werth, 1996, p. 62):

1. Consultation with a mental health professional who can make an assessment of mental competence (which would include the absence of treatable major depression)
2. Nonimpulsive consideration of all alternatives
3. Consideration of the congruence of the act with one's personal values
4. Consideration of the impact on significant others
5. Consultation with objective others (e.g., medical and religious professionals) and with significant others

DIFFERENTIAL DIAGNOSIS

Margaret Battin has developed an excellent questionnaire that, for our purposes as clinicians, provides a good reminder of the relevant issues to cover in determining a diagnosis. I have included those questions, with her permission, in Table 27.1 (Battin, 1994a). Other resources include this author's previous article (Holtby, 1996b) and George Burnell's article, "Psychiatric Assessment of the Suicidal Terminally Ill." A caution from Dr. Burnell:

> Many depressive symptoms are similar to those of the medical illness (fatigue, weakness, weight loss) and can wax and wane as the illness progresses. Diagnostic criteria in the psychiatric nosology have been generally inadequate when applied to terminally ill patients. (Burnell, 1995, p. 512)

Some of the major distinctions between symptoms of suicidal depression and a desire to die due to medical illness include the following:

1. *Self-esteem:* This is typically lowered in an individual who is suicidally depressed, but for the terminally ill individual choosing the manner of death, it may be the final act of assertive will (Supreme Court, 1996, p. 18).
2. *Feelings of guilt and shame:* These are present with depression but not with those appropriately seeking a hastened death.
3. *Suicidal motivation:* For those who are depressed, the motivations include psychic or interpersonal conflict, whereas with hastened death, the motivation is to end suffering, indignity, and pain specifically related to the terminal condition.
4. *Means of suicide:* For those who are clinically depressed, the means of suicide is often seized upon impulsively, poorly planned, and involving a violent method, with little regard for who finds them (or an unconscious desire to act out their anger at loved ones). With those appropriately seeking a hastened death, none of these elements are true.
5. *Depressive history:* The clinically depressed individual is likely to have a history of depressive episodes prior to the current illness. In addition, a history of previous suicide attempts is often evident. These are not significantly apparent with the terminally ill individual seeking a hastened death.
6. *Interpersonal history and relationships:* The individual seeking an appropriate hastened death is likely to have close relationships with

friends and family, whereas the depressed individual is much more likely to have dysfunctional, conflicted relationships and/or be socially withdrawn. The depressed individual's interpersonal behavior is manipulative, showing a lack of regard for the feelings of others.

7. *Timing of death:* Dr. Margaret Battin has pointed out that those who are rationally considering hastening their death are concerned with timing their demise. They do not want to lose what may be left of quality time, but yet they do not want to wait until it is too late (due to dementia or other factors) and then have to endure prolonged, painful, or undesirable late-stage disease processes. This is different from individuals who are depressed—usually ASAP is their preferred time. There is no reason, in their mind, to savor the time left (Battin, 1994b).

TABLE 27.1. Battin Questionnaire

__ Is the person making a request for help?	__ How accurate are other nonmedical facts cited in the request?
__ Why is the person consulting a physician or mental health professional?	__ Is the suicide plan financially motivated?
__ What has kept the person from attempting or committing suicide so far?	__ Has the person considered the effects of his or her suicide on other persons?
__ Is the request for help in suicide a request for someone else to decide?	__ Does the person fear becoming a burden?
__ How stable is the request?	__ What cultural influences are shaping the person's choice?
__ Is the request consistent with the person's basic values?	__ Are the person's affairs in order?
__ How far in the future would the suicide take place?	__ Has the person picked a method of committing suicide?
__ Are the medical facts cited in the request accurate?	__ Would the person be willing to tell others about his or her suicide plan?
	__ Does the person see suicide as the only way out?

THE CLINICIAN'S ROLE BEYOND ASSESSMENT

It would be very short-sighted for our role to be limited to gatekeeper—one more hoop to jump through for an already exhausted client. Our interventions can go well beyond assessment. Ideally, our first involvement is not assessing the validity of a hastened death. That is just one part of a long, ongoing process of support and therapy with an individual facing a life-threatening illness. However, to facilitate this specific decision, we can do the following:

1. Advise clients as to the resources available in terms of palliative care, doctors, support groups, legal considerations, and sources of more information, etc. An excellent book to recommend to clients and their caregivers is *Final Acts of Love*, by Stephen Jamison (1995).
2. Help our clients consider alternatives such as palliative care, better pain control, and the use of antidepressants.
3. Through self-hypnosis, we can give clients another way to deal with physical and emotional pain and insomnia.
4. Collaborate with the client's physician to ascertain the best guess as to progression probabilities and end-stage complications to aid the client in timing his or her death through adequate information (Battin, 1994a).
5. Help clients devise a plan that will minimize tragedy, violence, or disability instead of death.
6. Make sure all the bases are covered: living wills, estate planning, memorial services, and so forth.
7. Explore the client's emotional pain as it relates to anticipatory grief, unresolved relationships, and life regrets.
8. Help clients deal with their family and friends and consider what impact their death will have on others and what emotional closure and processing is necessary.
9. Facilitate communications between clients and their loved ones, with additional skills and an appropriate setting, if possible.
10. Provide a safe place for the client to discuss existential concerns:

    a. What happens after one dies?
    b. What is life's spiritual meaning?
    c. How does one wish to be remembered?

A Postscript: Freud's Hastened Death

Clinicians might find it of particular interest that Freud, dying of cancer, asked his personal physician Max Shur to help him die. He had previously prepared the physician by discussing the matter and extracting the doctor's promise that he would help. When Freud determined his cancer was no longer bearable, Dr. Shur gave him an injection of morphine, and the father of psychoanalysis fell into a coma from which he never awoke (Stone, 1997).

NOTES

1. Frederick Abrahms quoted by author (Martin, 1997).
2. John Stansell quoted by author (Guthrie, 1996).
3. Randy Shilts quoted by author (Stolberg, 1996).
4. Peter Bradley quoted by author (Henry, 1997).
5. Richard Wagner quoted by author (Stolberg, 1996).
6. Dr. Werth uses a more expanded criteria than I have outlined here that includes more than just those who are terminal and in the end-stages of their disease: "The person considering suicide has an unremitting 'hopeless' condition. 'Hopeless' conditions include, but are not necessarily limited to, terminal illnesses, severe physical and/or psychological pain, physically or mentally debilitating and/or deteriorating conditions, or quality of life no longer acceptable to the individual" (Werth, 1996, p. 62).

REFERENCES

Battin, M. P. (1994a). Assisting in suicide: Seventeen questions physicians and mental health professionals should ask. *The least worst death*, M. Battin (Ed.). New York: Oxford Press, pp. 145-162.

Battin, M. P. (1994b). Going early, going late: The rationality of decisions about suicide in AIDS. *The Journal of Medicine and Philosophy, 19*(6), 571-594.

Burnell, G. (1995). Psychiatric assessment of the suicidal terminally ill. *Hawaii Medical Journal, 54*(5), 510-513.

Centers for Disease Control (1997). CDC update trends in AIDS incidence, deaths and prevalence—United States, 1996. *Morbidity and Mortality Weekly Report* (February 28), *46*(8), 165-173.

Guthrie, J. (1996). AIDS activists will defy suicide ban. *San Francisco Examiner,* October 2, A1.

Hedge, B. (1991). Psychological aspects of HIV infection. *AIDS Care, 3*(4), 409-412.

Henry, S. (1997). The death with dignity debate. *Family Therapy Networker, 1*(1), 14-15.

Holtby, M. E. (1996b). HIV/AIDS and suicide: Be open. *Social Work, 41*, 324.

Jamison, S. (1995). *Final acts of love: Family, friends, and assisted dying.* New York: Putnam's Sons.

Laane, H. M. (1995). Euthanasia, assisted suicide and AIDS. *AIDS Care, 7*(2), 163-167.

Leiser, R. J., Mitchell, T. F., Hahn, J., Slome, L., Mandel, N., Townley, D., and Abrams, D. (1996). Nurses' attitudes toward assisted suicide in AIDS (citing UCSF study of 136 couples). Presented at the Eleventh International Conference on AIDS, Vancouver, Canada, July 10.

Martin, C. (1997). Choosing life or death. *Denver Post,* February 17, E1-2.

Marzuk, P. M., Tierney, H., Tardiff, K., Gross, E. M., Morgan, E. B., Hsu, M., and Mann, J. J. (1988). Increased risk of suicide in persons with AIDS. *Journal of the American Medical Association, 259*(9), 1333-1337.

Moncoske, R. J., Wadsworth, C. M., Dugas, D. S., and Hansney, J. A. (1995). Suicide risk among people living with AIDS. *Social Work, 40*(6), 783-787.

National Association of Social Workers (1994). Client self-determination in end-of-life decisions. *Social Work Speaks.* Washington, DC: NASW Press, pp. 58-61.

Ogden, R. (1994). *Euthanasia, assisted suicide and AIDS.* New Westminster, BC: Peroglyphics Publications.

Passik, S., McDonald, M., Rosenfeld, B., and Brietbart, W. (1996). End of life issues in patients with AIDS: Clinical and research considerations. In M. Battin and A. Lipman (Eds.), *Drug Use in Assisted Suicide and Euthanasia.* Binghamton, NY: The Haworth Press, pp. 91-111.

Preston, T. and Mero, R. (1996). Observations concerning terminally ill patients who choose suicide. *Journal of Pharmaceutical Care in Pain and Symptom Control, 4*(1/2), 183-192.

Slome, L. R., Mitchell, T. F., Charlebois, E., Benevedes, J. M., Abrams, D. (1997). Physician-assisted suicide and patients with human immunodeficiency virus disease. *The New England Journal of Internal Medicine, 33*(6), 417-421.

Solomon, G. F. and Temoshok, L. (1987). A psychoneuroimmunologic perspective on AIDS research: Questions, preliminary findings and suggestions. *Journal of Applied Social Psychology, 17*, 286-308.

Span, P. (1996). A matter of life and death: The court to hear arguments for and against physician-assisted suicide. *Washington Post,* November 14, B101.

Stephenson, J. (1996). Experts say AIDS pain "dramatically under treated." *JAMA: Medical News and Perspectives, 276*(17), 1369-1370.

Stolberg, S. (1996). Ending life on their own terms. *Los Angeles Times*, October 1, 1,1.

Stone, A. (1997). Physician-assisted suicide and the psychiatric profession, *The Harvard Mental Health Letter,* January 1,4.

Supreme Court of the United States (1996). Brief of the Washington State Psychological Association, the American Counseling Association, the Association for Gay, Lesbian, and Bisexual Issues in Counseling, and a Coalition of Mental Health Professionals as amici curiae in support of the respondent: *State of*

Washington et al. v. Harold D. Glucksberg, MD, et al., and *Dennis C. Vacco, Attorney General of the State of New York, et al. v. Timothy E. Quill, MD, et al.*

Werth, J. L. (1996). *Rational suicide? Implications for mental health professionals.* Washington, DC: Taylor and Francis.

Chapter 28

Coming Out Positive?
HIV Prevention for Gay, Lesbian,
and Bisexual Youths

Peter A. Newman

Due to massive prevention efforts, often on the impetus of lesbian, gay, and bisexual (LGB) communities, rates of new seroconversions for HIV are declining among adult gay men. We have not fared so well, however, regarding LGB youths, for whom rates of new seroconversions continue to rise. This chapter will address the critical importance of LGB-affirmative HIV/AIDS education and prevention targeting LGB youths, along with issues and risk factors particular to coming out in an often hostile or denigrating larger social environment. Programmatic suggestions for effective prevention will be offered. A central theme of this chapter is that effective HIV prevention for LGB youths must be conceptualized and implemented as part of a comprehensive and affirmative programmatic response to the distinct needs of this population. The major issues to be addressed are as follows:

1. Most young people are having sex and are at risk for HIV.
2. LGB youths are at greater risk for HIV/AIDS than heterosexual youths, in part due to additional psychosocial risk factors.
3. Ethnic minority LGB youths are at a particularly high risk for HIV.
4. Developmental issues and coming out are integral to HIV risk and prevention.
5. HIV prevention must be part of a broader, LGB-affirmative programmatic response to the social, cognitive, and emotional needs of LGB youths.
6. Components of effective HIV prevention for LGB youths are presented.

YOUTHS AND HIV/AIDS

A recent White House report estimated that one in four new seroconversions for HIV is among youths ages thirteen to twenty (Fleming, 1996). Fully two-thirds of adolescents in the United States have had sexual intercourse by age nineteen, although less than 10 percent report regular condom use (Flora and Thoresen, 1989). A marker of a youth being at high risk for HIV is that sexually active adolescents have the highest rates of sexually transmitted diseases (STDs) of all age groups (Hein, 1993; Perry and Sieving, 1991). If one takes into account the average ten- to eleven-year-lag between initial infection and AIDS diagnosis—when considering that AIDS is the leading cause of death among twenty-five to forty-four-year-olds in the United States (Centers for Disease Control [CDC], 1996)—it is also evident that many adults become HIV positive during adolescence and young adulthood. In sum, young people are clearly at risk for HIV/AIDS.

LGB Youths and HIV/AIDS

Although all young people are potentially at risk for HIV, 70 percent of HIV-positive adolescents and young adults are male; one-third of HIV-positive adolescent males ages thirteen to nineteen and 63 percent ages twenty to twenty-four years old are reported to have contracted HIV through male-to-male sexual contact (CDC, 1996). It is likely that male-to-male sex is underreported by youths so seroprevalence data provide a low estimate of the latter as a risk factor. Several surveys of gay and bisexual male youths have found that upward of 70 percent report being sexually active, while only 10 to 15 percent consistently use condoms for oral or anal sex (Rotheram-Borus and Koopman, 1991; Rotheram-Borus et al., 1992). Studies contrasting older and younger gay males have reported higher rates of unprotected anal sex among the younger group (Hayes, Kegeles, and Coates, 1990; Stall et al., 1992). Additionally, condom use is a preventive behavior that correlates negatively with most risk behaviors (Ku, Sonnenstien, and Pleck, 1992). This means that those young people who engage in the most sexual encounters or who are substance abusers are also least likely to use condoms.

Together, these statistics point to an alarming risk for HIV among gay and bisexual male youths. Although gay and bisexual male youths are disproportionately represented in rates of HIV, young lesbians and bisexual women are increasingly at risk. In the last decade, the incidence of new cases of HIV in women has doubled from 9 percent to 18 percent, with younger women at the greatest risk (CDC, 1996). More than twice as many new cases of AIDS in 1995 were among women ages thirteen to nineteen (40 percent) as compared to women over twenty-five (18 percent).

Despite the disproportionate risk for HIV infection among gay and bisexual male youths, however, and the increasing risk among young lesbians and bisexual young women, the meager sex education and condom information offered to youths is most often based on a heterosexual model. Most research on HIV/AIDS, specifically in adolescents and young adults, also denies the existence of lesbian, gay, and bisexual youths among this population (Sussman and Duffy, 1996). This is a recipe for disaster.

There are several substantive reasons for the elevated risk for HIV/AIDS among LGB youths as compared to their heterosexual counterparts. Understanding the nature and mechanisms of these risks is essential to developing effective prevention strategies and allows one to appreciate the necessity of broad programmatic responses targeting these populations.

LGB youths, as contrasted with heterosexuals, experience intense cognitive, social, and emotional isolation (Hetrick and Martin, 1987; Malyon, 1981). These forms of isolation have specific relevance to HIV-related, sexual risk-taking behaviors among young people and present obstacles to prevention as well. Cognitive isolation refers to a lack of accurate information about what it means to be lesbian, gay, or bisexual and a lack of positive role models. Social isolation results from a sense of feeling different from the "norm" and distancing from peers and family. Being unable to openly share feelings about sexuality with family and friends results in emotional isolation as well. The experience of isolation and stigma is common among LGB youths.

Specifically with regard to HIV/AIDS, cognitive isolation results in a dearth of accurate information about HIV and its transmission. This isolation may distance one from feeling oneself at risk and may promote the belief that HIV is a disease only of adults. Alternatively, the equation of gay men and AIDS may lead gay male youths to believe AIDS is inevitable. For lesbian youths, there may exist the erroneous belief that they cannot contract HIV, even though they may at times have sex with men. Lesbian youths may experiment with unprotected sex with gay men, both unconsciously believing gay people cannot become pregnant (Hunter and Schaecher, 1994). One pilot study found that 75 percent of young lesbians engaged in intercourse with young, often gay, men as well as sex with other women (Hunter, Rosario, and Rotheram-Borus, 1993, cited in Hunter and Schaecher, 1994). Another risk factor is that young people may use anal sex as a form of birth control, even if it presents a risk of HIV transmission (Catania et al., 1989). Confusion also arises for bisexual male youths, who may believe that because they are not gay they are not at risk for HIV. Lack of access to accurate information and lack of forums to discuss these issues and their sexuality may greatly increase the risk of contracting HIV for LGB young people.

Social and emotional isolation render both lesbian and gay young people vulnerable. It is important, however, to address the differential developmental paths of lesbians and gay men. For young women, loneliness and isolation may result in their seeking out a relationship with another woman and then withdrawing into the relationship to the exclusion of other friends and sources of support (Krestan and Bepko, 1980). Particularly for young women who do not have available a lesbian community, and who lack social support, more dependent and enmeshed relationships may result (Lewis, 1984). This may lead in turn to further isolation from peers and render the relationship itself quite vulnerable, with potentially deleterious effects on social support. Not only may young women who self-identify as lesbians experiment sexually with men, but pregnancy may at times function as a means to hide sexual orientation (Hunter and Schaecher, 1994).

Differences in the psychosocial developmental trajectories of gay and lesbian youths have distinct ramifications for HIV-related risk behavior (Hunter and Schaecher, 1994). Social and emotional isolation for gay and bisexual male youths may lead to their going to bars or other venues in which they have heard other gay and bisexual men can be found. Their cognitive isolation gives greater credibility to homophobic media depictions of all gay men as hypersexual and of gay male relationships as nonexistent. At times, the meetings in these venues may promote sexual contact. With this sexual contact, seen as the only means for affirmation of their sexual identity, these young gay and bisexual men, even if they know about safer sex, may give in to having unsafe sex with other, sometimes older, men to avoid further rejection. Gay and bisexual male youths, some of whom may seek out sexual intimacy (much as their heterosexual peers), may fear being stigmatized and ostracized, in addition to outright violence, if they are seen with male companions in their schools, neighborhoods, or homes. This may lead to more furtive and underground sexual encounters that generally entail greater risk of unsafe sex than situations in which sexual negotiation and refusal are greater possibilities.

Ethnic Minority LGB Youths and HIV/AIDS

African-American, Latino, Asian-American, and other ethnic minority LGB youths face all of the isolation described of other LGB youths, but their experience is often compounded by living among three worlds (Chan, 1989; Icard, 1986; Morales, 1990). First, they face the homophobia and discrimination of the dominant heterosexual culture, compounded with racism. Second, as opposed to heterosexual ethnic youths of color who may greatly benefit from the support of their ethnically similar parents and the larger ethnic community, LGB youths may feel a sense of alienation from their own ethnic community due to homophobia. They may experience support concerning their ethnic identity but not in being LGB and may either hide their sexual orientation or distance themselves from their ethnic community. Third, ethnic minority youths frequently do not experience the larger LGB community as home, due to the racism that exists in this often European-American dominated culture.

The confluence of these negative social phenomena, and the feeling of not wholly belonging anywhere, may exacerbate the process of identity development and may render self-esteem and social support particularly difficult for some ethnic minority LGB young people. AIDS knowledge may be substantial but the motivation and capacity to act on that knowledge may be negatively affected by feelings of alienation, low self-esteem, and lack of social support. It is also necessary to consider that some LGB youths of color may have developed considerable resiliency, having earlier dealt with ethnic identity development in a largely hostile society. Another possibility for some youths of color is that LGB issues may not be as salient, nor as stressful, as compared to living in a racist society. However, feeling compelled at times to declare one's allegiance (e.g., "Are you black or are you gay?") is a stressor not faced by European-American LGB youths (Washington, 1995). The variety of psychosocial stressors and social vulnerabilities experienced by ethnic minority lesbian and gay youths likely contributes to the overrepresentation of African-American and Hispanic youths and young adults in HIV/AIDS statistics (CDC, 1996; Rotheram-Borus et al., 1995).

HIV prevention and education must differentially target LGB youths of color, who may not relate to messages developed for European-American youths. LGB youths of color may have distinct experiences, some of which alienate them from the dominant culture. One significant factor is that more African-American and Latino men who have sex with men may identify as bisexual than European-American men (Rogers and Williams, 1987), suggesting that bisexual men must be specifically targeted as at risk in these populations. There also exists a legitimate and historically based mistrust of the dominant European-American culture, and of the health care system in particular, that must be addressed for prevention to be effective (e.g., the Tuskegee Syphilis Study) (Thomas and Quinn, 1991).

Research has specifically underscored the distinct language and meanings concerning sex and sexuality used by African-American gay men and the need to make HIV prevention culturally relevant (Mays et al., 1992).

Issues concerning language and acculturation are also strongly relevant for Latinos, Asian Americans, and Native Americans, necessitating targeted prevention. Latinos who are more acculturated have more accurate knowledge about AIDS (Marin and Marin, 1990), even though they also evidence increased HIV-related risk behavior, such as drinking (Caetano, 1987), as compared to less acculturated Latinos. There are also culture- and gender-specific obstacles to prevention (as well as strengths) among Latinas, as assessed in a survey of Chicana/Latina university youths (Flores-Ortiz, 1994), that must be addressed in culturally competent interventions.

The field of social work, and HIV prevention in particular, must be increasingly challenged to address multiculturalism, not only across different individuals, but in the intersections of multiple social identities in each and every one of us (Reed et al., 1997). This entails moving beyond simple additive models that neglect the dynamic interactions among race, ethnicity, social class, gender, sexual orientation, age, and ability. Culturally appropriate HIV-prevention programs acknowledge the intersections of these multiple layers of social identity in addressing the cultures of participants and seek to work within and across those cultures to identify behaviors and values that reduce risk (Freudenberg, 1994; McLean, 1994; Schinke et al., 1990; Singer et al., 1990).

COMING OUT AND HIV-RELATED RISK-TAKING BEHAVIOR

A critical aspect of LGB identity development, and one which is distinct from that of heterosexuals, is coming out. The coming-out process has several ramifications for HIV-related risk behavior and its prevention. Coming out is usually understood as psychologically beneficial, in that LGB people eliminate, or lessen, the dissonance caused by the lack of congruence between public and private personas (Vincke et al., 1993). There are several aspects of this process, including recognizing oneself as lesbian, gay, or bisexual, making one's social and emotional attraction to persons of the same sex public, the reactions of one's social environment, and the subsequent adjusting of social relationships. The development of LGB identity and the need to express one's newfound identity are part of the coming-out process.

Although the internal psychological adjustment that accompanies coming out may indeed be positive, coming out to a hostile social environment can also bring with it a variety of new stressors. On the one hand, coming out can decrease risk-taking behavior because one who is less psychologically vulnerable, with a more intact sense of self-esteem, is more likely to practice health-promoting behaviors (Vincke et al., 1993). Alternatively, coming out can expose one to greater stress, which increases sexual risk-taking behavior—particularly if sex is perceived as the primary expression of one's newfound gay identity, as is characteristic for some gay youths (Rotheram-Borus and Fernandez, 1995; Vincke et al., 1993). One may also experience increased social ostracism and the loss of social support, which may cause greater drug use and increased sexual risk-taking behavior.

Coming out, then, must be conceptualized as a transactional process between the person and the environment and one in which LGB-affirmative social support is crucial. Social support is correlated with greater self-esteem as well as the implementation of preventive behaviors for HIV in gay and bisexual male youths (Rotheram-Borus et al., 1995). Greater social support has been found to be directly linked to decreased risk for HIV among African-American adolescents (St. Lawrence et al., 1994).

A distinct challenge that has not been faced by previous cohorts of LGB youths is that of coming out in the age of AIDS. For young gay men, the belief may exist that AIDS is an inevitability. I have argued elsewhere that, tragically, for some gay youths who have never known adolescent and young adult life without AIDS and who have witnessed the decimation of the older gay community, becoming HIV positive may represent a normative milestone in the coming-out process (Newman, 1998). In the context of AIDS, coming out and seeking intimacy is vastly complicated by fears of illness and death that manifest for the individual, as well as for family, significant others, and friends (Paradis, 1991). Some gay youths "now perceive themselves as potential carriers of death, and others have become severely anxious about contracting the disease" (Isay, 1989, p. 68). Interventions must combat the correlation of being gay and having AIDS, in addition to providing social support and HIV-negative, adult, gay male role models for HIV-negative gay youths.

A final and critical aspect of coming out of relevance to HIV prevention lies in its developmental trajectory. The median age of first male-male sexual intercourse is fifteen years old (van Griensven, Koblin, and Osmond, 1994), while the median age of coming out (acknowledging and revealing one's sexual orientation) is most often in later adolescence or early adulthood. Although there is considerable variability in the ages at which these developmental milestones are attained (MacDonald, 1983)—in part as a function of societal changes over time—generally, coming out for gay men has been found to follow the first sexual experience by roughly four years (Roesler and Deisher, 1972). Gay men are also reported to first act on their sexual feelings an average of five years earlier than lesbians (Riddle and Morin, 1977).

It cannot be emphasized enough that many LGB youths experiment with opposite-sex activity and engage in same-sex sexual behavior well before self-identifying as lesbian, gay, or bisexual (de Monteflores and Schulz, 1978). Additionally, some young gay men who engage in sex with men and who dismiss their sexuality may also deny the risks of their sexual behavior (Coleman and Remafedi, 1989).

The implications of the coming-out trajectory regarding sexual behavior are critical. To the extent that HIV/AIDS education and prevention is situated solely in LGB-designated programs, it will often be accessed too late. Sadly, many LGB young adults feel compelled to come out in response to receiving an HIV-positive test result rather than in the natural course of identity development, without the fear of impending illness. Thus, although it is imperative that HIV prevention be included in LGB programs, and be made accessible and affirmative for LGB youths, HIV education and prevention that is lesbian and gay affirmative must also occur as part of other medical, psychosocial, and educational programs that recognize the variable nature of sexual behavior, particularly among young people, who may not seek out, or may assiduously avoid, LGB-designated programs.

HIV PREVENTION FOR LGB YOUTHS

Given the often intense isolation experienced by LGB youths, and the various aspects, both positive and potentially conflicted, of the normative coming-out process, it becomes imperative that HIV prevention for LGB youths be situated as just one aspect of a larger programmatic response to the distinct needs of this population. Research confirms the potential for negative sequelae of the coming-out process, including increased alcohol and drug use and increased sexual risk behaviors (Vincke et al., 1993). These possible negative outcomes are best understood as resulting from stigmatization and decreased social support, when coming out is undergone in a hostile environment, rather than as individual psychological problems experienced in a social vacuum.

Further confirmation of the importance of LGB-affirmative social support is reported in a study of young gay men (under age twenty-five).

Researchers found that young gay men who did not belong to a gay organization had significantly higher levels of unprotected sex than young gay men who were connected to a gay organization (Ridge, Plummer, and Minichiello, 1994). These findings underscore the critical nature of LGB-affirmative social support—and positive LGB identity—for LGB youths and link social support directly to sexual risk-taking behavior and prevention.

Implications for HIV Prevention for LGB Youths

Effective HIV prevention and education for youths includes cognitive, affective, behavioral, and environmental components (Flora and Thoresen, 1989). AIDS knowledge and condom awareness alone have consistently been found to be insufficient in effecting behavior change (Hingson et al., 1990; Kegeles, Adler, and Irwin, 1988; Rickert et al., 1989). In addition to the development of accurate knowledge, components of successful prevention programs include the building of behavioral skills in condom use, building and practicing sexual negotiation and sexual refusal skills (for which role-play is essential), open dialogue, social and emotional support, and teaching how to enjoy safer sex.

Peer-facilitated programs are integral to effective HIV prevention for LGB young people. The use of peers helps LGB youths to personalize AIDS information, to perceive the threat to themselves—that they are potentially at risk (Hansen, Hahn, and Wolkenstein, 1990; Hunter and Schaecher, 1994). LGB peer educators and counselors promote the diffusion of prevention messages among other LGB youths (Fisher, 1988; Kelly et al., 1991). LGB peer involvement in HIV prevention also has salubrious effects on peer norms. Research consistently reveals the significance of peer norms in influencing the behavior of youth and safer-sex behaviors in particular (Fishbein and Middlestadt, 1989; Jemmott, Jemmott, and Fong, 1992). Limited research comparing peer-led and adult-led AIDS education programs has also found that although adult and peer leaders were both effective in promoting knowledge gains and attitude change, more questions were asked of peer educators (Rickert, Jay, and Gottlieb, 1991). Dialogue and interaction is a critical dimension of engendering safer-sex behavior.

Given the different developmental trajectories and life experiences of lesbians, bisexuals, gay men, and LGB persons of color, differential targeting of these populations is necessary to make the messages relevant, affirmative, comprehensible, and culturally appropriate. To these ends, the target population of the intended intervention needs to be involved across all stages of intervention planning and implementation.

General sex education, anatomy and physiology, and STD education are also imperative for prevention efforts, particularly since much sex education to which young people have been previously exposed was presented via a heterosexist and nondialogical model. The inculcation of shame and guilt is contrary to supporting self-esteem and discourages frank and open discussion of actual sexual behavior and the difficulties that may accompany safer sex.

The availability of condoms is crucial to HIV-prevention efforts. Positive attitudes toward condoms are meaningless if one lacks access to them. The distribution of free condoms by community-based organizations, community and student health services, and LGB organizations, in the context of health and prevention programs, also serves an important symbolic function in acknowledging the reality of youths' sexual behavior and fostering discussion about sex and AIDS.

Given the developmental trajectory of coming out, and the fact that sexual experimentation may precede self-identifying as gay, lesbian, or bisexual (or heterosexual) by many years, the availability of nonhomophobic and, moreover, LGB-affirmative medical and psychosocial support is essential for both those who are HIV negative and those who are HIV positive. Access to a community of LGB young people and "out" LGB adult role models is also essential, as coming out is a transactional process between person and environment. Social support and modeling are critical environmental components of effective prevention.

In addition to medical and social services, anonymous HIV-antibody testing, with the provision of pre- and posttest counseling, should be available and accessible to youth. Overreliance on testing as a cornerstone of prevention, however, may be counterproductive, as it may in effect communicate that seroconversion is an inevitability (Odets, 1994).

HIV prevention also necessitates the availability and accessibility of alcohol and substance abuse education and treatment. Although sharing unsterilized needles during injection drug use can directly transmit HIV, noninjection drug use and alcohol use are strongly implicated in greater sexual risk-taking behavior among adolescents and young adults (Bowser, Fullilove, and Fullilove, 1990; Johnson, 1990-1991; Koopman, Rosario, and Rotheram-Borus, 1994; Stall et al., 1986). The higher incidence of substance abuse among LGB youths as compared to their heterosexual counterparts, underscores the importance of LGB-affirmative education and treatment regarding drug and alcohol use. Related education also offers benefits by linking substance use with sexual risk-taking behavior and by offering harm-reduction strategies.

Overall, effective prevention is best understood not as a one-shot deal, but as a sustained and integrated effort. The stresses of being a young LGB person in an ambient culture of homophobia are ongoing. Coming out, rather than a discrete event, is also an ongoing process. Prevention, too, should be ongoing. Additionally, statistics indicating a return to unsafe sex by some gay men who previously practiced only safer sex also underscore the need for sustained prevention strategies (Hart et al., 1992; Stall et al., 1990). The ongoing stress often experienced by LGB youths may also be compounded for LGB youths of color, who are also faced with negotiating a society permeated by racism and white supremacism and who, as a result, are also more likely to live in poverty.

Finally, as well-meaning social workers involved in AIDS education and prevention, we benefit immensely from periodically reassessing our own views and prejudices regarding LGB youths, sex, intimacy, and HIV/AIDS. It may be humbling to remember that as adults we have myriad difficulties with sexual relationships, sexual negotiation, and safer sex. Many of us are products of a homophobic and erotophobic culture and are at different stages of working through our prejudices.

CONCLUSION

This chapter has presented HIV-related risk-taking behavior and HIV prevention in a person-in-environment framework that is central to social work. Frequently, health promotion efforts, and HIV prevention in particular, are divorced from sociocultural context. Prevention strategies are often based on individual-level models of decision making and risk behavior. Nowhere is this less appropriate than in dealing with LGB youths. In acknowledging the social context of isolation and discrimination and the transactional nature of the coming-out process, and in underscoring the power of social support, it is clear that social- as well as individual-level aspects of HIV-related risk-taking behavior must be addressed for prevention to be relevant and effective. From this perspective, it is also evident that HIV prevention must be instituted as a sustained component of a comprehensive and proactive programmatic initiative to facilitate the overall health and well-being of LGB youths.

In acknowledging the social context of LGB identity development and of sex and HIV/AIDS, one must not, however, assume the individual to be a passive subject. The framework of this chapter advocates that we address the relationship between individual and social conceptualizations of health behavior and sexual behavior from a balanced and transactional perspective. Within the context of social and environmental forces, individuals make choices—some more or less informed and free than others. As difficult as it may be, with even the best prevention programs and the greater experience and knowledge we as social workers and concerned adults may wish to impart in earnestly wanting to help, decisions as to sexual behavior lie with the youths with whom we work—not with us. It is our role as social workers to offer accurate information, to encourage open dialogue concerning beliefs and values about life, sex, and intimacy, and to offer appropriate counseling, confrontation, and reframing of issues, but ultimately, young people must make their own decisions as to what constitutes an acceptable level of risk (Odets, 1994). Being overly directive or authoritarian serves to disempower young people—the opposite of what is aimed for in helping them to be reflective decision makers. Our role is to empower LGB youths to make the most informed and beneficial choices for themselves.

REFERENCES

Bowser, B. P., Fullilove, M. T., and Fullilove, R. E. (1990). African-American youth and AIDS high-risk behavior: The social context and barriers to prevention. *Youth and Society, 22*(1), 54-66.

Caetano, R. (1987). Acculturation and drinking patterns among U.S. Hispanics. *British Journal of Addictions, 82*(7), 789-799.

Catania, J. A., Dolcini, M. M., Coates, T. J., Kegeles, S. M., Greenblatt, R. M., Puckett, S., Corman, M., and Miller, J. (1989). Predictors of condom use and multiple partnered sex among sexually-active adolescent women: Implications for AIDS-related health interventions. *The Journal of Sex Research, 26*(4), 514-524.

Centers for Disease Control (CDC). (1996). *HIV/AIDS surveillance report.* Atlanta, GA: U.S. Government.

Chan, C. S. (1989). Issues of identity development among Asian-American lesbians and gay men. *Journal of Counseling and Development, 68*(1), 16-20.

Coleman, E. and Remafedi, G. (1989). Gay, lesbian, and bisexual adolescents: A critical challenge to counselors. *Journal of Counseling & Development: Special Issue: Gay, Lesbian, and Bisexual Issues in Counseling, 68*(1), 36-40.

de Monteflores, C. and Schultz, S. J. (1978). Coming out: Similarities and differences for lesbians and gays. *Journal of Social Issues, 34*(3), 59-72.

Fishbein, M. and Middlestadt, S. (1989). Using the theory of reasoned action as a framework for understanding and changing AIDS-related behaviors. In Mays, V., Albee, G., and Schneider, S. (Eds.). *Primary prevention of AIDS—Psychological approaches.* Newbury Park, CA: Sage, 93-110.

Fisher, J. D. (1988). Possible effects of reference group-based social influence on AIDS-risk behavior and AIDS prevention. *American Psychologist, 43*(11), 914-920.

Fleming, P. (1996). *Youth and HIV/AIDS: A White House report.* Washington, DC: U.S. Government Printing Office.

Flora, J. A. and Thoresen, C. E. (1989). Reducing the risk of AIDS in adolescents. *American Psychologist, 43*(11), 965-970.

Flores-Ortiz, Y. G. (1994). The role of cultural and gender values in alcohol use patterns among Chicana/Latina high school and university students: Implications for AIDS prevention. *International Journal of the Addictions, 29*(2), 1149-1171.

Freudenberg, N. (1994). Towards a new agenda for HIV prevention and services for young people: Seven dilemmas that divide AIDS workers serving adolescents. *The Networker,* (5), 5-9.

Hansen, W. B., Hahn, G. L., and Wolkenstein, B. H. (1990). Perceived personal immunity: Beliefs about susceptibility to AIDS. *Journal of Sex Research, 27*(4), 622-628.

Hart, G., Boulton, M., Fitzpatrick, R., McLean, J., and Dawson, J. (1992). "Relapse" to unsafe sexual behavior among gay men: A critique of recent behavioral HIV/AIDS research. *Sociology of Health and Illness, 14*(2), 216-232.

Hayes, R. B., Kegeles, S. M., and Coates, T. J. (1990). High HIV risk-taking among young gay men. *AIDS, 4*(9), 901-907.

Hein, K. (1993). "Getting real" about HIV in adolescents. *American Journal of Public Health, 83*(4), 492-494.

Hetrick, E. and Martin, A. D. (1987). Developmental issues and their resolution for gay and lesbian adolescents. *Journal of Homosexuality, 14*(1-2), 25-43.

Hingson, R. W., Strunin, L., Berlin, B. M., and Heeren, T. (1990). Beliefs about AIDS, use of alcohol and drugs, and unprotected sex among Massachusetts adolescents. *American Journal of Public Health, 80*(3), 295-299.

Hunter, J. and Schaecher, R. (1994). AIDS prevention for lesbian, gay, and bisexual adolescents. *Families in Society: The Journal of Contemporary Human Services, 75*(6), 346-354.

Icard, L. (1986). Black gay men and conflicting social identities: Sexual orientation versus racial identity. *Journal of Social Work and Human Sexuality, 4*(1-2), 83-93.

Isay, R. A. (1989). *Being homosexual: Gay men and their development.* New York: Farrar, Straus, Giroux.

Jemmott, J. B., Jemmott, L. S., and Fong, G. T. (1992). Reductions in HIV risk-associated sexual behaviors among black male adolescents: Effects on an AIDS prevention intervention. *American Journal of Public Health, 82*(3), 372-377.

Johnson, J. L. (1990-1991). Preventive interventions for children at risk: Introduction. *International Journal of the Addictions, 25*(4-A), 429-434.

Kegeles, S. M., Adler, N. E., and Irwin, C. E. (1988). Sexually active adolescents and condoms: Changes over one year in knowledge, attitudes, and use. *American Journal of Public Health, 78*(4), 460-461.

Kelly, J. A., St. Lawrence, J. S., Diaz, Y. E., Stevenson, L. Y., Hauth, A. C., Brasfield, T. L., Kalichman, S. C., Smith, J. E., and Andrew, M. E. (1991). HIV risk behavior reduction following intervention with key opinion leaders of population: An experimental analysis. *American Journal of Public Health, 81*(2), 168-171.

Koopman, C., Rosario, M., and Rotheram-Borus, M. J. (1994). Alcohol and drug use and sexual behaviors placing runaways at risk for HIV infection. *Addictive Behaviors, 19*(1), 95-103.

Krestan, J. A. and Bepko, C. S. (1980). The problem of fusion in the lesbian relationship. *Family Process, 19*(3), 277-289.

Ku, L., Sonnenstein, F. L., and Pleck, J. H. (1992). Patterns of HIV risk and preventive behaviors among teenage men. *Public Health Reports, 107*(2), 131-138.

Lewis, L. A. (1984). The coming-out process for lesbians: Integrating a stable identity. *Social Work, 29*(5), 464-469.

MacDonald, G. B. (1983). Exploring sexual identity: Gay people and their families. *Sex Education Coalition News, 5,* 1, 4.

Malyon, A. K. (1981). The homosexual adolescent: Developmental issues and social bias. *Child Welfare, 60*(5), 321-330.

Marin, B. V. and Marin, G. (1990). Effects of acculturation on knowledge of AIDS and HIV among Hispanics. *Hispanic Journal of Behavioral Sciences, 12*(2), 110-121.

Mays, V. M., Cochran, S. D., Belliga, G., and Smith, R. G. (1992). The language of black gay men's sexual behavior: Implications for AIDS risk reduction. *The Journal of Sex Research, 29*(3), 425-434.

McLean, D. A. (1994). A model for HIV risk reduction and prevention among African-American college students. *Journal of American College Health, 42*(5), 220-223.

Morales, E. S. (1990). HIV infection and Hispanic gay and bisexual men. *Hispanic Journal of Behavioral Sciences, 12*(2), 212-222.

Newman, P. (1998). Discursive condoms in the age of AIDS: Queerying HIV prevention. *Journal of Gay and Lesbian Social Services 8*(1), 83-102.

Odets, W. (1994). AIDS education and harm reduction for gay men: Psychological approaches for the 21st century. *AIDS and Public Policy Journal, 9*(1), 3-19.

Paradis, B. A. (1991). Seeking intimacy and integration: Gay men in the era of AIDS. Special Issue: Men and men's issues in social work theory and practice. *Smith College Studies in Social Work, 61*(3), 260-274.

Perry, C. L. and Sieving, R. (1991). Peer involvement in global AIDS prevention among adolescents (report no. unpublished). Geneva, Switzerland: Global Programme on AIDS World Health Organization.

Reed, B., Newman, P., Suarez, Z., and Lewis, E. (1997). Interpersonal practice beyond diversity, and towards social justice: The importance of critical consciousness. In C. Garvin and B. Seabury (Eds.), *Interpersonal Practice in Social Work.* New York: Allyn and Bacon.

Rickert, V. I., Jay, M. S., and Gottlieb, A. (1991). Effects of a peer-counseled AIDS education program on knowledge, attitudes, and satisfaction of adolescents. *Adolescent Health, 12*(1), 38-43.

Rickert, V. I., Jay, M. S., Gottlieb, A., and Bridges, C. (1989). Females' attitudes and behaviors toward condom purchase and use. *Journal of Adolescent Health Care, 10*(4), 313-316.

Riddle, D. I. and Morin, S. F. (1977). Removing the stigma: Data from individuals. *APA Monitor,* (November), 7(11), 16, 28.

Ridge, D. T., Plummer, D. C., and Minichiello, V. (1994). Young and gay men and HIV: Running the risk? *AIDS Care, 6*(4), 371-378.

Roesler, T. and Deisher, R. W. (1972). Youthful male homosexuality: Homosexual experience and the process of developing homosexual identity in males aged 16 to 22 years. *JAMA: Journal of the American Medical Association, 219*(8), 1018-1023.

Rogers, M. and Williams, W. (1987). AIDS in blacks and Hispanics: Implication for prevention. *Issues in Science and Technology, 3*, 89-94.

Rotheram-Borus, M. J. and Fernandez, M. I. (1995). Sexual orientation and developmental challenges experienced by gay and lesbian youths. *Suicide and Life-Threatening Behavior, 25*, (supplement), 26-34.

Rotheram-Borus, M. J. and Koopman, C. (1991). Sexual risk behavior: AIDS among predominantly minority gay and bisexual male adolescents. *AIDS Education and Prevention, 3*(4), 305-312.

Rotheram-Borus, M. J., Meyer-Bahlburg, H. F., Rosario, M., and Koopman, C. (1992). Lifetime sexual behaviors among predominantly minority male runaways and gay/bisexual adolescents in New York City. *AIDS Education and Prevention,* (Fall supplement), 34-32.

Rotheram-Borus, M. J., Rosario, M., Reid, H., and Koopman, C. (1995). Predicting patterns of sexual acts among homosexual and bisexual youths. *American Journal of Psychiatry, 152*(4), 588-595.

Schinke, S. P., Botvin, G. J., Orlandi, M. A., and Schilling, R. F. (1990). African-American and Hispanic-American adolescents, HIV infection, and prevention intervention. *AIDS Education and Prevention, 2*(4), 305-312.

Singer, M., Flores, C., Davison, L., Burke, G., Castillo, Z., Scanlon, K., and Rivera, M. (1990). SIDA: The economic, social, and cultural context of AIDS among Latinos. *Medical Anthropology Quarterly, 4*(1), 72-114.

St. Lawrence, J. S., Brasfield, T. L., Jefferson, K. W., and Allyene, E. (1994). Social support as a factor in African-American adolescents' sexual risk behavior. *Journal of Adolescent Research, 9*(3), 292-310.

Stall, R., Burrett, D., Bye, L., Catania, J. A., Frutchey, C., Henne, J., Lemp, G., and Paul, J. (1992). A comparison of younger and older gay men's HIV risk-taking behaviors: The communication technologies 1989 cross-sectional survey. *Journal of Acquired Immune Deficiency Syndrome, 5*(7), 682-687.

Stall, R., Ekstrand, M., Pollack, L., McKusick, L., and Coates, T. J. (1990). Relapse from safer sex: The next challenge for AIDS prevention efforts. *Journal of Acquired Immune Deficiency Syndrome, 3*(12), 1181-1187.

Stall, R., McKusick, L., Wiley, J., and Coates, T. J. (1986). Alcohol and drug use during sexual activity and compliance with safe sex guidelines for AIDS: The AIDS behavioral research project. *Health Education Quarterly, 13*(4), 359-371.

Sussman, T. and Duffy, M. (1996). Are we forgetting about gay male adolescents in AIDS-related research and prevention? *Youth and Society, 27*(3), 379-393.

Thomas, S. and Quinn S. C. (1991). Implications for HIV education and AIDS risk education programs in the black community. *American Journal of Public Health, 81*(11), 1498-1504.

van Griensven, G., Koblin, B. A., and Osmond, D. (1994). Risk behavior and HIV infection among younger homosexual men. *AIDS, 8*(1), 125-130.

Vincke, J., Bolton, R., Mak, R., and Blank, S. (1993). Coming out and AIDS-related high-risk sexual behavior. *Archives of Sexual Behavior, 22*(6), 559-586.

Washington, J. (1995). Talk given at University of Michigan, Rackman School of Graduate Studies, Ann Arbor, MI (November 7).

Index

Page numbers followed by the letter "f" indicate figures; those followed by the letter "t" indicate tables.

Group affiliation, black men
and, 125-126
Group composition, GMHC
HIV-negative group, 90, 96
Group dynamics, PWA support
groups, 41
Group leader, PWA support groups,
40, 41
Group sessions, the WHEEL, 62-63
"Grow or go," Harper model, 224-226
Guilt
bereaved mothers, 47-48, 50
HIV-negative gay men, 86, 88, 100
and protease inhibitor therapy,
13, 38-39

Hall, Stuart, 126, 131
Hallucinations, HIV-associated
cognitive/motor complex,
289, 290-291
Harassment, response to, 113, 114
Harm reduction model, 330, 332
the WHEEL, 63
Harper, B. C., caregiver development
stages, 222-228
Harper, Phillip Brian, 131
Harris, Thomas Allen, 131
Hastened dying, criteria for, 342-343
Health care proxy, 192
Health care system, and people
of color, 10-11
"Health education," HIV-prevention
program, 64
Health professionals, assisted
suicide's impact on, 341-342
Heidi Chronicles, The, 101, 107
Hemlock Society, The, 209
Hermaphrodite, 161, 161t
Heroic measures, use of medical,
278-279
"Heterosexism," 180
Highly active antiretroviral therapy
(HAART), *xxiv*

Hispanics, AIDS in, 319-320. *See
also* Latinos, LGB youth
HIV Law Project, 259
*HIV Negative: How the Uninfected
Are Affected by AIDS,* 95
HIV status, and gay men's identity,
96, 97-98
HIV transmission, mixed-HIV-status
couples, 266, 268
HIV/AIDS
current research education, 322
diagnostic criteria, 237
education
LGB youth, 351, 355-356, 361
and training programs, 320-321
prevention
black men and, 125, 135-136
education needed on, 322
LGB youth, 351, 355-356,
358-361
risk factors
black men, 132-135, 133f, 134f,
135f
gay and male bisexual youths,
352
LGB youth, 352-353
testing, 237
transmission
black men, 133-135, 133f, 134f,
135f, 320
LGB youth, 353
"HIV/AIDS and Mental Hygiene,"
325
"HIV/AIDS Focus," newsletter,
323, 325
HIV-associated cognitive/motor
complex
diagnosis of, 285-286
prevalence of, 287
HIV-associated dementia complex,
286, 289
HIV-infected children, telephone
family support groups, 43

HIV-negative gay men
  and AIDS community, 88
  and gay community, 98, 109, 110
  primary prevention, 85
HIV-positive birth survival, 69
HIV-prevention programs, 58
Holistic approach, traditional folk
      healers, 120
Hollywood Access Center, drop
      in facility, 77
Home assignments, GMHC
      HIV-negative group, 91
Homelessness, and HIV, 77
Homophobia
  black community, 131, 132
  concept of, 180
  and health care delivery, *xxv*
  internalized, 105-106, 179-180,
      185
  minority LGB youth, 355
  unconscious internalized, 180,
      181, 183-184, 185
Homosexuality, conflation with
      AIDS, 182-183, 184
"Homosexualization of AIDS,"
      98, 99
Hormone treatments, transgendered
      individuals, 169-171
Hospice care, 194-195
  limitations of, 204
Hospital, AIDS work in, 228
Housing, loss of for PWAs, 80
Housing discrimination, black men,
      128
Hypophonia, 288

Idealizing self-objects needs,
      149, 153-155
Identification, in support groups, 52
Identity
  and HIV status, 96, 97-98
  HIV/AIDS services, 128, 129
  and work, 19, 20
Immigrants, HIV/AIDS, 255-263

Imposter syndrome, 151
Independent living skills
      programming, 68
Indinavir (Crixivan), 3, 15
Individuation, GMHC HIV-negative
      group, 92
Information processing, HIV-
      associated cognitive/motor
      complex, 287-288
"Institutional landscape," 212
Integrated services, women at risk
      for HIV infection, 64
Intellectualization, Harper model,
      222-223
Interactional/existential therapy,
      HIV-negative gay men, 86
Interpersonal pressure, and health
      transition, 25
Interventions, women sexual partners
      of injection drug users, 59
Intimacy, GMHC HIV-negative
      group, 93
Intimacy and closeness, 110
Intrapsychic homeostasis, 23
Invisible Epidemic, The, 237
Involuntary hospitalization,
      psychotherapists, 341
Isolation
  family of HIV-infected children, 44
  of HIV-negative gay men, 106
  in homeless, 80
  immigrants with HIV/AIDS,
      257, 259, 261
  LGB youth, 353, 358
  and medication failure, 37
  MFT transsexuals, 159, 160, 164
  mixed-HIV-status couples, 269-270,
      277
Its My Party, 340

Jacobs, Raymond, 321
Jamison, Stephen, 346
*Journal of the American Medical
      Association (JAMA),* 204, 338
Jungle Fever, 317

Order Your Own Copy of
This Important Book for Your Personal Library!

AIDS AND MENTAL HEALTH PRACTICE
Clinical and Policy Issues

_____ in hardbound at $34.95 (ISBN: 0-7890-0464-X)

COST OF BOOKS_____

OUTSIDE USA/CANADA/
MEXICO: ADD 20%_____

POSTAGE & HANDLING_____
*(US: $3.00 for first book & $1.25
for each additional book)
Outside US: $4.75 for first book
& $1.75 for each additional book)*

SUBTOTAL_____

IN CANADA: ADD 7% GST_____

STATE TAX_____
*(NY, OH & MN residents, please
add appropriate local sales tax)*

FINAL TOTAL_____
*(If paying in Canadian funds,
convert using the current
exchange rate. UNESCO
coupons welcome.)*

☐ **BILL ME LATER:** ($5 service charge will be added)
(Bill-me option is good on US/Canada/Mexico orders only;
not good to jobbers, wholesalers, or subscription agencies.)

☐ Check here if billing address is different from
shipping address and attach purchase order and
billing address information.

Signature _____

☐ **PAYMENT ENCLOSED: $**_____

☐ **PLEASE CHARGE TO MY CREDIT CARD.**

☐ Visa   ☐ MasterCard   ☐ AmEx   ☐ Discover
☐ Diner's Club

Account # _____

Exp. Date _____

Signature _____

Prices in US dollars and subject to change without notice.

NAME _____

INSTITUTION _____

ADDRESS _____

CITY _____

STATE/ZIP _____

COUNTRY _____ COUNTY (NY residents only) _____

TEL _____ FAX _____

E-MAIL_____
May we use your e-mail address for confirmations and other types of information? ☐ Yes   ☐ No

Order From Your Local Bookstore or Directly From
The Haworth Press, Inc.
10 Alice Street, Binghamton, New York 13904-1580 • USA
TELEPHONE: 1-800-HAWORTH (1-800-429-6784) / Outside US/Canada: (607) 722-5857
FAX: 1-800-895-0582 / Outside US/Canada: (607) 772-6362
E-mail: getinfo@haworthpressinc.com
PLEASE PHOTOCOPY THIS FORM FOR YOUR PERSONAL USE.

Discover the effects of AIDS on specific subpopulations and the possibilities for future prevention, intervention, and coping!

AIDS AND MENTAL HEALTH PRACTICE
Clinical and Policy Issues
Edited by Michael Shernoff NEW!
This book will provide professionals in the field and students in training with the most current practice information about mental health practice and HIV/AIDS, and will help you understand the diverse needs of individuals with HIV/AIDS and organize programs to serve these populations.
Over 300 Pages!
$34.95 hard. ISBN: 0-7890-0464-X.
Text price (5+ copies): $24.95.
Available Winter 1998/99.
Approx. 344 pp. with Index.
Features case studies and interviews, tables/figures, diagnostic criteria, questionnaires and tests, and appendixes.

AIDS AND DEVELOPMENT IN AFRICA
A Social Science Perspective
Edited by Kempe Ronald Hope, Sr., PhD NEW!
Goes beyond the usual analyses of demographic impact to much more substantial assessments and analyses of the burden on peoples, economies, and health care systems of African countries.
Over 225 Pages!
$39.95 hard. ISBN: 0-7890-0638-3.
Text price (5+ copies): $24.95.
Available Spring 1999. Approx. 231 pp. with Index.

AIDS CAPITATION
Edited by David A. Cherin, PhD, and George J. Huba, PhD NEW!
AIDS Capitation explores end-stage care reform in HIV/AIDS care. You'll discover descriptive and evaluative aspects of the model of care as well as the program that funds national demonstration projects.
(A monograph published simultaneously as Home Health Care Services Quarterly, Vol. 17, No. 1.)
$34.95 hard. ISBN: 0-7890-0654-5.
Text price (5+ copies): $19.95.
Available Fall 1998. 115 pp. with Index.

LOVE AND ANGER
Essays on AIDS, Activism, and Politics
Peter F. Cohen NEW!
One of the first books to take an interdisciplinary approach to AIDS activism and politics by looking at the literary response to the disease, class issues, and the AIDS activist group ACT UP.
$39.95 hard. ISBN: 0-7890-0455-0.
$16.95 soft. ISBN: 1-56023-930-1.
1998. Available now. 194 pp. with Index.
Features interviews, recommended readings, a bibliography, and analyses of plays and books.

 Take 20% Off Each Book! SPECIAL OFFER

WOMEN, DRUG USE, AND HIV INFECTION
Edited by Sally J. Stevens, PhD, Stephanie Tortu, PhD, and Susan L. Coyle, PhD NEW!
This book focuses on research conducted within the context of a national, multi-site Cooperative Agreement funded by the *National Institute on Drug Abuse.*
Over 225 Pages!
(A monograph published simultaneously as Women & Health, Vol. 27, Nos. 1/2.)
$49.95 hard. ISBN: 0-7890-0351-1.
$24.95 soft. ISBN: 0-7890-0527-1.
1998. Available now. 237 pp. with Index.

HIV AND SOCIAL WORK
A Practitioner's Guide
Edited by David M. Aronstein, MSW, and Bruce J. Thompson, PhD NEW!
There are things you can do—very specific kinds of help you can offer—that can make an enormous difference in the lives of people with HIV/AIDS and those who love and care for them.
Over 550 Pages!
$89.95 hard. ISBN: 0-7890-0180-2.
$49.95 soft. ISBN: 1-56023-906-9.
1998. Available now. 586 pp. with Index.
Includes case studies, recommended readings, 3 tables, and an appendix.
Special Discount: TAKE 30% OFF!
(Not good with any other discount.)

NEW INTERNATIONAL DIRECTIONS IN HIV PREVENTION FOR GAY AND BISEXUAL MEN
Edited by Michael T. Wright, LICSW, B. R. Simon Rosser, PhD, MPH, and Onno de Zwart, MA NEW!
Researchers, practitioners, and community organizations will be challenged to examine current assumptions and to consider neglected aspects of risk behavior such as love, trust, and the dynamics of sexual intimacy.
(A monograph published simultaneously as the Journal of Psychology & Human Sexuality, Vol. 10, Nos. 3/4.)
$49.95 hard. ISBN: 0-7890-0538-7.
$22.95 soft. ISBN: 1-56023-116-5.
1998. Available now. 167 pp. with Index.

THE HIV-NEGATIVE GAY MAN
Developing Strategies for Survival and Emotional Well-Being
Edited by Steven Ball, MSW, ACSW NEW!
Addresses divisions within the gay community between men who are HIV-negative and those who are infected with HIV or ill with AIDS.
(A monograph published simultaneously as the Journal of Gay & Lesbian Social Services, Vol. 8, No. 1.)
$29.95 hard. ISBN: 0-7890-0522-0.
$12.95 soft. ISBN: 1-56023-114-9.
1998. Available now. 115 pp. with Index.

The Haworth Press, Inc.
10 Alice Street
Binghamton, New York 13904-1580 USA

DRY BONES BREATHE

Gay Men Creating Post-AIDS Identities and Cultures
Eric Rofes

Learn how social, political, and biomedical changes are dramatically transforming gay identities and cultures.
$49.95 hard. ISBN: 0-7890-0470-4.
$24.95 soft. ISBN: 1-56023-934-4.
1998. Available now. 352 pp. with Index.
Features interviews, personal revelations, and article and book reviews.

HIV/AIDS AND THE DRUG CULTURE

Shattered Lives
Elizabeth Hagan, RN, BSN, ACRN, and Joan Gormley, RN, BSN

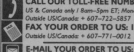

Explores interventions for decreasing the rate of HIV infection among injection drug users.
$39.95 hard. ISBN: 0-7890-0465-8.
$14.95 soft. ISBN: 0-7890-0554-9.
1998. Available now. 191 pp. with Index.
Features case studies, treatment regimes, diagnostic criteria, a bibliography, and a glossary.

NOBODY'S CHILDREN

Orphans of the HIV Epidemic
Steven F. Dansky, CSW

By the year 2000, an estimated 82,000 to 125,000 children will become orphans of the human immunodeficiency virus (HIV). This book shows how caregivers and the community can meet the ever-increasing social and economic needs of these children.
$39.95 hard. ISBN: 1-56023-855-0.
$14.95 soft. ISBN: 1-56023-923-9. 1997. 178 pp. with Index.

Textbooks are available for classroom adoption consideration on a 60–day examination basis. You will receive an invoice payable within 60 days along with the book. **If you decide to adopt the book, your invoice will be cancelled.** Please write to us on your institutional letterhead, indicating the textbook you would like to examine as well as the following information: course title, current text, enrollment, and decision date.

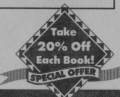

FOR OTHER AVAILABLE BOOKS AND JOURNALS ON HIV/AIDS AND RELATED TOPICS :
VISIT OUR WEB SITE AT:
http://www.haworthpressinc.com

Take 20% Off Each Book!
SPECIAL OFFER

CALL OUR TOLL-FREE NUMBER: 1–800–HAWORTH
US & Canada only / 8am–5pm ET; Monday–Friday
Outside US/Canada: + 607–722–5857
FAX YOUR ORDER TO US: 1–800–895–0582
Outside US/Canada: + 607–771–0012
E-MAIL YOUR ORDER TO US:
getinfo@haworthpressinc.com
VISIT OUR WEB SITE AT:
http://www.haworthpressinc.com

Order Today and Save!

TITLE	ISBN	REGULAR PRICE	20%–OFF PRICE

- Discount available only in US, Canada, and Mexico and not available in conjunction with any other offer.
- Individual orders outside US, Canada, and Mexico must be prepaid by check, credit card, or money order.
- In Canada: Add 7% for GST after postage & handling.
- Outside USA, Canada, and Mexico: Add 20%.
- MN, NY, and OH residents: Add appropriate local sales tax.

Please complete information below or tape your business card in this area.

NAME _____

ADDRESS _____

_____

CITY _____

STATE_____ZIP_____

COUNTRY_____

COUNTY (NY residents only) _____

TEL _____ FAX _____

E-MAIL_____
May we use your e-mail address for confirmations and other types of information?
( ) Yes ( ) No. We appreciate receiving your e-mail address and fax number. Haworth would like to e-mail or fax special discount offers to you, as a preferred customer. We will never **share, rent, or exchange** your e-mail address or fax number. We regard such actions as an invasion of your privacy.

POSTAGE AND HANDLING:	
If your book total is:	Add
up to	$29.95	$5.00
$30.00 – $49.99	$6.00
$50.00 – $69.99	$7.00
$70.00 – $89.99	$8.00
$90.00 – $109.99	$9.00
$110.00 – $129.99	$10.00
$130.00 – $149.99	$11.00
$150.00 and up	$12.00

- US orders will be shipped via UPS; Outside US orders will be shipped via Book Printed Matter. For shipments via other delivery services, contact Haworth for details. Based on US dollars. Booksellers: Call for freight charges. • If paying in Canadian funds, please use the current exchange rate to convert total to Canadian dollars. • Payment in UNESCO coupons welcome. • Please allow 3–4 weeks for delivery after publication. • Prices and discounts subject to change without notice. • Discount not applicable on books priced under $15.00.

☐ **BILL ME LATER** ($5 service charge will be added).
(Bill-me option available on US/Canadian/Mexican orders only. Not available for subscription agencies. Service charge is waived for booksellers/wholesalers/jobbers.)

Signature _____

☐ **PAYMENT ENCLOSED** _____
(Payment must be in US or Canadian dollars by check or money order drawn on a US or Canadian bank.)

☐ **PLEASE CHARGE TO MY CREDIT CARD:**
☐ VISA ☐ MASTERCARD ☐ AMEX ☐ DISCOVER ☐ DINERS CLUB

Account # _____ Exp Date _____

Signature _____
May we open a confidential credit card account for you for possible future purchases? ( ) Yes ( ) No

The Haworth Press, Inc.
10 Alice Street, Binghamton, New York 13904-1580 USA

(34) 10/98 BBC98

WILLIAM F. RUSKA LIBRARY
BECKER COLLEGE